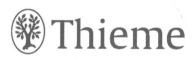

Top 3 Differentials in Musculoskeletal Imaging

A Case Review

Jasjeet Bindra, MBBS
Associate Professor of Radiology
Division of Musculoskeletal Imaging
Department of Radiology
University of California, Davis School of Medicine
Sacramento, California

Robert D. Boutin, MD
Clinical Professor of Radiology
Co-Director of Musculoskeletal Imaging Fellowship
Department of Radiology
Stanford Medical School
Stanford, California

Series Editor:

William T. O'Brien, Sr., DO, FAOCR
Director, Pediatric Neuroradiology Fellowship
Cincinnati Children's Hospital Medical Center
Associate Professor of Radiology
University of Cincinnati College of Medicine
Cincinnati, Ohio

424 illustrations

Thieme
New York • Stuttgart • Delhi • Rio de Janeiro

Library of Congress Cataloging-in-Publication Data

Names: Bindra, Jasjeet, author, editor. | Boutin, Robert D., author, editor.

Title: Top 3 differentials in musculoskeletal imaging : a case review / [edited by] Jasjeet Bindra, Robert D. Boutin.

Other titles: Top three differentials in musculoskeletal imaging

Description: New York : Thieme, [2021] | Includes bibliographical references and index. | Summary: "Top 3 Differentials in Musculoskeletal Imaging: A Case Review by Jasjeet Bindra, Robert D. Boutin, and expert contributors is one in a series of radiology case books mirroring the format of the highly acclaimed O'Brien classic, Top 3 Differentials in Radiology: A Case Review. The book is organized in 10 parts: trauma, bone tumors, upper extremity, lower extremity, arthropathies, infection, soft tissue tumors, metabolic musculoskeletal conditions, spine, and pediatric/developmental musculoskeletal conditions"—Provided by publisher.

Identifiers: LCCN 2020043380 | ISBN 9781626233485 (paperback) | ISBN 9781626233652 (ebook)

Subjects: MESH: Musculoskeletal Diseases—diagnostic imaging | Musculoskeletal System—diagnostic imaging | Musculoskeletal System—injuries | Diagnosis, Differential | Atlas | Case Reports

Classification: LCC RC925.7 | NLM WE 17 | DDC 616.7/075—dc23

LC record available at https://lccn.loc.gov/2020043380.

Thieme Publishers New York
333 Seventh Avenue, New York, NY 10001 USA
+1 800 782 3488, customerservice@thieme.com

Georg Thieme Verlag KG
Rüdigerstrasse 14, 70469 Stuttgart, Germany
+49 [0]711 8931 421, customerservice@thieme.de

Thieme Publishers Delhi
A-12, Second Floor, Sector-2, Noida-201301
Uttar Pradesh, India
+91 120 45 566 00, customerservice@thieme.in

Thieme Publishers Rio de Janeiro
Thieme Publicações Ltda.
Edifício Rodolpho de Paoli, 25º andar
Av. Nilo Peçanha, 50 – Sala 2508
Rio de Janeiro 20020-906 Brasil
+55 21 3172 2297 / +55 21 3172 1896

Cover design: Thieme Publishing Group
Typesetting by DiTech Process Solutions, India

Printed in USA by King Printing Company, Inc.   5 4 3 2 1

ISBN 978-1-62623-348-5

Also available as an e-book:
eISBN 978-1-62623-365-2

Important note: Medicine is an ever-changing science undergoing continual development. Research and clinical experience are continually expanding our knowledge, in particular our knowledge of proper treatment and drug therapy. Insofar as this book mentions any dosage or application, readers may rest assured that the authors, editors, and publishers have made every effort to ensure that such references are in accordance with **the state of knowledge at the time of production of the book.**

Nevertheless, this does not involve, imply, or express any guarantee or responsibility on the part of the publishers in respect to any dosage instructions and forms of applications stated in the book. **Every user is requested to examine carefully** the manufacturers' leaflets accompanying each drug and to check, if necessary in consultation with a physician or specialist, whether the dosage schedules mentioned therein or the contraindications stated by the manufacturers differ from the statements made in the present book. Such examination is particularly important with drugs that are either rarely used or have been newly released on the market. Every dosage schedule or every form of application used is entirely at the user's own risk and responsibility. The authors and publishers request every user to report to the publishers any discrepancies or inaccuracies noticed. If errors in this work are found after publication, errata will be posted at www.thieme.com on the product description page.

Some of the product names, patents, and registered designs referred to in this book are in fact registered trademarks or proprietary names even though specific reference to this fact is not always made in the text. Therefore, the appearance of a name without designation as proprietary is not to be construed as a representation by the publisher that it is in the public domain.

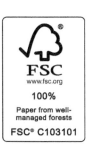

To my dear parents who remain my source of inspiration and who raised me with all the love and kindness in the world.

To Ramit for his love and support.

To my daughters, Suhela and Mehr, who light up my life.

—Jasjeet Bindra, MBBS

To my Dad, Frank,

Thank you for showing me the wonderful world of medicine.

To my Mom, Charlotte,
Thanks for showing me that there is more to life than medicine.

To my wife, Kristen,
Thanks for being 110% patient, 25 hours every day.

To my daughters, Tess and Lila,
Listen to your mother!

—Robert D. Boutin, MD

Contents

Series Foreword

The original "Top 3" concept was something engrained during my residency training in the military. From day 1, our program emphasized the importance of having gamut-based differentials as part of our daily readout sessions, as well as during didactic and clinical case-based conferences. The bulk of residency training was then centered around learning the key clinical and imaging manifestations of each entity on the list of differentials to be able to distinguish one from another, when possible. To avoid providing clinicians with a laundry list of differentials that would be of little value, we were encouraged to consider the "Top 3" differentials and any other important considerations based upon the specific clinical scenario or imaging finding(s) presented. I found that concept and approach to radiology so useful that I continue to utilize it to this day.

One thing I have learned throughout my radiology career, especially as a residency program director, is that not every individual learns or processes information in the same manner. Some individuals can read through a traditional textbook that is organized by pathology (i.e., developmental abnormalities, infectious processes, neoplasms, etc.) and readily recognize that the developmental abnormality in Chapter 1 is in the same differential for the infectious process in Chapter 2 and a few neoplasms in Chapter 3. Others, like me, best learn from gamut-based resources where content is organized based upon the key imaging findings, similar to how we practice radiology. If you are part of the latter group, then the "Top 3" approach may be the right fit for you. The intent of the series is to provide a comprehensive case-based alternative to traditional subspecialty textbooks where the focus remains on differential diagnoses. After all, when the dust settles and the core and certifying exams are nothing but distant (and hopefully pleasant) memories, this is what radiology is all about.

The Musculoskeletal (MSK) Imaging Top 3 book is edited by Dr. Jasjeet Bindra and Dr. Robert D. Boutin of the University of California, Davis (UC Davis), and Stanford University, respectively. I have known Dr. Bindra since residency and was thrilled when she agreed to serve as MSK editor for the second edition of the original Top 3 book a few years ago. Her contributions of teaching cases and pearls were truly exceptional. Dr. Boutin was instrumental in my MSK training, both as a faculty at UC Davis during my residency training, as well as through his involvement with the University of California, San Francisco, radiology review courses. Their combined clinical and teaching experience comes across beautifully in this high-yield resource.

Top 3 Differentials in Musculoskeletal Imaging is organized into 10 parts: trauma, bone tumors, upper extremity, lower extremity, arthropathies, infection, soft tissue tumors, metabolic musculoskeletal conditions, spine, and pediatric or developmental musculoskeletal conditions. As with the original Top 3 book, the emphasis is on differential-based cases with the addition of Roentgen Classics where appropriate.

It is my sincere hope that you find this subspecialty Top 3 book both enjoyable and educational.

William T. O'Brien, Sr., DO, FAOCR

Foreword

It is my great pleasure to write the foreword for this book entitled *Top 3 Differentials in Musculoskeletal Imaging: A Case Review* written by my colleague and good friend Jasjeet Bindra, MBBS, Associate Professor of Radiology at the University of California (UC), Davis, Sacramento and co-edited by Robert D. Boutin, MD, Clinical Professor of Radiology at Stanford Medical School. Jasjeet received her MD diploma from the medical school, Lady Harding Medical College of University of Delhi, New Delhi, India, followed by residency in Radiology and fellowship in Musculoskeletal Imaging at the UC Davis Medical Center, Sacramento, California. She is well-known in radiologic circles for her leadership in the musculoskeletal training program which involves medical students, radiology and orthopedic residents and fellows. An extension of her teaching passion, which she carried on to the higher level, is this publication that emulates the idea of the very popular book written in 2009 by William T. O'Brien, Sr., *Top 3 Differentials in Radiology: A Case Review*. Robert, an established educator, is well recognized in the field of musculoskeletal imaging and has published numerous scientific articles and chapters on this subject. Their combined work has resulted in this outstanding resource.

This book follows a specific format, practical from the point of view of the differential case-based references, and contingent on the key findings on the presented unknown cases. This form of a gamut, providing clinical history, imaging findings, and followed by the top three differential diagnostic possibilities and additional differential considerations, is directed towards the idea of helping trainees prepare for the American Board of Radiology examination. A very helpful feature is the inclusion of *Pearls* at the end of each case.

The book, as explained in the Preface, is organized and divided into 10 parts that include anatomical sites such as upper and lower extremity and spine, and various clinical entities of musculoskeletal disorders such as trauma, bone and soft-tissue tumors, arthropathies, infections, metabolic conditions, and developmental anomalies, comprising 146 cases. Each case is concentrated on the specific imaging finding, such as aggressive periosteal reaction, focal cortical thickening, diffuse increased bone density, focal periphyseal edema, acro-osteolysis, and many others. The cases are written clear, focused, and informative manner. The chosen images, which include radiographs, CTs, and MRIs, are of a very good quality and have been meticulously selected. The presentation of various cases provides the reader with a guide to make a correct diagnosis, based on the specific imaging finding or findings, and awareness of the most common differential possibilities. The list of references is short but pertinent and up to date.

In summary, this book is an excellent, well-organized, and concise guide, composed of valuable sources of information. Although it is primarily intended for radiology residents and fellows, the book may prove to be a resource of useful diagnostic pearls for any physician interested in musculoskeletal disorders. I earnestly recommend this book, which should be a welcome addition to any personal or departmental library.

Adam Greenspan, MD, FACR
Professor Emeritus of Radiology and Orthopedic Surgery
Department of Radiology
University of California, Davis School of Medicine
Sacramento, California

Preface

It is a distinct pleasure and honor to present *Top 3 Differentials in Musculoskeletal Imaging: A Case Review*. This book is primarily intended for radiology residents, musculoskeletal radiology fellows, and practicing physicians. We believe that the book will not only help prepare radiology trainees for core and certifying examinations but also provide a useful framework for all those who utilize musculoskeletal radiology in their practice.

The book is organized into the following 10 parts: trauma, bone tumors, upper extremity, lower extremity, arthropathies, infection, soft-tissue tumors, metabolic musculoskeletal conditions, spine, and pediatric/developmental musculoskeletal conditions. Each part contains a series of common and important imaging gamuts. We have followed the *Top 3 Differentials* series format, which was first used by Dr. William T. O'Brien, Sr., in his 2009 publication. The book includes unknown differential-based cases. The illustrative cases are meant to highlight a key finding or gamut, which is the basis for the case discussion. The final diagnosis for each case is by no means the focus of this review book. The differentials and discussions are based on the key finding or gamut and not necessarily on the illustrative cases that are shown. The discussion section provides a list of differentials broken down into *Top 3* and additional differential diagnoses, with a brief review of important imaging findings for the differentials. *Pearls* are provided at the end of each case for a quick review of key points.

We sincerely hope that you find this book useful and it proves to be a welcome addition to the *Top 3 Differentials* series.

Jasjeet Bindra, MBBS
Robert D. Boutin, MD

Contributors

M. Jason Akers, MD
Chief Radiologist
St Mary's Medical Center
Radiology, Inc.
Huntington, West Virginia

Cyrus Bateni, MD
Associate Professor and Chief
Division of Musculoskeletal Imaging
Department of Radiology
University of California, Davis School of Medicine
Sacramento, California

Jasjeet Bindra, MBBS
Associate Professor of Radiology
Division of Musculoskeletal Imaging
Department of Radiology
University of California, Davis School of Medicine
Sacramento, California

Robert D. Boutin, MD
Clinical Professor of Radiology and Co-Director
Musculoskeletal Imaging Fellowship
Department of Radiology
Stanford Medical School
Stanford, California

James S. Chalfant, MD
Clinical Instructor
Department of Radiology
University of California
Los Angeles, California

Jennifer Chang, MD
Assistant Clinical Professor, Neuroradiology
Program Director—Radiology Residency
University of California, Davis School of Medicine
Sacramento, California

Eva M. Escobedo, MD
Professor of Radiology, Musculoskeletal Imaging
Associate Residency Program Director
Department of Radiology
University of California, Davis School of Medicine
Sacramento, California

Philip Granchi, MD
President
Mother Lode Diagnostic Imaging
Sutter Amador Hospital
Jackson, California;
Mad River Community Hospital
Arcata, California

Leslie E. Grissom, MD
Clinical Professor of Radiology and Pediatrics
Nemours duPont Hospital for Children
Thomas Jefferson University (Retired)
Wilmington, Delaware

John Hunter, MD
Professor of Radiology, Musculoskeletal Imaging
Department of Radiology
University of California, Davis School of Medicine
Sacramento, California

Paulomi K. Kanzaria, MD
Associate Program Director
Radiology Elective Director
Department of Radiology
St. Vincent Hospital
Templeton, Massachusetts

Wonsuk Kim, MD
Staff Radiologist
Department of Radiology
Beth Israel Deaconess Medical Center
Boston, Massachusetts

Jennifer L. Nicholas, MD, MHA
Assistant Professor of Pediatric Radiology
University Hospitals Rainbow Babies and Children's
    Hospital
Cleveland, Ohio

William T. O'Brien, DO, FAOCR
Chief of Neuroradiology
Director, Pediatric Neuroradiology Fellowship
Cincinnati Children's Hospital Medical Center
Associate Professor of Radiology
University of Cincinnati College of Medicine
Cincinnati, Ohio

Geoffrey M. Riley, MD
Clinical Professor of Radiology
Director of Community Radiology
Director of Radiology Continuing Medical Education
Department of Radiology
Stanford University School of Medicine
Stanford, California

Rebecca Stein-Wexler, MD
Professor and Chief Pediatric Radiology
Department of Radiology
University of California, Davis School of Medicine
Sacramento, California

Michael A. Tall, MD
Associate Professor
Department of Musculoskeletal Radiology
University of Texas Health Science Center at San Antonio
San Antonio, Texas

Adrianne K. Thompson, MD
Division of Body Imaging
South Texas Veterans Health Care System
San Antonio, Texas

Robert J. Wood, MD
University of San Diego
San Diego, California

Sandra L. Wootton-Gorges[†], MD
Professor of Pediatric Radiology
Director of Pediatric Imaging
University of California, Davis Medical Center and
Children's Hospital
Sacramento, California

[†]Deceased

Part 1

Trauma

Case 1

Eva Escobedo

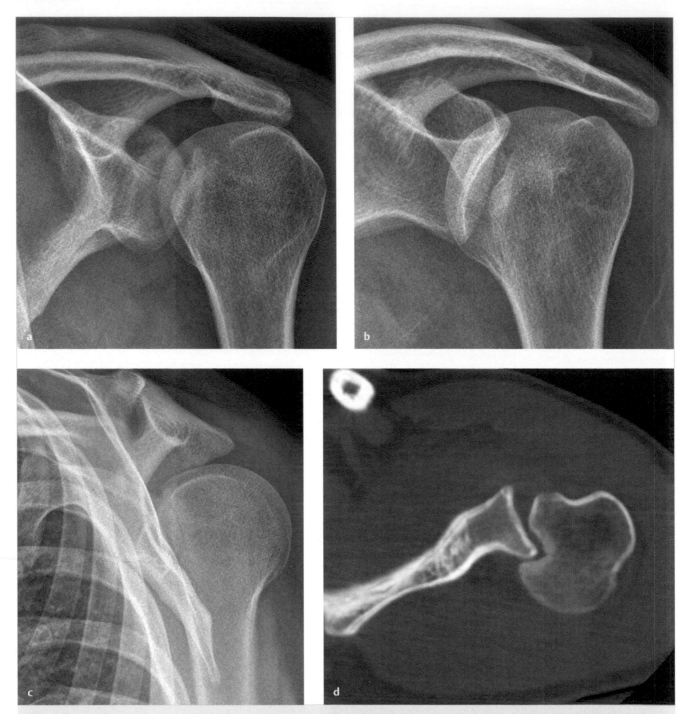

Fig. 1.1 AP radiograph of the shoulder **(a)** shows apparent widening of the glenohumeral joint, and a linear sclerotic area on the humeral head, adjacent to the posterior rim of the glenoid. Grashey view **(b)** shows overlap of the humerus on the glenoid. Transcapular "Y" view **(c)** shows the humeral head dislocated with respect to the glenoid. Axial CT image **(d)** reveals humeral head impacted posterior to the glenoid, with compression deformity on the anteromedial humeral head.

■ **Clinical History**

A 36-year-old male with shoulder pain after motor vehicle accident (▶ Fig. 1.1).

■ Key Finding

Shoulder dislocation.

■ Top 3 Differential Diagnoses

- **Anterior shoulder dislocation:** A large majority of shoulder dislocations are anterior in direction, and typically occur with external rotation and abduction of the humerus. Complications include bony or soft tissue avulsion from the anterior inferior glenoid (Bankart lesion) and compression injury of the posterior humeral head (Hill–Sachs lesion). Greater tuberosity fracture is more common in older patients. Although diagnosis is usually apparent on frontal radiographs, an axillary view or transcapular "Y" view helps confirm the presence and direction of dislocation.

- **Posterior shoulder dislocation:** Posterior dislocations are rare, accounting for less than 5% of shoulder dislocations. Many cases are initially missed on radiographs. Common causes are high-energy trauma with force on a shoulder in flexed, adducted, and internally rotated position, seizure, electrocution, and falls on an outstretched hand. The humeral head is locked in internal rotation, which is a sign noted both clinically and radiographically. An axillary view or transcapular "Y" will confirm presence. The compression deformity on the anteromedial humeral head is termed "reverse Hill–Sachs" lesion. Similarly, a posterior labral tear and posterior glenoid rim fracture are termed soft tissue and osseous "reverse Bankart" lesions, respectively.

- **Luxatio erecta:** This is a rare form (less than 1%) of shoulder dislocation secondary to hyperabduction. The arm is characteristically locked in an elevated position, with the humeral head inferior to the glenoid on radiographs. This type of dislocation is frequently associated with neurovascular and musculoskeletal injuries, with rotator cuff tears and greater tuberosity fractures more prevalent than in the other types.

■ Additional Diagnostic Considerations

- **Pseudosubluxation/pseudodislocation:** Inferior subluxation of the humeral head due to hemarthrosis or joint effusion may mimic posterior dislocation on AP view, but axillary or transcapular view shows no dislocation.

- **Rotator cuff tear:** Superior subluxation of humeral head is seen with large chronic rotator cuff tears. No dislocation is apparent on axillary or transcapular views.

■ Diagnosis

Posterior shoulder dislocation.

✓ Pearls

- Axillary or transcapular view are essential in diagnosing shoulder dislocations.
- Failure to see the joint articulation on a true AP (Grashey) view is a sign of dislocation.
- Signs to look for on the AP view with posterior dislocation include the "lightbulb" appearance of the humeral head due to fixed internal rotation of the humerus, widened glenohumeral joint due to lateral displacement of the humeral head, and "trough" sign secondary to bony impaction.
- Associated bony and soft tissue injuries are not well-evaluated on radiographs. CT and MRI are more sensitive for evaluation of bone and soft-tissue injuries.

■ Suggested Readings

Cicak N. Posterior dislocation of the shoulder. J Bone Joint Surg Br. 2004; 86(3): 324–332

Cutts S, Prempeh M, Drew S. Anterior shoulder dislocation. Ann R Coll Surg Engl. 2009; 91(1):2–7

Hassanzadeh E, Chang CY, Huang AJ. CT and MRI manifestations of luxatio erectahumeri and a review of the literature. Clin Imaging. 2015; 39(5):876–879

Kowalsky MS, Levine WN. Traumatic posterior glenohumeral dislocation: classification, pathoanatomy, diagnosis, and treatment. Orthop Clin North Am. 2008; 39 (4):519–533, viii

Case 2

Jasjeet Bindra

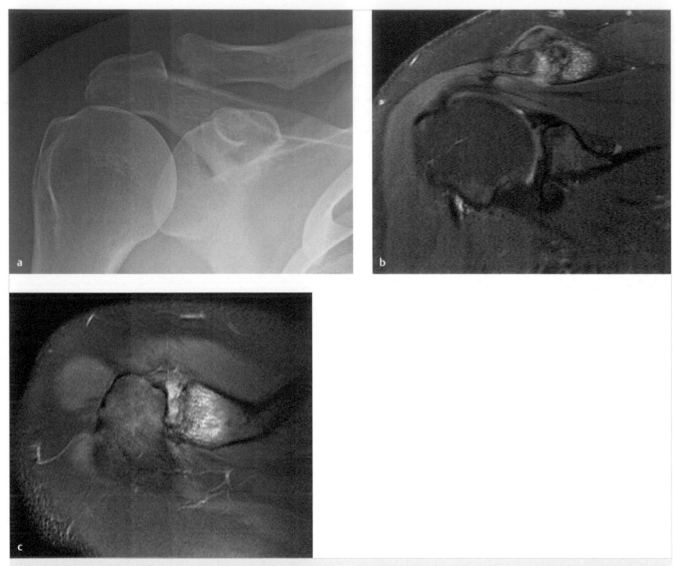

Fig. 2.1 Frontal radiograph of the shoulder **(a)** shows distal clavicular erosion. Corresponding coronal oblique fat-saturated proton density-weighted MR image of the shoulder **(b)** demonstrates erosive change of distal clavicle with adjacent fluid signal. Axial fat-saturated proton density-weighted MR image **(c)** of the shoulder shows distal clavicular edema.

■ **Clinical History**

A 32-year-old female with shoulder pain (▶ Fig. 2.1).

■ Key Finding

Distal clavicular erosion.

■ Top 3 Differential Diagnoses

- **Trauma:** Stress osteolysis of distal clavicle can occur when repeated forces are applied to the acromioclavicular (AC) joint. This is classically seen in weightlifters. Symptoms begin with aching pain in the AC region which are exacerbated by weight training (e.g., bench presses, push-ups, dips on the parallel bars, overhead activities, and horizontal adduction). The most accepted etiology is that repetitive microtrauma causes subchondral stress fractures and remodeling in the distal clavicle. Acromion is spared in this entity.
- **Rheumatoid arthritis (RA):** Rheumatoid arthritis can cause distal clavicular resorption identical to other etiologies. Presence of other findings of inflammatory arthropathy including periarticular osteopenia, erosions of acromion, glenohumeral joint space narrowing, and erosions of the glenohumeral joint can help in pinpointing the diagnosis.
- **Hyperparathyroidism:** Besides the distal clavicular erosion, another finding that can be seen in hyperparathyroidism on the shoulder or clavicular radiographs is subligamentous resorption at the site of coracoclavicular ligament on the clavicle. Generalized bone demineralization is a uniform feature of all types of hyperparathyroidism. Subchondral bone loss can also be seen at sacroiliac, sternoclavicular and temporomandibular joints, and at symphysis pubis, in addition to the AC joint.

■ Additional Diagnostic Considerations

- **Scleroderma:** Scleroderma is a multisystem disease. Radiographically, acro-osteolysis and soft tissue calcifications are commonly seen. Erosions can occur but arthritis is not a prominent feature.
- **Infection:** Septic arthritis should always be entertained as a possibility in distal clavicular erosion.

■ Diagnosis

Posttraumatic osteolysis.

✓ Pearls

- Posttraumatic distal clavicular osteolysis is most commonly associated with weight training involving upper extremities.
- In RA, presence of other findings like periarticular osteopenia, glenohumeral joint space narrowing and erosions can help in narrowing the differential.
- Hyperparathyroidism will also demonstrate other findings like generalized osteopenia, subligamentous, and subperiosteal resorption.

■ Suggested Readings

Currie JW, Davis KW, Lafita VS, et al. Musculoskeletal mnemonics: differentiating features. Curr Probl Diagn Radiol. 2011; 40(2):45–71

Manaster BJ, May DA, Disler DG. Musculoskeletal Imaging, The Requisites. 4th ed. Philadelphia: Mosby Elsevier; 2013

Schwarzkopf R, Ishak C, Elman M, Gelber J, Strauss DN, Jazrawi LM. Distal clavicular osteolysis: a review of the literature. Bull NYU Hosp Jt Dis. 2008; 66(2):94–101

Case 3

Eva Escobedo and Jasjeet Bindra

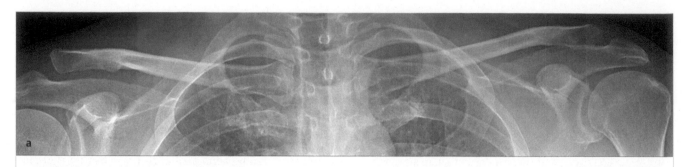

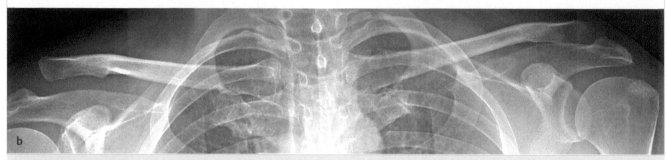

Fig. 3.1 Radiograph of bilateral acromioclavicular (AC) joints **(a)** shows mild widening of AC joint and superior subluxation of clavicle on the right side. Radiograph of bilateral AC joints with 10-pound weights attached to the wrists **(b)** shows increase in degree of widening of the joint and superior displacement of the clavicle.

■ Clinical History

A 32-year-old male with shoulder pain after 6-foot fall onto right shoulder (▶ Fig. 3.1).

■ Key Finding

Widening of acromioclavicular (AC) joint.

■ Top 3 Differential Diagnoses

- **Trauma:** AC injuries are more common in men and are caused by contact sports, heavy overhead manual labor, and falls on outstretched hand. An AC interval greater than 6 to 7 mm or a difference in AC interval of greater than 2 to 3 mm between the two sides are considered pathologic. AC joint separation is categorized using the Rockwood classification. Type I involves sprain or partial tear of the AC ligaments. Radiographically, the AC joint is normal. In type II AC separation, the AC ligaments are completely torn, and coracoclavicular ligaments sprained. Radiographically, the AC joint is widened, and there may be mild elevation of the clavicle. Type III injuries show complete disruption of both AC and coracoclavicular ligaments. The clavicle is more significantly elevated and the coracoclavicular interspace is 25 to 100% increased. Type IV to VI occur in more severe injuries.

- **Distal clavicle erosion:** Distal clavicle erosion can present as widening of the AC joint on radiographs. More common causes include posttraumatic osteolysis, rheumatoid arthritis, and hyperparathyroidism. With posttraumatic osteolysis, there is commonly a history of repetitive trauma such as weightlifting. Rheumatoid arthritis and hyperparathyroidism are systemic diseases, thus most often present bilaterally.

- **Postsurgical change:** Distal clavicular resection or Mumford procedure can be performed as part of subacromial decompression. Subacromial decompression consists of enlarging the subacromial space with osseous burring or excision of the undersurface of acromion. Concomitant symptomatic AC joint arthrosis is treated with resection of the AC joint and up to 1 cm of distal clavicle. The AC joint thus appears widened, even up to 2.5 cm.

■ Diagnosis

Type III acromioclavicular separation.

✓ Pearls

- Less than 15% of shoulder girdle injuries involve injury to the AC joint.
- The most common grading system for AC joint injuries used is the Rockwood classification system, which grades injury from type I to VI, with the most common being types I–III.
- Simultaneous view of bilateral AC joints helps to distinguish pathologic widening from normal variation.

- Stress views of the AC joints with 10 to 15 pounds of weight suspended from each forearm can reveal more severe injuries than originally apparent. They are especially helpful in distinguishing Type II from Type III injuries.
- MRI can be used to assess injury of coracoclavicular ligaments and deltoid and trapezius tendon insertions; thus, it is helpful in more accurately grading injuries.

■ Suggested Readings

Alyas F, Curtis M, Speed C, Saifuddin A, Connell D. MR imaging appearances of acromioclavicular joint dislocation. Radiographics. 2008; 28(2):463–479, quiz 619

Ha AS, Petscavage-Thomas JM, Tagoylo GH. Acromioclavicular joint: the other joint in the shoulder. AJR Am J Roentgenol. 2014; 202(2):375–385

Macdonald PB, Lapointe P. Acromioclavicular and sternoclavicular joint injuries. Orthop Clin North Am. 2008; 39(4):535–545, viii

Melenevsky Y, Yablon CM, Ramappa A, Hochman MG. Clavicle and acromioclavicular joint injuries: a review of imaging, treatment, and complications. Skeletal Radiol. 2011; 40(7):831–842

Case 4

Eva Escobedo

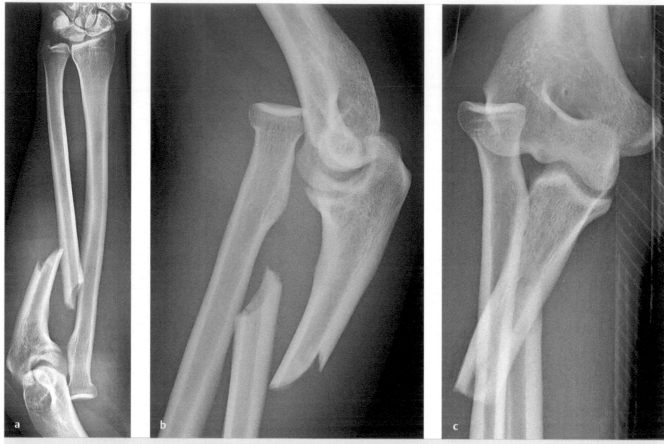

Fig. 4.1 Single radiograph of the forearm **(a)** and lateral and AP radiographs of the elbow **(b, c)** show a displaced fracture of the proximal ulna and dislocation of the radial head.

■ Clinical History

A 23-year-old male after fall on an outstretched arm (▶ Fig. 4.1).

■ Key Finding

Fracture dislocation of forearm.

■ Top 3 Differential Diagnoses

- **Galeazzi fracture:** The Galeazzi fracture is a fracture through the distal radius (between the middle and distal thirds) with disruption of the distal radioulnar joint (DRUJ). With distal radial fractures, care must be taken to evaluate the distal radioulnar joint both clinically and radiographically. Thus, evaluation requires both forearm and wrist radiographs. Evidence of DRUJ disruption include widening of the DRUJ space, lack of overlap of the ulnar head on the distal radius on PA view, dislocation of the ulnar head relative to the radius on a true lateral view, or shortening of the distal radius by more than 5 mm. Treatment of this injury is almost always surgical.
- **Monteggia fracture:** The Monteggia fracture is a fracture of the proximal third of the ulna with associated radial head dislocation. With proximal ulna fractures, attention should be paid to radiocapitellar joint alignment. A line drawn through the center of the proximal radius should intersect the capitellum on all the views. Injuries may involve the deep branch of the radial nerve (posterior interosseous nerve) which is intimately associated with the radial head at the elbow.
- **Essex–Lopresti fracture:** This rare but often overlooked injury is the combination of a comminuted radial head fracture with disruption of the interosseous membrane, resultant dislocation of the distal radioulnar joint, and proximal migration of the distal radius. Because the dislocation at the DRUJ is often missed both clinically and radiographically, it is important to obtain dedicated wrist views with attention to this area. Failure to address these injuries will lead to poor outcome.

■ Additional Diagnostic Consideration

- **"Nightstick" fracture:** This is an isolated fracture of the ulna with no joint or radius involvement. Unlike the fracture dislocations of the forearm, which typically occur with an axial load such as a fall on an outstretched hand, the nightstick fracture is caused by a direct blow, thus being an exception to the forearm "ring rule," which states that injury to one part of the forearm should result in a second fracture or dislocation elsewhere.

■ Diagnosis

Monteggia fracture.

✓ Pearls

- Most forearm injuries from axial load follow the "ring rule," that is, an injury of one bone or joint is often associated with fracture or dislocation in a second location. An exception to this rule is the "nightstick" fracture.
- With a distal radius or comminuted radial head fracture, wrist radiographs should be obtained to evaluate the distal radioulnar joint.
- With a fracture of the proximal ulna, elbow films should be obtained to evaluate radial head dislocation. A line drawn through the proximal radius can confirm a dislocation, as this should always intersect the capitellum of the humerus.
- If a Galeazzi, Monteggia, or Essex–Lopresti fracture is missed, long-term disability and pain often result.

■ Suggested Readings

Bock GW, Cohen MS, Resnick D. Fracture-dislocation of the elbow with inferior radioulnar dislocation: a variant of the Essex-Lopresti injury. Skeletal Radiol. 1992; 21(5):315–317

Gyftopoulos S, Chitkara M, Bencardino JT. Misses and errors in upper extremity trauma radiographs. AJR Am J Roentgenol. 2014; 203(3):477–491

Perron AD, Hersh RE, Brady WJ, Keats TE. Orthopedic pitfalls in the ED: Galeazzi and Monteggia fracture-dislocation. Am J Emerg Med. 2001; 19(3):225–228

Case 5

Eva Escobedo

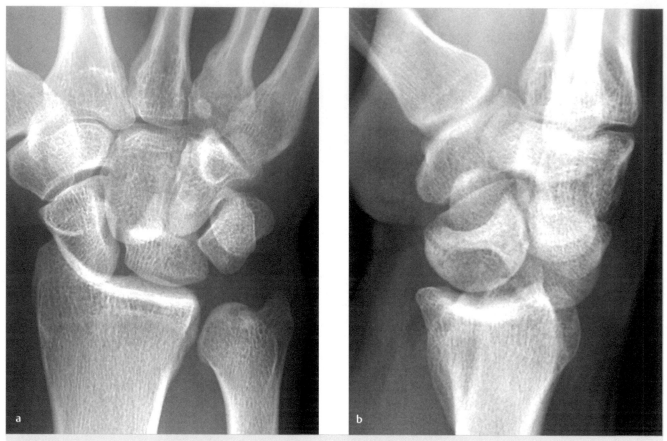

Fig. 5.1 PA view of the wrist **(a)** shows triangular-shaped lunate and nonvisualization of the capitolunate articulation. Lateral view of the wrist **(b)** shows normal position of the lunate; however, there is dorsal dislocation of capitate along with other carpal bones.

■ **Clinical History**
....
A 29-year-old male after fall on an outstretched hand (▶ Fig. 5.1).

Key Finding

Carpal dislocation.

Top 3 Differential Diagnoses

- **Perilunate dislocation:** Perilunate injuries result from forced hyperextension of the wrist with ulnar deviation and carpal supination. They occur in a sequence of ligamentous disruptions termed "progressive perilunar instability," which extends from a radial to ulnar direction. The perilunate dislocation is an intermediate stage in this sequence. On PA radiograph of the wrist, the lunate will appear triangular in shape, and a normal capitolunate articulation will not be visible. On lateral radiograph, the lunate articulates normally with the distal radius, but the capitate is dorsally dislocated.
- **Lunate dislocation:** This injury occurs as the last stage of "progressive perilunar instability." With increasing hyperextension force, a perilunate dislocation may become a lunate dislocation, as the dislocated capitate forces the lunate ventrally, disrupting its ligamentous attachment to the radius. Thus, the capitate becomes realigned with the distal radius, and the lunate is dislocated in a palmar direction. As with the perilunate dislocation, PA view of the wrist will show an abnormally shaped lunate, without a normal articulation between the lunate and capitate.
- **Midcarpal dislocation:** The intermediate stage between perilunate and lunate dislocation, the midcarpal dislocation is a result of ligamentous injury at the lunotriquetral joint. The PA view of the wrist is similar to that of perilunate and lunate dislocations. However, lateral view of the wrist typically shows dorsal dislocation of the capitate, and volar tilt and subluxation of the lunate. Thus, neither the lunate nor the capitate is normally positioned in relation to the distal radius.

Additional Diagnostic Consideration

- **"SLAC" wrist:** Scapholunate advanced collapse (SLAC) is a progressive form of wrist osteoarthritis most commonly secondary to trauma or calcium pyrophosphate dihydrate (CPPD) crystal deposition disease. Beginning with scapholunate dissociation, there is a progressive pattern of involvement with osteoarthritic changes initially occurring at the radioscaphoid joint and eventually affecting capitolunate joint with proximal migration of the capitate, causing more pronounced separation of the scapholunate interspace.

Diagnosis

Perilunate dislocation.

✓ Pearls

- Perilunate instability has been classified into four stages of ligamentous injury, starting at the scapholunate joint, progressing through the capitolunate and lunotriquetral joint (resulting in perilunate and midcarpal dislocation), with the final stage resulting in lunate dislocation.
- Perilunate injuries may either be purely ligamentous (lesser arc injuries) or be associated with fractures (greater arc injuries), most commonly through the scaphoid (transscaphoid perilunate dislocation).
- Review of the lateral wrist radiograph is essential in detecting and classifying these injuries.
- Detection of perilunate injuries is important because early treatment can prevent the complications of chronic carpal instability and posttraumatic arthritis.

Suggested Readings

Grabow RJ, Catalano L, III. Carpal dislocations. Hand Clin. 2006; 22(4):485–500, abstract vi–vii

Kaewlai R, Avery LL, Asrani AV, Abujudeh HH, Sacknoff R, Novelline RA. Multidetector CT of carpal injuries: anatomy, fractures, and fracture-dislocations. Radiographics. 2008; 28(6):1771–1784

Kennedy SA, Allan CH. In brief: Mayfield et al. Classification: carpal dislocations and progressive perilunar instability. Clin Orthop Relat Res. 2012; 470(4):1243–1245

Scalcione LR, Gimber LH, Ho AM, Johnston SS, Sheppard JE, Taljanovic MS. Spectrum of carpal dislocations and fracture-dislocations: imaging and management. AJR Am J Roentgenol. 2014; 203(3):541–550

Case 6

Eva Escobedo

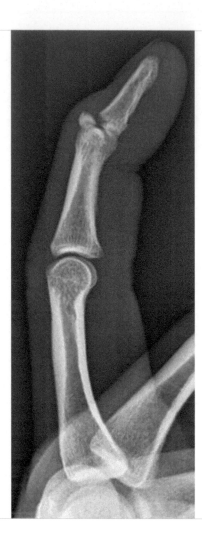

Fig. 6.1 Lateral radiograph of the index finger shows an intra-articular fracture of the dorsal aspect of the base of the distal phalanx.

■ **Clinical History**

A 22-year-old male jammed finger while playing basketball
(▶ Fig. 6.1).

■ Key Finding

Avulsion fracture of finger.

■ Top 3 Differential Diagnoses

- **Terminal extensor tendon avulsion**: The "mallet finger" is the most common closed tendon injury seen in sports, usually secondary to a direct blow (often baseball or basketball), which forcibly flexes an extended finger. This may result in a tendinous or bony avulsion of the extensor tendon. Clinically, the patient is unable to actively extend the distal interphalangeal (DIP) joint, and radiographs often show flexion of the DIP joint. If left untreated, the imbalance in extensor forces may lead to a swan neck deformity.
- **Volar plate avulsion**: The volar plate, a fibrocartilaginous structure that reinforces the joint capsule, is present at the proximal interphalangeal (PIP) and metacarpophalangeal (MCP) joints. The term volar plate avulsion is used most commonly for PIP injuries, and is secondary to hyperextension, with avulsion of the volar plate from the base of the middle phalanx. Pure ligamentous or bony avulsions can occur, and injury may be associated with dorsal dislocation. Fracture involvement of greater than 40% of the articular surface is considered unstable.
- **Flexor digitorum profundus avulsion**: Avulsion of the profundus tendon ("jersey finger") is caused by forceful hyperextension of a flexed DIP joint, most commonly of the ring finger. Most avulsions are tendinous and invisible on radiographs, thus requiring US or MRI for definitive diagnosis. A bony fragment may avulse in some cases and be visualized radiographically.

■ Additional Diagnostic Considerations

- **Central slip rupture**: Acute central slip ruptures occur most commonly with forced flexion of an extended PIP joint, with injury at or near the dorsal insertion on the base of the middle phalanx. Other mechanisms include blow to the dorsum of the middle phalanx, or volar dislocation of the PIP joint. Avulsion fractures are much less common than ligamentous injury. An unrecognized injury often results in a boutonniere deformity.
- **Collateral ligament avulsion**: Collateral ligament injury is caused by forced ulnar or radial deviation, and it can occur at the MCP or any interphalangeal joint, most commonly the PIP joint. Radiography may show an avulsion fracture at the insertion. Treatment is based on size of fragment and stability.

■ Diagnosis

Extensor tendon avulsion ("mallet finger").

✓ Pearls

- Tendinous and ligamentous avulsions of the fingers may be soft-tissue injuries or bony avulsion fractures.
- Avulsion fractures of the fingers commonly seen on radiographs include terminal extensor tendon avulsions "mallet finger," volar plate avulsions, flexor digitorum profundus avulsions "jersey finger," and collateral ligament avulsions.
- Stability is often based on the size of the fracture fragment or percentage of articular surface involved.
- Although seemingly insignificant, many of these injuries, if not addressed, can result in deformities and altered function.

■ Suggested Readings

Alla SR, Deal ND, Dempsey IJ. Current concepts: mallet finger. Hand (N Y). 2014; 9 (2):138–144

Clavero JA, Alomar X, Monill JM, et al. MR imaging of ligament and tendon injuries of the fingers. Radiographics. 2002; 22(2):237–256

Leggit JC, Meko CJ. Acute finger injuries: part I. Tendons and ligaments. Am Fam Physician. 2006; 73(5):810–816

Perron AD, Brady WJ, Keats TE, Hersh RE. Orthopedic pitfalls in the emergency department: closed tendon injuries of the hand. Am J Emerg Med. 2001; 19 (1):76–80

Case 7

John C Hunter and Jasjeet Bindra

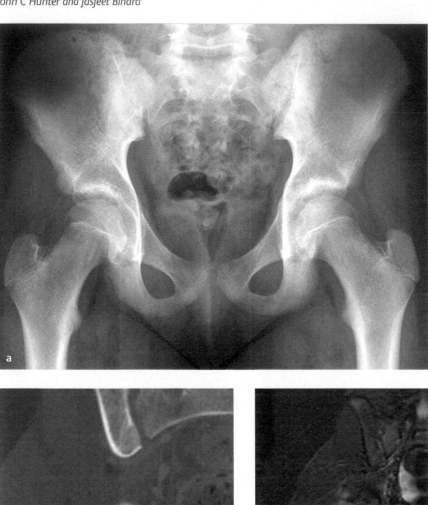

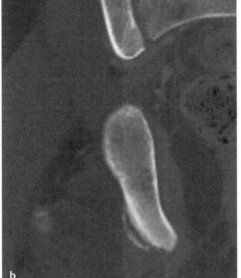

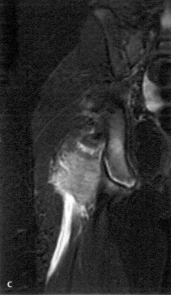

Fig. 7.1 AP view of the hip **(a)** shows subtle curvilinear density along the right ischial tuberosity. Coronal reformation CT image **(b)** shows the avulsion fragment to a better advantage, and coronal STIR MR image of the pelvis **(c)** shows fluid at the site of fracture and edema surrounding this region.

■ **Clinical History**

A 15-year-old male soccer player with right posterior hip pain after a game (▶ Fig. 7.1).

▪ Key Finding

Avulsion fracture of the pelvis.

▪ Top 3 Differential Diagnoses

- **Avulsion of the anterior inferior iliac spine (AIIS):** AIIS avulsion occurs secondary to a forceful pull of the rectus femoris muscle on an open apophysis during trauma or athletic activity. Like most pelvic avulsions, it occurs in adolescents. The AIIS is the site of origin of the straight head of rectus femoris muscle. Avulsion fragments can be seen proximal and lateral to the acetabular rim. Small fragments may be overlooked on AP views; however, oblique views are more sensitive for small and nondisplaced fragments.
- **Avulsion of ischial tuberosity:** This fracture occurs at the site of origin of the hamstring group of muscles (semimembranosus, semitendinosus, and biceps femoris), which is the most common avulsion fracture of the pelvis. Avulsion is caused by extreme active contraction of hamstrings which usually

occurs before the closure of apophysis. At radiography, healing avulsions can have an aggressive appearance, including lysis and destruction. In such cases, history and CT may be helpful in diagnosis. Depending on the degree of displacement, acute injuries may require open reduction and internal fixation for treatment.
- **Avulsion of the anterior superior iliac spine (ASIS):** The ASIS is the site of origin of the sartorius muscle and some fibers of tensor fascia latae. Avulsion occurs with a strong sudden pull of the sartorius, with the hip in extension and the knee in flexion, most commonly in sprinters and other running athletes. Radiographs demonstrate a triangular-appearing avulsion fragment at the ASIS.

▪ Additional Diagnostic Considerations

- **Avulsion of the lesser trochanter:** The lesser trochanter is the site of insertion of the iliopsoas muscle. This injury occurs mostly in adolescent soccer players and is caused by violent contraction of iliopsoas while the thigh is extended. In adults, this type of injury results in strain or tear at the distal musculotendinous junction of iliopsoas. Isolated nontraumatic

avulsion of lesser trochanter in adults is usually a pathologic fracture related to an underlying lesion, most commonly metastatic disease.
- **Avulsion of the greater trochanter:** The greater trochanter is the site of attachment of hip rotators, and avulsions can occur with abrupt directional changes.

▪ Diagnosis

Avulsion of ischial tuberosity.

✓ Pearls

- In many series, soccer and gymnastics are the most common sports of patients with pelvic avulsions.
- The same mechanism of injury that results in avulsion in young patients usually results in a musculotendinous muscle injury in an adult patient.
- Lesser trochanter avulsions in adolescents are nearly all traumatic; in adults, many are pathologic fractures, most commonly from an underlying metastatic lesion.

- If the patient presents even a few weeks after the initial injury, the appearance of a healing avulsion fracture may be confused with a more ominous process such as osteosarcoma on both imaging and pathologic examination. Such cases require evaluation by a team of clinicians, radiologists, and pathologists experienced with these entities to avoid serious errors.

▪ Suggested Readings

Fernbach SK, Wilkinson RH. Avulsion injuries of the pelvis and proximal femur. AJR Am J Roentgenol. 1981; 137(3):581–584

James SL, Davies AM. A traumatic avulsion of the lesser trochanter as an indicator of tumour infiltration. Eur Radiol. 2006; 16(2):512–514

Metzmaker JN, Pappas AM. Avulsion fractures of the pelvis. Am J Sports Med. 1985; 13(5):349–358

Wood DG, Packham I, Trikha SP, Linklater J. Avulsion of the proximal hamstring origin. J Bone Joint Surg Am. 2008; 90(11):2365–2374

Case 8

Jasjeet Bindra

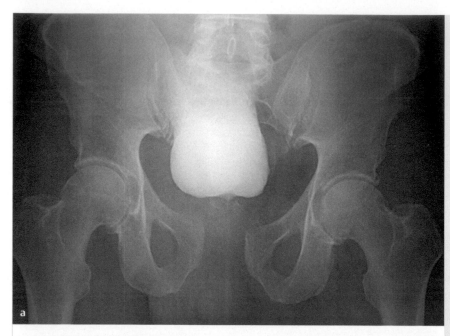

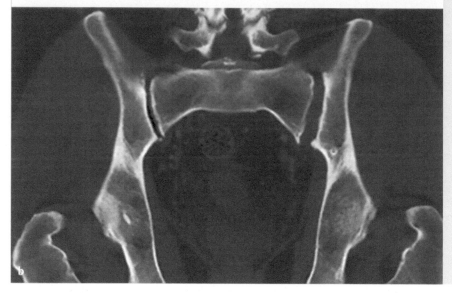

Fig. 8.1 AP view of the pelvis **(a)** shows marked widening of the symphysis pubis. Coronal reformatted CT image of the pelvis **(b)** in the same patient reveals widening of bilateral sacroiliac joints, more on the left.

■ Clinical History

A 48-year-old male status post motor vehicle accident (▶ Fig. 8.1).

■ Key Finding

Widened pubic symphysis.

■ Top 3 Differential Diagnoses

- **Trauma:** Trauma is a very common cause of pubic symphysis widening. Pubic symphysis is the weakest link in the pelvic ring. In AP compression injuries of pelvis, the first point of failure is the pubic symphysis, which is either disrupted or surrounded by vertical fractures through one or both pairs of pubic rami. In AP compression type 1 injuries, diastasis of pubic symphysis is less than 2.5 cm and without rupture of the posterior pelvic ligaments. However, pure AP compression type 1 injuries are rare and patients with any degree of traumatic symphysis diastasis should be treated as if a posterior pelvic injury is present until it is proved otherwise. In AP compression type 2 injuries, there is more than 2.5 cm diastasis of symphysis along with widening of anterior sacroiliac (SI) joints due to injury to anterior SI complex. In AP compression type 3 injuries, there is complete disruption of posterior SI ligament with separation of iliac wing from sacrum. The distinction between anterior and posterior SI diastasis is best made on axial CT images. Symphysis diastasis can also be seen with vertical shear injuries, but the key finding in these injuries is cephalad displacement of iliac crest of the injured hemipelvis relative to the other side.

- **Peripartum widening:** During pregnancy, under the influence of hormones, particularly relaxin, there can be mild widening of symphysis pubis. Frank diastasis of more than 10 mm can sometimes be seen prenatally, or as a result of rapid or prolonged vaginal delivery or assisted forceps delivery. In symptomatic cases, there is suprapubic pain, difficulty in ambulation and, occasionally, bladder dysfunction.

- **Osteitis pubis:** Osteitis pubis is a chronic inflammatory response to mechanical stresses on pubic symphysis and results in osteitis and periostitis of the pubic bones. It is common in athletes who subject symphysis to repetitive shear and distraction forces during sports such as football. Radiographs may show mild irregularity of the articular surfaces. In some cases, gross erosions can develop, leading to symphyseal widening. Productive changes like sclerosis and osteophyte formation can also be seen.

■ Additional Diagnostic Considerations

- **Exstrophy of bladder:** Patients are born with their bladder mucosa exposed to the environment through a lower abdominal wall defect. There is widening of symphysis pubis, with external rotation of innominate bones on radiographs.

- **Prune belly syndrome:** Prune belly syndrome is a rare disorder characterized by marked dilatation of the ureters, cryptorchidism, and significant deficiency of abdominal musculature.

■ Diagnosis

Trauma with anteroposterior compression injury.

✓ Pearls

- Posttraumatic pubis symhysis diastasis is usually associated with posterior pelvic injury.
- Peripartum symphysis widening can vary from mild widening to frank diastasis.
- Osteitis pubis, common in athletes, can be associated with erosions and symphysial widening.

■ Suggested Readings

Budak MJ, Oliver TB. There's a hole in my symphys is: a review of disorders causing widening, erosion, and destruction of the symphysis pubis. Clin Radiol. 2013; 68 (2):173–180

Khurana B, Sheehan SE, Sodickson AD, Weaver MJ. Pelvic ring fractures: what the orthopedic surgeon wants to know. Radiographics. 2014; 34(5):1317–1333

Case 9

John C. Hunter and Jasjeet Bindra

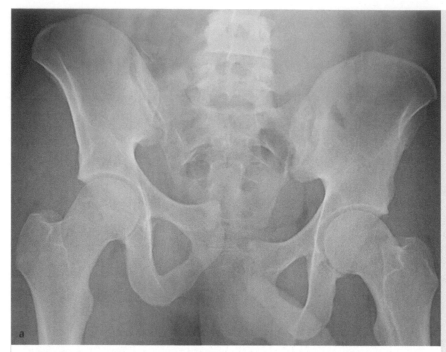

Fig. 9.1 AP radiograph of the pelvis **(a)** shows pubic symphysis diastasis, widening of the left sacroiliac joint, disruption of right sacral arcuate lines, and vertical superior displacement of right hemipelvis. Axial CT image **(b)** of the pelvis shows right sacral fracture and left sacroiliac joint widening to a better advantage.

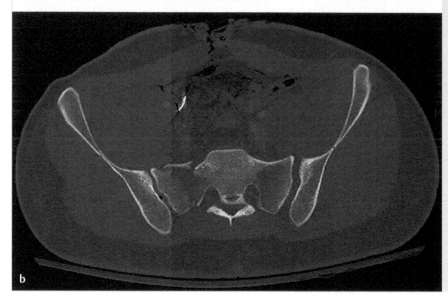

■ Clinical History

A 22-year-old male status post motor vehicle accident (▶ Fig. 9.1).

Key Finding

Pelvic ring disruption.

Top 3 Differential Diagnoses

- **Anteroposterior compression (APC) injury:** APC injuries are also called "open book" pelvic fractures. The first injury occurs in the anterior pelvis, with either diastasis of the pubic symphysis or vertical fractures through one or both sets of pubic rami. If the compression stops here, an APC I injury results. If the compressive force continues, the anterior sacroiliac (SI) ligaments are next to give way, resulting in unilateral or bilateral anterior SI diastasis. This pattern is termed APC II. Finally, in APC III injury, the posterior SI ligaments are disrupted, thereby completely separating the hemipelvis. The distinction between anterior and posterior diastasis is best appreciated on axial CT images. Substantial hemorrhage is most prevalent with AP compression injuries, as the pelvic volume can expand and there is no tamponade.
- **Lateral compression (LC) injury:** Lateral compression injury is the most common type of pelvic ring injury. The force in this pattern comes from a direct blow to the iliac crest or hip, usually in the side-impact vehicular accident. This is a crushing injury which causes internal rotation of the hemipelvis, and the pelvic volume is decreased. In LC injuries, the anterior pubic rami fractures are typically transverse; the degree of posterior pelvic involvement determines the grade of injury. LC-I injuries involve sacral impaction. These commonly occur in elderly patients as a result of falls in the setting of osteoporosis. The sacral alar fractures are difficult to identify on pelvic radiographs, making it necessary to pay close attention to arcuate lines. In LC-II injuries, the hemipelvis rotates internally and rather than crushing the sacrum, the strong posterior sacroiliac ligaments avulse a crescent-shaped fragment of the posterior ilium. LC-III injuries involve a contralateral APC type injury in addition to LC-I or LC-II injury on the side of the impact.
- **Vertical shear:** Vertical shear injuries are one of the most severe forms of pelvic ring disruptions. The characteristic feature is vertical and/or posterior displacement of the disrupted hemipelvis. Due to the anterior tilt of the pelvic ring, inlet and outlet views often provide better assessment of the displacement than the AP view alone. Anteriorly, there is symphysis diastasis or vertical fractures through one or both obturator rings. Posteriorly, there is disruption of the SI joints or fractures through the ilium or sacrum.

Additional Diagnostic Consideration

- **Combined or complex fractures:** Certain severe pelvic disruptions do not easily fit into the classification schemes. The combined category has fractures that demonstrate elements of more than one pattern.

Diagnosis

Vertical shear injury.

✓ Pearls

- The classifications utilized by orthopedic surgeons include description of the mechanism of injury and assessment of pelvic stability.
- Pubic symphysis diastasis, particularly greater than 2.5 cm, implies disruption of not only the symphysis but also of one or both SI ligaments.
- Transverse or overriding obturator ring fractures raise the suspicion for a LC type of injury.
- If the patient has been wrapped in a compressive binding, diastasis may be reduced and difficult to identify.

Suggested Readings

Khurana B, Sheehan SE, Sodickson AD, Weaver MJ. Pelvic ring fractures: what the orthopedic surgeon wants to know. Radiographics. 2014; 34(5):1317–1333

Stambaugh LE, III, Blackmore CC. Pelvic ring disruptions in emergency radiology. Eur J Radiol. 2003; 48(1):71–87

Case 10

Eva Escobedo and Jasjeet Bindra

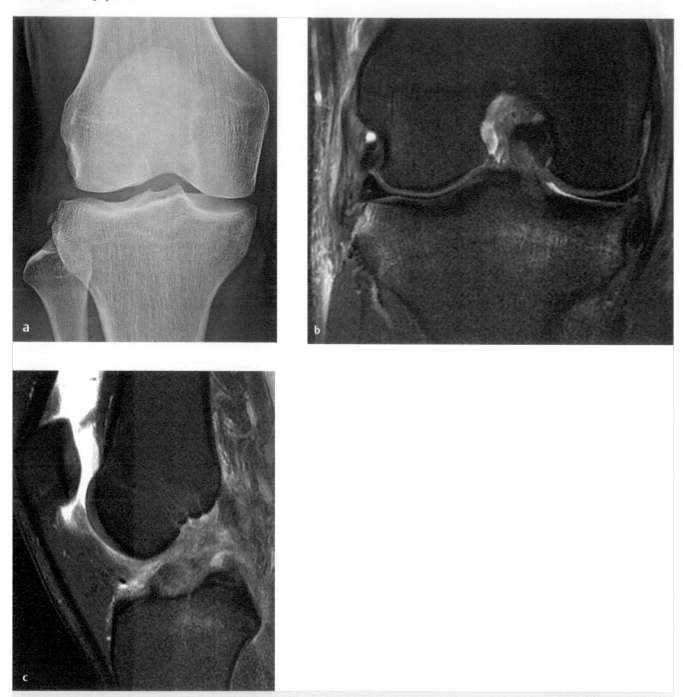

Fig. 10.1 AP radiograph of the knee **(a)** demonstrates a small avulsion fracture fragment from the lateral aspect of tibial plateau. Coronal fat-suppressed proton density-weighted MR image of the knee **(b)** shows mild osseous edema at the donor site of the fracture fragment and sagittal fat-suppressed proton density-weighted image of the knee **(c)** shows disruption of anterior cruciate ligament.

■ **Clinical History**

A 23-year-old female with knee injury while playing flag football (▶ Fig. 10.1).

■ Key Finding

Avulsion fracture at the knee.

■ Top 3 Differential Diagnoses

- **Segond fracture:** The Segond fracture is typically a vertically oriented, curvilinear, or elliptic bone fragment off the lateral aspect of the tibial plateau, best seen on AP radiographs. It is highly associated with tear of the anterior cruciate ligament (ACL). The fracture has been most commonly attributed to avulsion of the middle third of the lateral capsular ligament. Recently, the anterior lateral ligament has been described as a distinct ligament attaching to the Segond fracture, with one study showing major contributions from the iliotibial band and lateral capsule. MRI is advised when a Segond fracture is seen due to concomitant meniscal and ligamentous injuries.
- **Tibial spine avulsion:** A fracture of the anterior medial tibial eminence usually indicates an avulsion of the ACL. These are most common in skeletally immature patients between the ages of 8 to 14 years. The fracture fragment may be difficult to see in children due to the presence of cartilage. CT scan is useful in assessing fracture anatomy and degree of displacement. MRI is useful in outlining the nonosseous concomitant injuries like meniscal injury, cartilage injury, and other ligamentous injury.
- **Fibular head avulsion:** A fracture of the styloid process of the fibular head (the "arcuate sign") is an indication of injury to the arcuate complex. Fractures at the lateral aspect of the fibular head indicate lateral collateral ligament and/or the biceps femoris tendon avulsions. These posterolateral corner injuries are highly associated with cruciate ligament injuries, most commonly the posterior cruciate ligament (PCL).

■ Additional Diagnostic Considerations

- **Medial patellar avulsion:** This injury occurs with transient lateral patellar dislocation along with avulsion of the medial patellofemoral ligament. It is best seen with CT, but the soft-tissue injury is better assessed on MRI.
- **Reverse Segond fracture:** This elliptic fragment represents an avulsion of the deep capsular component of the medial collateral ligament. It is known to be associated with PCL and medial meniscal tears.
- **PCL avulsion:** Fractures at the posterior tibia plateau, near the posterior tibial eminence, may represent an avulsion of the PCL. These usually occur with hyperextension or with posterior forces on the tibia such as falling on a flexed knee or "dashboard" injuries. These are best seen on lateral radiographs.

■ Diagnosis

Segond fracture.

✓ Pearls

- MRI is recommended for Segond fractures because, in addition to the associated ACL tear, there is a high-rate of meniscal and other ligamentous injury.
- Small bony avulsions at the knee can be an indication of much more severe ligamentous injury and meniscal tears. MRI is useful in evaluating these associated injuries.
- Avulsion fractures of the fibular head indicate posterolateral corner injuries. If not addressed at the time of surgery for the associated cruciate ligament tears, it may result in chronic instability and graft failure.

■ Suggested Readings

Gottsegen CJ, Eyer BA, White EA, Learch TJ, Forrester D. Avulsion fractures of the knee: imaging findings and clinical significance. Radiographics. 2008; 28 (6):1755–1770

Shaikh H, Herbst E, Rahnemai-Azar AA, et al. The Segond fracture is an avulsion of the anterolateral complex. Am J Sports Med. 2017; 45(10):2247–2252

Venkatasamy A, Ehlinger M, Bierry G. Acute traumatic knee radiographs: beware of lesions of little expression but of great significance. Diagn Interv Imaging. 2014; 95(6):551–560

Case 11

Eva Escobedo

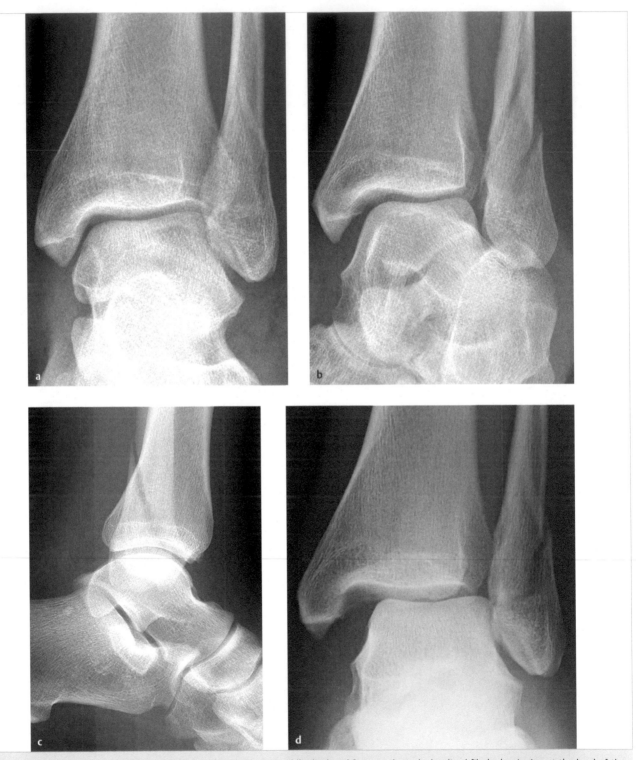

Fig. 11.1 Anteroposterior **(a)** and Mortise **(b)** views of ankle show a mildly displaced fracture through the distal fibula, beginning at the level of the joint and extending proximally. Lateral view **(c)** shows the fracture running obliquely from anterior inferior to posterior superior aspect of distal fibula. Gravity stress view **(d)** shows marked widening of the medial clear space and tibiofibular syndesmosis.

■ **Clinical History**

A 25-year-old man twisted ankle while playing soccer (▶ Fig. 11.1).

■ Key Finding

Distal fibular fracture.

■ Top 3 Differential Diagnoses

- **Weber A fracture:** The Danis–Weber classification of ankle fractures is one of the most commonly used and is based on the location of the distal fibular fracture in relation to the syndesmosis. A Weber A fracture occurs distal to ankle joint (below syndesmosis). It usually occurs due to avulsion from supination of the foot. There may be an associated oblique or vertically oriented medial malleolar fracture. The deltoid ligament and syndesmosis remain intact; thus, this injury is usually stable.
- **Weber B fracture:** A Weber B fracture is the most common type of ankle fracture, and it is secondary to supination and external rotation. It begins at the level of the syndesmosis, extending proximally and laterally up the fibula. More than half of them are associated with syndesmotic injury, and there may be an associated medial malleolus, deltoid ligament, or posterior malleolus injury. Stability varies, depending on the associated ligamentous injuries. Because the deep deltoid ligament is a major stabilizing structure, stress views are often taken to assess for widening of the medial clear space, which would indicate injury to this ligament and/or the syndesmosis.
- **Weber C fracture:** A Weber C fracture occurs above the level of the syndesmosis. The mechanism of injury is pronation and external rotation or pronation and abduction. The syndesmosis is assumed to be torn distal to the fracture, as is usually evidenced by widening of the distal tibiofibular articulation. In almost all cases, there is either a medial malleolus fracture or deltoid ligament injury. The Maissoneuve fracture, which presents with a high-fibular fracture, is included in this category. This is an unstable injury and requires surgical intervention.

■ Additional Diagnostic Considerations

- **Fibular stress fracture:** Fibular stress fractures are much less common than tibial fractures, as the fibula is not load-bearing in nature. The mechanism may involve muscle traction and torsional forces. It most commonly occurs in runners at the distal third of the fibula. Findings on radiographs may be subtle and initially be normal or show subtle periosteal reaction.
- **Pilon fracture:** A pilon fracture is a comminuted and impacted fracture of the tibial plafond secondary to high-energy axial load. The majority of these fractures are associated with distal fibular fractures.

■ Diagnosis

Weber B fracture.

✓ Pearls

- The most common classification systems for ankle fractures are the Danis–Weber and Lauge–Hansen systems. The Danis–Weber system is based on location of the distal fibular fracture, with more proximal injuries at greater risk of syndesmosis disruption and instability. The Lauge–Hansen system is based on the mechanism of injury.
- Weber B fractures fall under the supination external rotation (SER) category of Lauge–Hansen system.
- The Maissoneuve fracture should be considered when a medial malleolus fracture is present without an associated lateral malleolus injury, or if there is evidence of deltoid or syndesmotic injury. Tibial–fibular films should be obtained to evaluate high-fibular fracture.

■ Suggested Readings

Bugler KE, White TO, Thordarson DB. Focus on ankle fractures. J Bone JointSurg. 2012; 94:1107–1112

Dhillon MS, Kumar L, Sharma S, Mehta N. The Lauge–Hansen classification for ankle fractures: is it relevant in 2017? J Foot Ankle Surg (Asia-Pacific). 2017; 4(2): 53–56

Donatto KC. Ankle fractures and syndesmosis injuries. Orthop Clin North Am. 2001; 32(1):79–90

Hermans JJ, Wentink N, Beumer A, et al. Correlation between radiological assessment of acute ankle fractures and syndesmotic injury on MRI. Skeletal Radiol. 2012; 41(7):787–801

Case 12

Eva Escobedo and Jasjeet Bindra

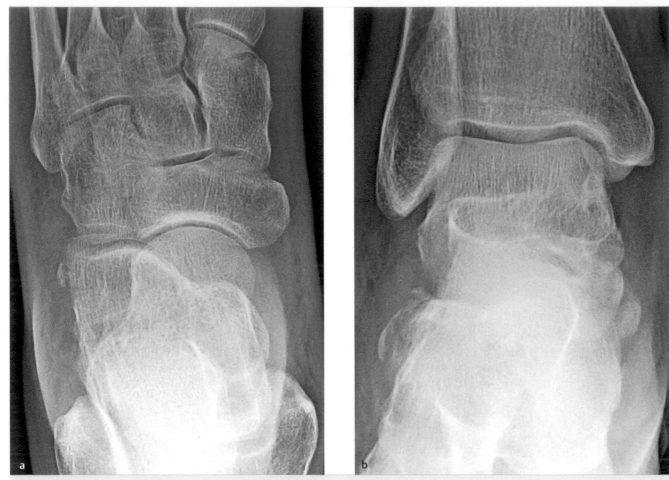

Fig. 12.1 Anteroposterior (AP) view of the foot **(a)** shows a fracture of the distal lateral aspect of the calcaneus. AP view of the ankle **(b)** shows the fracture, which is larger than it appeared on AP view of the foot.

■ Clinical History

A 45-year-old female with history of twisting ankle, and persistent pain (▶ Fig. 12.1).

■ Key Finding

Calcaneal avulsion fracture.

■ Top 3 Differential Diagnoses

- **Calcaneal tuberosity avulsion fracture:** Avulsion fractures of the calcaneal tuberosity are rare and tend to occur in two distinct populations. In the elderly, these are most commonly secondary to osteoporosis or diabetes. In young males, mechanisms include a forced dorsiflexion while the gastrocnemius and soleus are contracted, such as falling on a plantar-flexed foot; sudden contraction of the Achilles tendon on a fixed heel; or direct trauma. Propensity for these fractures may be related to a more extensive insertion of the Achilles tendon on the calcaneus. Surgery is the treatment of choice unless the fracture is nondisplaced or minimally displaced.
- **Anterior process avulsion fracture:** Anterior process fractures are usually caused by tension on the bifurcate ligament during forced inversion and plantar flexion of the foot. The bifurcate ligament is a Y-shaped ligament with calcaneonavicular and calcaneocuboid limbs and attaches proximally to the anterior process of calcaneus. The other mechanism of this fracture is impaction of this process from cuboid and talus during eversion and dorsiflexion, which is referred to as a "nutcracker" lesion. Patients often present with localized pain but without deformity. The fracture is best seen on lateral view of the ankle or oblique view of the foot. These fractures can be radiographically occult, and CT or MRI are required to confirm the diagnosis in many cases.
- **Extensor digitorum brevis (EDB) avulsion:** This injury is most commonly secondary to forced inversion of the foot. Radiographs show a fragment of bone arising from the dorsolateral aspect of the distal calcaneus, best visualized on a frontal view of the foot or AP view of the ankle. Patients present with pain and swelling at the dorsolateral midfoot.

■ Additional Diagnostic Consideration

- **Medial process of the calcaneal tuberosity fracture:** Fractures of the medial process usually occur after a fall from a height or a direct blow. The fracture is well seen on an axial calcaneal radiograph, but it may also be seen on a lateral view. CT is helpful in assessing intra-articular or sustentacular extension. Rarely, an avulsion of the medial plantar process may occur with forceful tension on the plantar fascia insertion. A small bony fragment or cortical discontinuity may be seen on lateral radiographs at the inferior surface of the calcaneal tuberosity.

■ Diagnosis

Extensor digitorum brevis avulsion fracture.

✓ Pearls

- Avulsion fractures of the calcaneus are uncommon but significant injuries that are often missed and should be included in the radiographic search pattern for foot and ankle injuries.
- Avulsion fracture of the extensor digitorum brevis is best seen (often only seen) on a frontal radiograph of the foot or AP view of the ankle.
- CT is useful in evaluating these fractures if the diagnosis is in question, and helpful in evaluating any additional associated fractures.
- MRI may be helpful in evaluating injury to muscles, tendons, and ligaments that may be involved.

■ Suggested Readings

Daftary A, Haims AH, Baumgaertner MR. Fractures of the calcaneus: a review with emphasis on CT. Radiographics. 2005; 25(5):1215–1226

Norfray JF, Rogers LF, Adamo GP, Groves HC, Heiser WJ. Common calcaneal avulsion fracture. AJR Am J Roentgenol. 1980; 134(1):119–123

Yu SM, Yu JS. Calcaneal avulsion fractures: an often forgotten diagnosis. AJR Am J Roentgenol. 2015; 205(5):1061–1067

Case 13

Eva Escobedo and Jasjeet Bindra

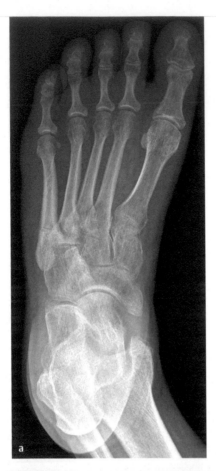

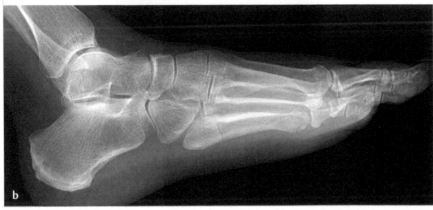

Fig. 13.1 AP and lateral radiographs of the foot (**a, b**) show a fracture at the junction of metaphysis and diaphysis of the fifth metatarsal.

■ **Clinical History**

A 45-year-old female with ankle and foot pain after fall (▶ Fig. 13.1).

■ Key Finding

Fracture at the base of the fifth metatarsal.

■ Top 3 Differential Diagnoses

- **Avulsion fracture of the tuberosity:** These are, by far, the most common fractures at the base of the fifth metatarsal. Avulsion fractures of the tuberosity are categorized as Zone I fractures. These fractures are caused by inversion injury with traction of either the peroneus brevis tendon or lateral cord of the plantar fascia. The fracture may extend to the fifth tarsometatarsal joint. These fractures are typically treated conservatively with good outcome.
- **"Jones" fracture:** The Jones fracture occurs at the junction of the metaphysis and diaphysis of the proximal fifth metatarsal involving, but not extending distal to the intermetatarsal joint. These are categorized as Zone II fractures, and usually occur with adduction force applied to the forefoot with the ankle in plantar flexion. They are slower to heal than Zone I

fractures, and have a higher incidence of delayed union, nonunion, and refracture. Operative treatment is advised for athletically active patients, and for nonunited or displaced fractures.
- **Proximal diaphyseal/stress fracture:** These occur distal to the fourth–fifth intermetatarsal joint in the proximal diaphyseal part of the bone. The majority of these fractures are stress fractures but can be related to blunt trauma. The mechanism of this injury is believed to be a repetitive load applied under the metatarsal head over a short period of time. The typical appearance on radiographs is a radiolucent line with surrounding sclerosis and cortical thickening at the lateral aspect of the bone. The treatment is similar to Zone II fractures.

■ Additional Diagnostic Consideration

- **Normal apophysis:** This secondary ossification center at the base of the fifth metatarsal is usually present between the ages of 9 and 14 years. The lucent cartilage line between the apophysis and the fifth metatarsal base runs vertically, parallels

the metatarsal shaft at the lateral margin, and does not extend to the joint. It is important to distinguish this from a fracture line which is usually transversely oriented.

■ Diagnosis

Jones fracture.

✓ Pearls

- The most common fracture at the base of the fifth metatarsal is the avulsion fracture of the tuberosity.
- Because the avulsion fracture is secondary to an inversion injury and can clinically present as an ankle injury, it is important to include at least one view of the base of the fifth metatarsal on every ankle series to exclude this injury.

- A Jones fracture occurs at the level of the fourth–fifth intermetatarsal joint. They are slower to heal than avulsion fractures, and surgery is the treatment of choice for athletically active individuals and delayed union.
- Fracture through the proximal diaphysis is typically a stress fracture related to repetitive loading.

■ Suggested Readings

Cheung CN, Lui TH. Proximal fifth metatarsal fractures: anatomy, classification, treatment and complications. Arch Trauma Res. 2016; 5(4):e33298

Chuckpaiwong B, Queen RM, Easley ME, et al. Distinguishing Jones and proximal diaphyseal fractures of the fifth metatarsal. ClinOrthopRelat Res. 2008; 466: 1966–1970

Mehlhorn AT, Zwingmann J, Hirschmüller A, Südkamp NP, Schmal H. Radiographic classification for fractures of the fifth metatarsal base. Skeletal Radiol. 2014; 43 (4):467–474

Quill GE, Jr. Fractures of the proximal fifth metatarsal. Orthop Clin North Am. 1995; 26(2):353–361

Part 2

Bone Tumors

Case 14

Jasjeet Bindra

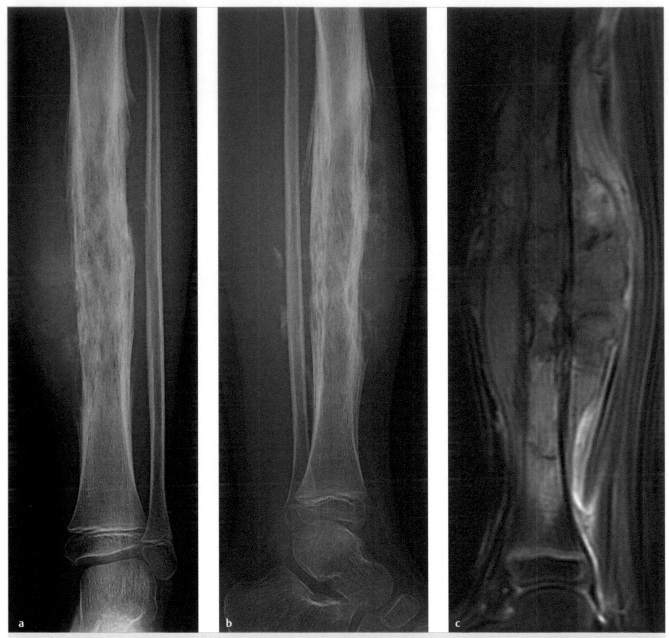

Fig. 14.1 AP **(a)** and lateral **(b)** radiographs of tibia and fibula show a lytic permeative lesion in the mid diaphysis of tibia with aggressive periosteal reaction, including a mix of Codman's triangle, lamellated, and spiculated patterns. Sagittal, fat-saturated, T2-weighted MR image **(c)** demonstrates the intramedullary lesion and intermediate- to high-signal intensity periosteal reaction.

■ Clinical History

A 6-year-old boy with leg pain (▶ Fig. 14.1).

■ Key Finding

Aggressive periosteal reaction.

■ Top 3 Differential Diagnoses

- **Primary bone malignancies:** Aggressive patterns of periosteal reaction are seen with osteosarcoma, Ewing's sarcoma, and chondrosarcoma. High-grade conventional intramedullary osteosarcomas have rapid doubling times and tend to invade the cortex without expanding it. Codman's triangle, lamellated or spiculated (hair-on-end and sunburst) patterns of periosteal reaction are seen. Codman's triangle forms when a portion of the periosteum is lifted off the cortex by a lesion. In lamellated or onion skin pattern, multiple layers of new bone are formed concentrically around the cortex. Spicules of bone form perpendicular (hair-on-end) or radiate in a divergent pattern (sunburst) from the surface of bone in spiculated pattern. Ewing's sarcomas also typically have aggressive periosteal reaction, with hair-on-end subtype being characteristic of them. In conventional chondrosarcoma, the cortex responds to maintain the lesion in the medullary canal, leading to cortical remodeling, thickening and periosteal reaction.
- **Hematologic malignancies:** In leukemia, lamellated appearance is common with hair-on-end appearance being less frequent. Lymphoma can produce aggressive and disorganized periosteal reaction with associated soft tissue mass that is larger than the area of bone destruction.
- **Osteomyelitis:** Various periosteal reaction patterns that can be seen with infection include disorganized, lamellated, and spiculated. In the acute phase, Codman triangle can also develop.

■ Additional Diagnostic Considerations

- **Benign bone tumors:** Calvarial hemangiomas can present as lucent lesions with spiculated sunburst pattern. Enplaque meningiomas usually provoke hyperostosis with rough spiculated margins in adjacent sphenoid ridge. Aneurysmal bone cysts (ABC) can show shell type periosteal reaction; however, intracortical or subperiosteal forms of ABC can also show spiculated pattern.
- **Metastases:** Prostatic osseous metastases can occasionally show sunburst-type reaction. Hypervascular lesions like renal cell metastases can be associated with shell-like pattern.

■ Diagnosis

Ewing's sarcoma.

✓ Pearls

- Osteosarcoma and Ewing's sarcoma are typically associated with various patterns of aggressive periosteal reaction.
- Lymphoma can be associated with aggressive periosteal reaction and a soft-tissue mass that is larger than the area of bone destruction.
- Osteomyelitis, especially in acute phase, can have aggressive periosteal reaction and other features, making it difficult to distinguish from a malignancy based on imaging. Clinical features, laboratory tests, and tissue sampling will help to distinguish.

■ Suggested Readings

Bisseret D, Kaci R, Lafage-Proust MH, et al. Periosteum: characteristic imaging findings with emphasis on radiologic-pathologic comparisons. Skeletal Radiol. 2015; 44(3):321–338

Rana RS, Wu JS, Eisenberg RL. Periosteal reaction. AJR Am J Roentgenol. 2009; 193(4): W259:7–12

Case 15

Jasjeet Bindra

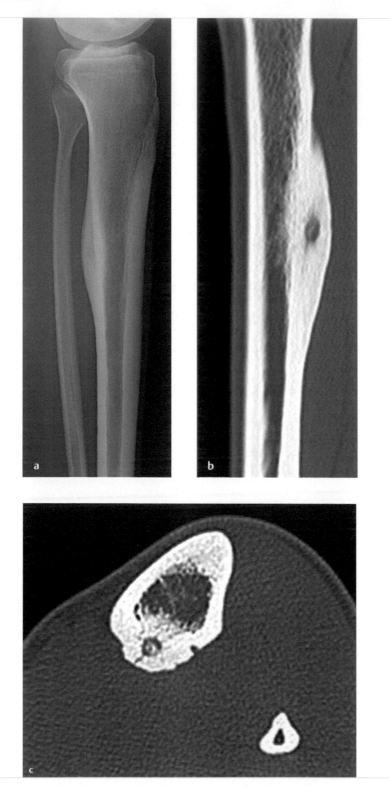

Fig. 15.1 Lateral view of tibia and fibula (a) shows focal cortical thickening along the posterior proximal tibia. Sagittal reformatted CT image (b) reveals a small round focal lucency within the focal area of cortical thickening. Axial CT image of the same lesion (c) shows the radiolucent nidus with a small internal mineralization to better advantage.

■ Clinical History

An 18-year-old male with leg pain (▶ Fig. 15.1).

■ Key Finding

Focal cortical thickening.

■ Top 3 Differential Diagnoses

- **Osteoid osteoma:** Osteoid osteoma is a benign bone tumor usually seen in boys and men between 7 and 25 years of age. The appearance of an osteoid osteoma may vary according to its location. Cortical osteoid osteoma, the most common variety, typically demonstrates fusiform sclerotic thickening in the shaft of a long bone, especially the tibia and femur. A characteristic radiolucent nidus representing the lesion itself is located in the center of osteosclerosis. The reaction can be so dense that the central nidus may be masked on plain films. CT is more sensitive than radiography for detection of the nidus, which may be entirely radiolucent or contain variable amount of mineralization. The reactive periosteal bone is usually solid but may be laminated.
- **Stress fracture:** Another common cause of focal cortical thickening or uninterrupted periosteal reaction is stress fracture. The periosteal reaction and endosteal thickening develop in an attempt to buttress the weakened cortex initially. As damage increases, a true fracture line may appear. These injuries typically involve the shaft of a long bone and are common in the posterior cortex of tibia in runners. In cases with atypical clinical and radiographic presentation, CT is excellent at demonstrating the presence of subtle lucent fracture lines and longitudinal fracture lines. The sclerosis associated with osteoid osteoma is usually much greater than the reactive change seen in stress fracture. A stress fracture is more likely than an osteoid osteoma if the size of the cortical lesion decreases during a short follow-up period. Bone scintigraphy can also help differentiate as a stress fractures demonstrates intense, linear uptake, whereas osteoid osteoma displays the "double density" sign, in which intense central uptake is seen at the nidus and moderate uptake is seen in the surrounding area.
- **Chronic osteomyelitis or intracortical abscess:** Chronic osteomyelitis can also cause cortical thickening and a lucent lesion. At radiography, an intracortical abscess and an osteoid osteoma can be indistinguishable. However, it is easier to differentiate between the two on CT. In osteoid osteoma, the inner side of the nidus is smooth, and a round calcification is seen at the center of the nidus. In an intracortical abscess, the inner margin is irregular and the sequestrum is also irregular and eccentric. On CT, osseous tunneling is seen extending from the lucency, and presence of a soft-tissue abscess adjacent to the area of sclerosis can be seen with infection. On MR, the central part of the abscess does not enhance, whereas in osteoid osteoma, an unmineralized nidus of highly vascularized stroma enhances strongly.

■ Diagnosis

Osteoid osteoma.

✓ Pearls

- In osteoid osteomas, CT is more sensitive than radiography for detection of the central nidus.
- CT is also excellent at demonstrating subtle lucent fracture lines in cases of stress fractures.
- The central part of an intracortical abscess does not enhance, whereas the central nidus of an osteoid osteoma enhances avidly on MR.

■ Suggested Readings

Chai JW, Hong SH, Choi JY, et al. Radiologic diagnosis of osteoid osteoma: from simple to challenging findings. Radiographics. 2010; 30(3):737–749

Datir AP. Stress-related bone injuries with emphasis on MRI. Clin Radiol. 2007; 62(9):828–836

Case 16

Adrianne K. Thompson and Jasjeet Bindra

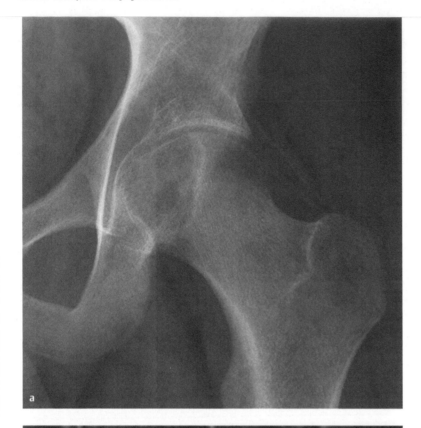

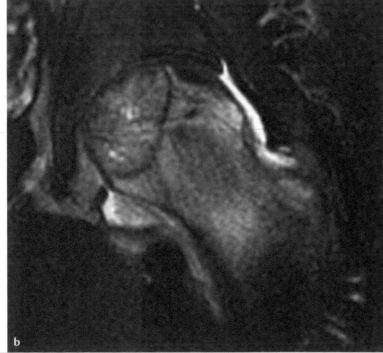

Fig. 16.1 Frontal radiograph of hip (a) demonstrates a circumscribed lucent lesion with thin sclerotic margins and a narrow zone of transition within the epiphyseal region of the femoral head. Coronal fat-suppressed, T2-weighted image (b) of the same hip reveals the lesion, surrounding osseous edema and a small hip joint effusion.

■ **Clinical History**

A 16-year-old male with hip pain (▶ Fig. 16.1).

■ Key Finding

Epiphyseal equivalent lucent lesion.

■ Top 3 Differential Diagnoses

- **Chondroblastoma:** Chondroblastomas are rare lesions that occur in the epiphyses of long bones and are usually seen before skeletal maturity. Most common locations include the humerus, tibia, and femur, as well as within epiphyseal equivalents such as the patella. On radiographs, chondroblastomas tend to be well-defined lucent lesions with a thin rim of sclerosis; calcifications can be seen in approximately 50% of cases. Periosteal reaction can occasionally be seen quite a distance away from the primary lesion. On MRI, they tend to show decreased signal intensity on T1 and variable signal intensity on T2-weighted sequences, depending upon the amount of chondroid matrix and calcification. However, chondroblastomas are associated with significant surrounding marrow edema that may extend into the soft tissues. They demonstrate increased uptake on nuclear medicine bone scans.
- **Giant cell tumor (GCT):** Giant cell tumors are locally aggressive bone tumors composed of giant cells, connective tissue, and stromal cells. They are most common in the third and fourth decades and more so in women than men. Its fundamental feature is extensive epiphyseal involvement and is usually seen after growth plate closure. GCT favors long tubular bones, but it can also be seen in the spine and flat bones such as the clavicles, ribs, and sternum. Radiographic evaluation shows a lucent, expansile, eccentric lesion, producing overlying cortical thinning. Margins can be well- or poorly defined. Approximately 5 to 10% of them may be malignant. They can also have recurrence after treatment.
- **Langerhans cell histiocytosis (LCH):** LCH typically occurs in children, adolescents and young adults, and has a 2:1 male predominance. Although LCH can be multiple, solitary lytic bone lesions predominate with a punched-out appearance; it commonly involves the skull ("punched out" lesion with beveled edges), mandible ("floating tooth"), spine (flattened vertebral body or vertebra plana), ribs, and long bones. These lesions occur in the epiphyses and can cross an open growth plate. LCH can mimic more aggressive processes such as infection or Ewing sarcoma both clinically and radiographically.

■ Additional Diagnostic Consideration

- **Intraosseous ganglion cyst:** These lesions tend to occur within the subchondral/subarticular regions of the shoulder, knee, ankle, hip, and carpal joints after skeletal maturation. On radiographs, they are well-defined lucent lesions with surrounding sclerotic margins. They demonstrate low-T1 and high-T2 signal intensity.

■ Diagnosis

Chondroblastoma.

✓ Pearls

- Chondroblastomas usually occur in epiphyses or epiphyseal equivalents before skeletal maturity.
- Chondroblastomas tend to be associated with a significant amount of marrow and soft-tissue edema.
- Giant cell tumors typically involve the epiphysis or epiphyseal equivalent only after skeletal maturity.
- LCH can occur in the epiphysis and can cross the growth plate.

■ Suggested Readings

Douis H, Saifuddin A. The imaging of cartilaginous bone tumours. I. Benign lesions. Skeletal Radiol. 2012; 41(10):1195–1212

Greenspan A, Jundt G, Remagen W. Differential Diagnosis in Orthopedic Oncology. 2nd ed. Lippincott Williams and Wilkins;2007

Resnick D, Kransdorf MJ. Bone and Joint Imaging. 3rd ed. Philadelphia, PA: Elsevier Saunders;2005

Case 17

Jasjeet Bindra

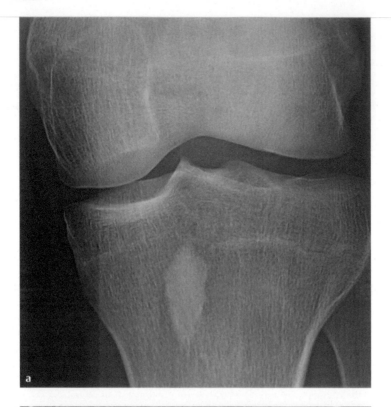

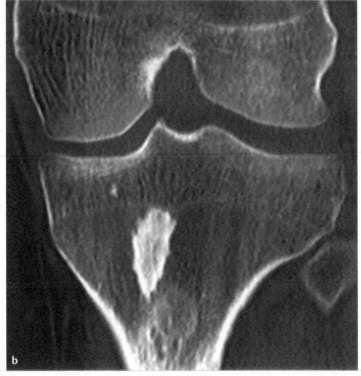

Fig. 17.1 AP view of the knee **(a)** shows an ovoid, sclerotic intramedullary lesion in the proximal tibia. Coronal reformatted CT image **(b)** reveals the same lesion with spiculated margins.

■ **Clinical History**

A 38-year-old female with knee pain (▶ Fig. 17.1).

■ Key Finding

Solitary focal sclerotic lesion.

■ Top 3 Differential Diagnoses

- **Bone island:** An enostosis, or bone island, is a benign entity that represents a focus of mature compact (cortical) bone within the cancellous bone. Radiography reveals a usually homogeneously dense, sclerotic focus within cancellous bone with spiculated margins or brush borders. Most lesions are between 2 mm and 2 cm in size and often oriented with the long axis of the bone. A lesion larger than 2 cm is termed "giant bone island." There is no destruction of cortex, soft-tissue mass or periosteal reaction. Their appearance is pathognomonic; however, if large in size, multiple, atypical in appearance, or in patients with history of a primary malignancy, they may need to be distinguished from other blastic lesions. On radionuclide imaging, they show no or occasionally low-grade activity.
- **Blastic metastasis:** Metastatic disease is a common cause of a sclerotic lesion, most commonly caused by prostate cancer in men and breast cancer in women. When presented with a sclerotic lesion, helpful features to suggest malignant disease include the following: 1) lesion borders which tend to be indistinct with a wide zone of transition, 2) presence of periosteal reaction, 3) soft tissue extension, and 4) size, as metastatic lesions tend to be larger and less uniform than those seen in benign conditions. Most blastic metastatic lesions show increased radiotracer uptake on bone scan.
- **Melorheostosis:** Melorheostosis (Leri disease) is a sporadic, sclerosing skeletal dysplasia that typically manifests in late childhood or early adulthood. It has a characteristic radiographic appearance consisting of cortical and medullary hyperostosis of a single bone or multiple adjacent bones. When a single bone is involved, the characteristic wavy appearance of hyperostosis that resembles melted wax dripping down the side of a candle, usually involving only one side of the bone, is helpful in making the diagnosis.

■ Additional Diagnostic Considerations

- **Low-grade intraosseous osteosarcoma:** Low-grade intraosseous osteosarcoma is an unusual variant of conventional osteosarcoma. It occurs most frequently in patients in the third decade of life, but patients have a wide age range. The most commonly affected sites are metaphyses of the femur and tibia (about the knee). At radiologic examination, the lesion may show well defined margins, sclerotic rim, prominent internal trabeculation, and diffuse sclerosis. However, radiologic evidence of a more aggressive process like focally indistinct margin, focal bone lysis, soft-tissue mass, and cortical destruction is apparent even if subtle.
- **Lymphoma:** Sclerotic lesions are rare in primary bone lymphoma compared to metastatic bone lymphoma. Hodgkin disease of bone tends to be sclerotic, and even in Hodgkin disease, lytic lesions predominate.

■ Diagnosis

Giant bone island.

✓ Pearls

- A bone island typically appears as a small, homogeneously sclerotic lesion within cancellous bone with spiculated margins.
- Blastic metastatic disease is commonly caused by prostate cancer in men and breast cancer in women.
- Melorheostosis has a characteristic "dripping candle wax" appearance of hyperostosis.

■ Suggested Readings

Ihde LL, Forrester DM, Gottsegen CJ, et al. Sclerosing bone dysplasias: review and differentiation from other causes of osteosclerosis. Radiographics. 2011; 31(7): 1865–1882

Manaster BJ, May DA, Disler DG. Musculoskeletal Imaging. The Requisites. 4th ed. Philadelphia: Mosby Elsevier; 2013

Case 18

Jasjeet Bindra

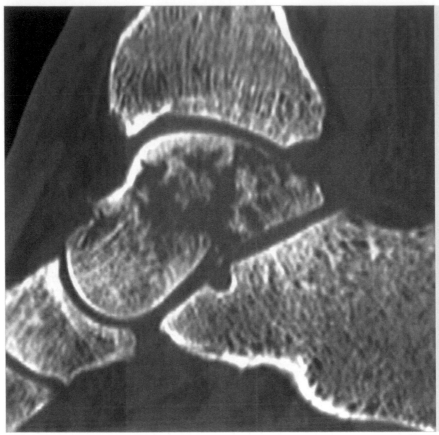

Fig. 18.1 Sagittal reformatted CT image of the ankle shows a permeative pattern of destruction in the talus. No other focal lesions were identified.

■ Clinical History

A 72-year-old male with ankle pain and weight loss (▶ Fig. 18.1).

■ Key Finding

Lesion with permeative or moth-eaten pattern.

■ Top 3 Differential Diagnoses

- **Multiple myeloma:** Multiple myeloma is a neoplastic monoclonal gammopathy that usually affects the axial skeleton and proximal portions of humerus and femur. The hallmark is detection of monoclonal protein in blood and/or urine. It can present as a solitary lesion, diffuse skeletal myelomatosis, diffuse osteopenia, and sclerosing myeloma. Diffuse osteopenia can change to more permeative destructive pattern.
- **Lymphoma:** Primary bone lymphoma occurs in a broad range of patients, from pediatric to elderly, with peak incidence in the sixth and seventh decades. Femur is the most common site. The most common radiographic appearance of primary bone lymphoma is permeative or moth-eaten pattern of lytic destruction. Secondary osseous lymphoma can present similarly.
- **Ewing's sarcoma:** Ewing's sarcoma is the second most common malignant bone tumor in children and adolescents. The most common sites are femur, ilium, and tibia. Bone destruction with moth-eaten to permeative pattern is seen in 76 to 82% of lesions with associated, often large, soft-tissue mass. Continuity between intraosseous and extraosseous components may be through large areas of cortical destruction or subtle channels through cortex.

■ Additional Diagnostic Considerations

- **Metastases:** Metastatic lesions can present as permeative or moth-eaten pattern of destruction. A history of known primary malignancy and multiplicity of lesions can help in making the diagnosis.
- **Infection:** Acute aggressive osteomyelitis can present with this pattern and be indistinguishable from a malignant lesion. Tissue sampling will be confirmatory, as even clinical picture can sometimes be confusing.

■ Diagnosis

Lymphoma.

✓ Pearls

- Permeative or moth-eaten pattern of bone destruction is indicative of an aggressive process.
- Multiple myeloma can present in a variety of forms. Serum and urine presence of monoclonal M protein is the hallmark.
- Round cell tumors such as lymphoma and Ewing's sarcoma can have relatively little cortical destruction in the presence of extensive marrow involvement and soft-tissue component.

■ Suggested Readings

Angtuaco EJ, Fassas AB, Walker R, Sethi R, Barlogie B. Multiple myeloma: clinical review and diagnostic imaging. Radiology. 2004; 231(1):11–23D

Krishnan A, Shirkhoda A, Tehranzadeh J, Armin AR, Irwin R, Les K. Primary bone lymphoma: radiographic-MR imaging correlation. Radiographics. 2003; 23(6): 1371–1383

Murphey MD, Senchak LT, Mambalam PK, Logie CI, Klassen-Fischer MK, Kransdorf MJ. From the radiologic pathology archives: ewing sarcoma family of tumors: radiologic-pathologic correlation. Radiographics. 2013; 33(3):803–831

Case 19

Jasjeet Bindra

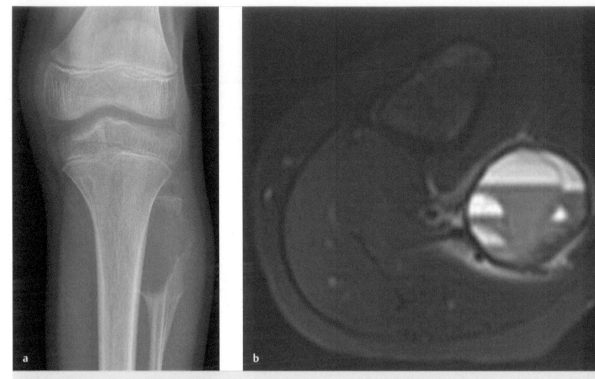

Fig. 19.1 Frontal radiograph of the knee **(a)** shows a lucent expansile lesion in the proximal fibula. Corresponding axial fat-saturated, T2-weighted MR image of the lesion **(b)** shows multiple fluid–fluid levels.

■ Clinical History

An 8-year-old male with knee pain (▶ Fig. 19.1).

■ Key Finding

Osseous lesion with fluid–fluid levels.

■ Top 3 Differential Diagnoses

- **Aneurysmal bone cyst:** An aneurysmal bone cyst (ABC) is an expansile bone lesion containing multiple, thin-walled, blood-filled cystic cavities. Most of the ABCs are found in patients from 5 to 20 years of age. Typical sites include metaphyses of long bones and posterior elements of the spine. Fluid–fluid levels occur whenever substances of different densities are contained within a cystic or compartmentalized structure. Fluid–fluid levels can be seen in ABCs with CT or MRI and are believed to represent sedimentation of red blood cells within the cystic cavities.
- **Simple bone cyst:** A simple bone cyst (SBC) or unicameral bone cyst (UBC) is a benign fluid-containing lesion that usually arises in the metaphyses of long bones. Proximal humerus and proximal femur are the most common sites. Majority of these lesions are seen in patients who are less than 20 years of age. On imaging, it is seen as a mildly expansile lesion, which has a narrow zone of transition with a thin sclerotic rim and no tumor matrix. It is often found incidentally or as a pathologic fracture. Fluid–fluid levels can be seen in SBCs usually associated with a pathologic fracture.
- **Telangiectatic osteosarcoma:** Telangiectatic osteosarcoma is a very aggressive type of osteosarcoma and is seen predominantly in the second and third decades of life. The lesions are expansile and destructive, and largely composed of cystic cavities containing necrosis and hemorrhage. Multiple aneurysmally dilated cystic cavities separated by septations are seen. Fluid–fluid levels are seen commonly. Nodularity can be seen along septations and periphery, which is a key feature to differentiate from ABCs.

■ Additional Diagnostic Considerations

- **Fibrous dysplasia:** Fibrous dysplasia is a noninherited bone disease characterized by replacement of normal lamellar cancellous bone by abnormal fibrous tissue. It can be monostotic or polyostotic. The radiographic appearance varies, with lesions containing greater fibrous content appearing more radiolucent and a characteristic ground glass appearance. Lesions with greater osseous content are more sclerotic. Fluid–fluid levels have been reported in cystic fibrous dysplasia.
- **Chondroblastoma:** Chondroblastoma is a benign cartilaginous tumor, mostly seen between the ages of 5 and 25 years and in epiphyses or apophyses of long bones. On imaging, it manifests as a geographic, lytic lesion that may contain chondroid matrix. They can show fluid–fluid levels.

■ Diagnosis

Aneurysmal bone cyst.

✓ Pearls

- ABCs commonly show fluid–fluid levels.
- SBCs can show fluid–fluid levels in association with a pathologic fracture.
- Telangiectatic osteosarcomas can show nodularity along septations and periphery which can be very helpful in distinguishing them from ABCs.

■ Suggested Readings

Keenan S, Bui-Mansfield LT. Musculoskeletal lesions with fluid-fluid level: a pictorial essay. J Comput Assist Tomogr. 2006; 30(3):517–524

Van Dyck P, Vanhoenacker FM, Vogel J, et al. Prevalence, extension and characteristics of fluid-fluid levels in bone and soft tissue tumors. Eur Radiol. 2006; 16(12): 2644–2651

Case 20

Jasjeet Bindra

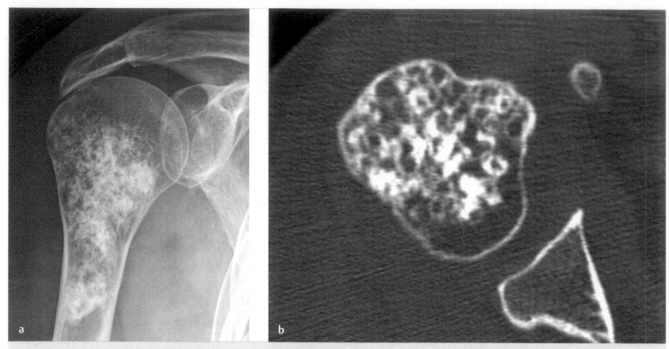

Fig. 20.1 Frontal radiograph of the shoulder **(a)** shows an intramedullary lesion with chondroid matrix and "rings and arcs" mineralizations in the right humerus. Axial CT image **(b)** of the same lesion demonstrates the mineralizations to a better advantage. No cortical breakthrough, deep endosteal scalloping, or soft tissue component were seen.

■ Clinical History

A 56-year-old female with incidentally discovered lesion on shoulder radiographs (▶ Fig. 20.1).

■ Key Finding

Focal lesion with chondroid matrix.

■ Top 3 Differential Diagnoses

- **Enchondroma:** Enchondroma is a benign chondroid lesion with a characteristic "arcs and rings" pattern of mineralization within an intramedullary lucent lesion. The lesions are common in the long tubular bones, particularly distal femur, proximal tibia and proximal humerus. They usually appear purely lucent in the short tubular bones of hands and feet, another common location. CT may show matrix calcifications to better advantage. On MRI, enchondromas are seen to be composed of high-T2 signal intensity lobules with thin intervening low-T2 signal intensity septations and mineralizations.
- **Chondrosarcoma:** Chondrosarcoma is the third most common primary malignant bone tumor. Chondroid matrix mineralization is seen in 60 to 78% of lesions. It can be challenging to

differentiate between low-grade chondrosarcomas and enchondromas on imaging alone. Features that would suggest chondrosarcoma include clinical symptom of pain, size greater than 6 cm, rapid growth, cortical breakthrough, deep endosteal scalloping (more than two-thirds of the overlying cortex), and soft-tissue component.
- **Chondroblastoma:** Chondroblastoma is an uncommon benign lesion occurring before skeletal maturity, characteristically presenting in the epiphyses of long bones like femur, and humerus and in epiphyseal equivalents like patella. These lesions can have chondroid matrix; however, young age of the patient, typical location, and smaller size help to differentiate these lesions from clear cell chondrosarcoma.

■ Additional Diagnostic Consideration

- **Bone infarct:** Medullary bone infarcts can sometimes mimic chondroid lesions on plain radiography. The key to differentiating the two is that calcifications are more central in chondroid lesions and more peripheral in bone infarcts which

show a serpentine margin. On MRI, bone infarcts present as geographic medullary lesions with central fat (bright on T1) and a margin that is hypointense on both T1- and T2-weighted sequences.

■ Diagnosis

Enchondroma.

✓ Pearls

- Enchondromas are common benign chondroid lesions with "rings and arcs" mineralizations.
- It is difficult to distinguish enchondromas and low-grade chondrosarcomas in long bones on imaging. Pain, deep

endosteal scalloping and other aggressive features favor chondrosarcoma.
- Bone infarcts have serpentine, calcified margins.

■ Suggested Readings

Brien EW, Mirra JM, Kerr R. Benign and malignant cartilage tumors of bone and joint: their anatomic and theoretical basis with an emphasis on radiology, pathology and clinical biology. I. The intramedullary cartilage tumors. Skeletal Radiol. 1997; 26(6):325–353

Murphey MD, Flemming DJ, Boyea SR, et al. Enchondroma versus chondrosarcoma in the appendicular skeleton: differentiating features. Radiographics. 1998; 18:1213–1237

Murphey MD, Walker EA, Wilson AJ, Kransdorf MJ, Temple HT, Gannon FH. From the archives of the AFIP: imaging of primary chondrosarcoma: radiologic-pathologic correlation. Radiographics. 2003; 23(5):1245–1278

Case 21

Jasjeet Bindra

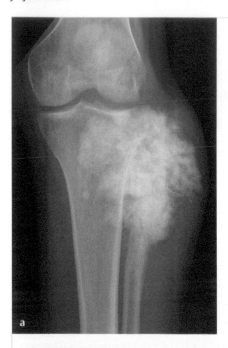
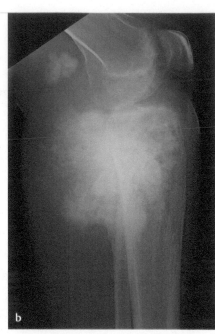

Fig. 21.1 Frontal and lateral radiographs of the knee **(a, b)** show extensive cloud-like mineralizations in the large mass arising from proximal fibula. Axial, T1-weighted MR image of the knee **(c)** demonstrates the large mass with mixed signal intensity arising from and surrounding the fibula.

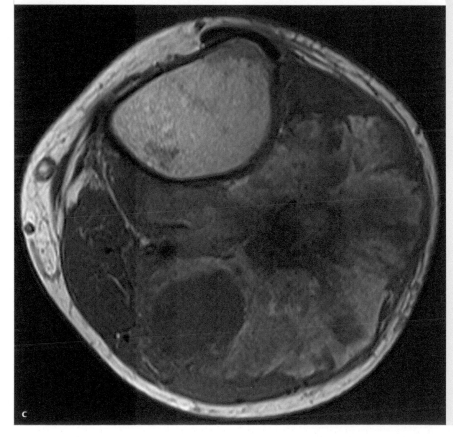

■ Clinical History

A 22-year-old male with pain and mass near the knee (▶ Fig. 21.1).

■ Key Finding

Osseous lesion with osteoid matrix.

■ Top 3 Differential Diagnoses

- **Osteosarcoma:** Osteosarcoma is the most common primary malignant tumor of bone in adolescents and young adults. Identification of osteoid matrix and aggressive features usually allow easy prospective radiologic diagnosis of this tumor. Intramedullary osteosarcomas frequently affect long bones, particularly about the knee. A vast majority of these lesions (90%) demonstrate fluffy, cloud-like opacities, which are characteristic of osteoid matrix, within the lesion. Occasionally, the lesion may be completely blastic or lytic. Ossifications may also be seen in metastases.
- **Osteoid osteoma:** Osteoid osteoma is a benign bone tumor seen in boys and men between 7 and 25 years of age. Typical findings include an intracortical nidus that may display a variable amount of mineralization, accompanied by cortical thickening and reactive sclerosis in the shaft of a long bone. CT is more sensitive than radiography for detection of the mineralized osteoid within the nidus.
- **Osteoblastoma:** Osteoblastoma is an uncommon benign bone-forming lesion that is histologically identical to osteoid osteoma. It has a predilection for the spine and is almost always in the posterior elements. Osteoblastoma displays progressive growth and may have malignant potential. At imaging, osteoblastoma is usually more expansile, larger than 2 cm, with more osteoid tissue formation, and has less surrounding sclerosis than osteoid osteoma. In spine, it can have a blowout appearance similar to aneurysmal bone cyst. Osteoblastomas can also have an aggressive appearance, simulating an osteosarcoma.

■ Additional Diagnostic Consideration

- **Enostosis:** Enostosis, or bone island, is a small benign lesion seen as round or oval focus of dense bone within medullary space. Spiculated margins or brush borders are seen classically. Their appearance is pathognomonic; however, if large in size, multiple or in patients with history of a primary malignancy, they may need to be distinguished from other blastic lesions with the help of radionuclide imaging on which they show no or occasionally low-grade activity.

■ Diagnosis

Osteosarcoma.

✓ Pearls

- Osteosarcomas with osteoid matrix and aggressive features usually do not pose a diagnostic challenge.
- CT is more sensitive for detection of mineralization in the central nidus of osteoid osteomas.
- Osteoblastomas can have a variety of appearances but are usually larger than 2 cm and with less surrounding sclerosis than osteoid osteomas.

■ Suggested Readings

Chai JW, Hong SH, Choi JY, et al. Radiologic diagnosis of osteoid osteoma: from simple to challenging findings. Radiographics. 2010; 30(3):737–749

Murphey MD, Robbin MR, McRae GA, Flemming DJ, Temple HT, Kransdorf MJ. The many faces of osteosarcoma. Radiographics. 1997; 17(5):1205–1231

Case 22

Jasjeet Bindra

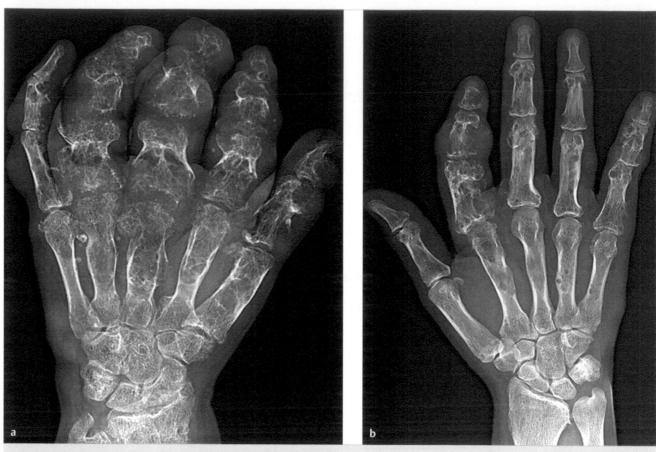

Fig. 22.1 PA radiographs of both hands **(a, b)** show multiple lytic expansile lesions in short tubular bones. Several phleboliths are also seen over the soft tissues of left hand.

■ Clinical History

A 30-year-old female with multiple masses in hands (▶ Fig. 22.1).

■ Key Finding

Polyostotic lesions–looks like a syndrome.

■ Top 3 Differential Diagnoses

- **Hereditary multiple exostoses (HME):** HME is characterized by multiple osteochondromas and shows an autosomal dominant inheritance pattern. Any bone can be involved except calvarium. The lesions are similar to solitary osteochondromas with cortical and medullary bone protruding and continuous with the underlying bone and can be pedunculated or sessile. Hyaline cap may show chondroid calcifications, has variable thickness and best measured by MRI. Various complications associated with osteochondromas include osseous deformity, vascular or neurologic compromise, bursa formation, and malignant transformation. The prevalence of malignant transformation is higher than with solitary osteochondromas.
- **Enchondromatosis:** Ollier disease or enchondromatosis is defined by presence of multiple enchondromas with asymmetric distribution of lesions which can be extremely variable (in terms of size, number, and evolution of enchondromas). Enchondromatosis associated with soft-tissue hemangiomas is called Maffucci syndrome. Both disorders appear spontaneously and are not inherited. Enchondromas are exclusively located in the metaphyses of long bones and in the small bones of hand and feet. They appear as multiple lucent lesions that may show chondroid calcifications. Growth abnormalities and deformities are common. Reported risk of malignant transformation varies from 5 to 50% of cases.
- **Polyostotic fibrous dysplasia:** Fibrous dysplasia is a benign skeletal disorder characterized by replacement of medullary bone with fibrous tissue. Polyostotic form may involve a few or many bones, most commonly skull, facial bones, pelvis, and spine. The lesions have varying degrees of density and may display characteristic ground glass appearance. Deformities like shepherd's crook may be seen. McCune–Albright syndrome consists of a triad of precocious puberty, café' au lait spots, and polyostotic fibrous dysplasia.

■ Additional Diagnostic Consideration

- **Neurofibromatosis (NF):** Multiple, well-defined, lucent expansile lesions with sclerotic margins may be seen with NF-1, possibly representing nonossifying fibromas.

■ Diagnosis

Maffucci syndrome.

✓ Pearls

- HME consists of multiple sessile or pedunculated osteochondromas.
- In enchondromatosis, growth abnormalities and deformities are common.
- Polyostotic fibrous dysplasia tends to involve larger segments of bone with severe deformities.

■ Suggested Readings

Fitzpatrick KA, Taljanovic MS, Speer DP, et al. Imaging findings of fibrous dysplasia with histopathologic and intraoperative correlation. AJR Am J Roentgenol. 2004; 182(6):1389–1398

Murphey MD, Choi JJ, Kransdorf MJ, Flemming DJ, Gannon FH. Imaging of osteochondroma: variants and complications with radiologic-pathologic correlation. Radiographics. 2000; 20(5):1407–1434

Silve C, Jüppner H. Ollier disease. Orphanet J Rare Dis. 2006; 1:3–7

Case 23

Jasjeet Bindra

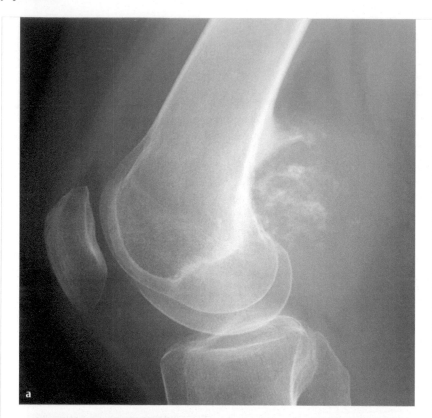

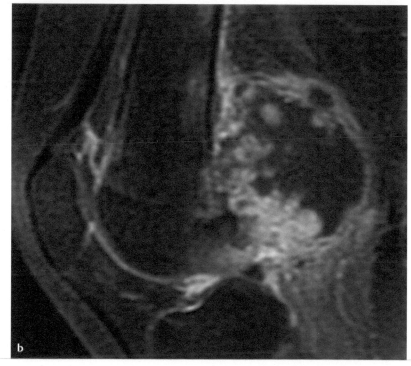

Fig. 23.1 Lateral view of the knee (**a**) shows a surface lesion along the posterior aspect of distal femur. The lesion has ill-defined mineralizations. Sagittal, fat-suppressed, postcontrast T1-weighted image of the knee (**b**) demonstrates irregular enhancement in the mass.

▪ Clinical History

A 60-year-old female with enlarging mass posterior to the knee (▶ Fig. 23.1).

■ Key Finding

Surface lesion of bone.

■ Top 3 Differential Diagnoses

- **Periosteal chondroma:** Periosteal chondroma is a rare benign tumor presenting on the surface of the cortex but deep to periosteum. It occurs in children as well as adults. It is usually seen at the metaphyseal region of long bones or in the small bones of hand and feet. Radiologic features include cortical scalloping, chondroid mineralizations, and thin periosteal shell.
- **Periosteal chondrosarcoma:** Periosteal chondrosarcoma is a rare malignant cartilaginous tumor usually presenting in the second to fourth decades. Metaphyseal regions of long bones like femur and humerus are the usual sites. The lesion is seen as a juxtacortical soft tissue mass with erosion, saucerization or thickening of underlying cortex and may have chondroid calcifications. It can be difficult to differentiate from periosteal chondroma. Periosteal chondroma tends to be smaller than 3 cm, whereas chondrosarcoma tends to be larger.
- **Periosteal osteosarcoma:** Periosteal osteosarcoma is a juxtacortical osteosarcoma, typically presenting in the second or third decades of life in a diaphyseal location of a long bone. Radiologically, it presents as a soft-tissue mass with underlying cortical erosion and thickening, and periosteal reaction that is perpendicular to the cortex.

■ Additional Diagnostic Consideration

- **Parosteal osteosarcoma:** This form of juxtacortical osteosarcoma manifests between the third and fourth decades of life. It usually occurs in the metaphyses of long bones, most commonly the posterior aspect of distal femur. It is classically seen as an exophytic mass with dense central ossification adjacent to the bone. A cleavage plane may be seen between the lesion and the underlying cortex.

■ Diagnosis

Periosteal chondrosarcoma.

✓ Pearls

- Periosteal chondroma typically shows cortical scalloping and thin periosteal shell.
- Periosteal chondrosarcomas tend to be larger than periosteal chondromas at presentation. Periosteal chondromas tend to be smaller than 3 cm.
- Periosteal osteosarcoma usually presents in a diaphyseal location with cortical erosion and periosteal reaction.

■ Suggested Readings

Chaabane S, Bouaziz MC, Drissi C, Abid L, Ladeb MF. Periosteal chondrosarcoma. AJR Am J Roentgenol. 2009; 192(1):W1–6

Douis H, Saifuddin A. The imaging of cartilaginous bone tumours. I. Benign lesions. Skeletal Radiol. 2012; 41(10):1195–1212

Yarmish G, Klein MJ, Landa J, Lefkowitz RA, Hwang S. Imaging characteristics of primary osteosarcoma: nonconventional subtypes. Radiographics. 2010; 30(6): 1653–1672

Case 24

Eva Escobedo

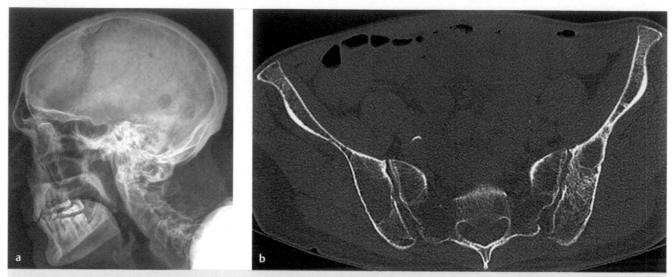

Fig. 24.1 Lateral radiograph of the skull **(a)** shows punched out lytic lesions of calvarium. Axial CT image of the pelvis **(b)** reveals multiple lytic lesions of bilateral iliac bones and of sacrum.

■ Clinical History

A 68-year-old female with diffuse bone pain (▶ Fig. 24.1).

■ Key Finding

Multiple lytic lesions.

■ Top 3 Differential Diagnoses in an Adult

- **Metastases:** Bone metastases can be either well- or poorly defined and may be difficult to distinguish from multiple myeloma. Purely osteolytic lesions originate from primary thyroid, renal, uterus, head and neck, and gastrointestinal (GI) sources. Mixed osteolytic/osteosclerotic lesions may arise from lung, breast, cervix, ovarian, and testicular malignancies. Metastases arising from thyroid and renal primaries may produce bone expansion.
- **Multiple myeloma:** Multiple myeloma, a plasma cell dyscrasia, is the most common primary bone malignancy in adults. The predominant pattern of bone involvement is osteolysis, and most commonly occurs at multiple sites, but can be solitary (plasmacytoma). The axial skeleton is the typical site of involvement, but extensive disease will affect the extremities

as well. The classic pattern of bone involvement is multiple discrete "punched out" lesions. Subcortical erosions of the endosteum may cause a characteristic "scalloped" appearance. The mandible is more commonly involved than with metastases.
- **Lymphoma:** Skeletal involvement is common in both Hodgkin and non-Hodgkin lymphomas. The most common manifestation of non-Hodgkin lymphoma is multiple osteolytic lesions with a moth-eaten or permeative pattern of bone destruction, sometimes with endosteal scalloping and cortical destruction. Osteosclerosis is more commonly seen in Hodgkin's lymphoma. Soft-tissue masses are common and may be seen in the absence of significant cortical disruption.

■ Top 3 Differential Diagnoses in a Child

- **Langerhans cell histiocytosis (LCH):** Bone lesions may be seen in any of the LCHs, but eosinophilic granuloma is the most common subtype, which manifests as single or multiple bone lesions in children or young adults. In the tubular bones, EG usually presents as a well-defined lucent lesion. As it enlarges, there may be associated periosteal reaction and cortical erosion. Characteristic radiographic appearances include "beveled edges" and "button sequestrum" in the skull, and "vertebra plana" of the spine.
- **Fibrous dysplasia:** Fibrous dysplasia is a sporadic disease of bone-forming mesenchyme with abnormal osteoblastic differentiation. The normal bone is replaced by immature,

woven bone and fibrous stroma. Lesions may be solitary or multiple, are typically well defined, and may have a lucent or hazy ("ground glass") matrix with sclerotic borders. They may be expansile or contain internal calcifications. Deformities may occur due to abnormal weakened bone or fractures. There is no associated periosteal reaction.
- **Chronic recurrent multifocal osteomyelitis (CRMO):** CRMO is a self limiting inflammatory disorder of unknown etiology of children. It affects predominately long bone metaphyses but can occur at any skeletal site. Although initially osteolytic, the hallmark is reactive sclerosis.

■ Diagnosis

Multiple myeloma.

✓ Pearls

- Osteolytic lesions may originate from thyroid and renal malignancy. Lung and breast may be mixed.
- The classic appearance of multiple myeloma is multiple discrete "punched-out" lytic lesions.

- Non Hodgkin lymphoma commonly demonstrates a moth-eaten or permeative pattern of bone destruction.
- LCH results in calvarial lesions with "beveled edges" and "button sequestrum" as well as vertebra plana.

■ Suggested Readings

Angtuaco EJ, Fassas AB, Walker R, Sethi R, Barlogie B. Multiple myeloma: clinical review and diagnostic imaging. Radiology. 2004; 231(1):11–23

Resnick D. Diagnosis of Bone and Joint Disorders. 4th ed. WB Saunders; 2002

Case 25

Adrianne K. Thompson and Jasjeet Bindra

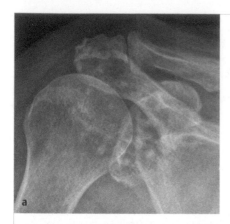
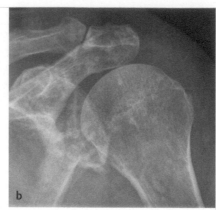
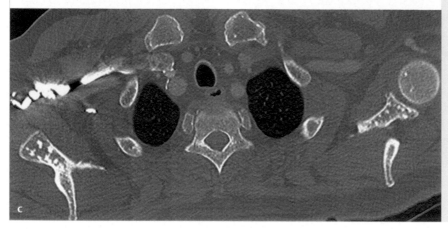

Fig. 25.1 AP radiographs of bilateral shoulders (**a, b**) demonstrate multiple small sclerotic lesions with symmetric distribution about both shoulders. Axial CT image through the upper chest (**c**) also shows similar but fewer foci in medial clavicles in addition to the sclerotic foci in both scapulae.

■ Clinical History

A 40-year-old female with incidental finding in bilateral shoulders radiographs (▶ Fig. 25.1).

■ Key Finding

Multiple sclerotic lesions.

■ Top 3 Differential Diagnoses

- **Osteopoikilosis:** Osteopoikilosis is an asymptomatic form of skeletal sclerotic dysplasia that occurs in both men and women. Cutaneous manifestations may be seen, such as keloids or fibrocollagenous infiltration of the skin. Imaging shows ovoid, well-defined, sclerotic foci, which are usually small and symmetrically distributed. Osteopoikilosis shows a predilection for long and short tubular bones, carpal and tarsal bones, pelvis, and scapulae. Usually, there is normal activity on bone scan. There may be an association with other osteosclerotic dysplasias such as osteopathia striata (Voorhoeve's syndrome) and melorheostosis.
- **Metastatic disease:** Metastatic disease is a common cause of sclerotic foci within the pelvis, most commonly caused by prostate cancer in men and breast cancer in women. When presented with sclerotic foci within the pelvis, helpful features to suggest malignant disease include: 1) lesion borders which tend to be indistinct with a wide zone of transition, 2) presence of periosteal reaction, 3) soft-tissue extension, 4) size, as metastatic lesions would be larger and less uniform than those seen in benign conditions, and 5) multiplicity, particularly when lesions are seen in bones outside of the pelvis.
- **Paget's disease:** Paget's disease is a disorder of bone metabolism seen in older patients with a slight male predilection and onset in the fifth and sixth decades. Numerous etiologies have been proposed, but the cause remains elusive. The disease shows increased bone remodeling, leading to an abnormal balance between bone resorption and replacement. Osteoblastic activity results in increased alkaline phosphatase, and increased osteoclastic activity leads to high-levels of hydroxyproline in urine. Most commonly affected bones include the pelvis, femurs, skull, tibiae, and spine. Radiographic findings reflect the cellular activity taking place at that phase; there are three main phases–osteolytic, mixed, and osteoblastic. In the osteolytic phase, bone resorption occurs, causing radiolucent changes in bone. In the calvarium, this results in bone destruction termed "osteoporosis circumscripta," while in the tibia, this results in a "blade of grass" appearance. The mixed phase shows both bone resorption and formation with prominent bony trabeculae and a "cottonwool" appearance. Finally, in the blastic phase, there is a drastic increase in bone density with cortical thickening and bony deformity. Specific changes within the pelvis include trabecular thickening of the iliopectineal/ilioischial lines, hemipelvic asymmetry, and enlargement. Complications include pathologic fractures, early degenerative joint disease, neurologic impingement, and malignant transformation.

■ Diagnosis

Osteopoikilosis.

✓ Pearls

- Osteopoikilosis is asymptomatic and usually demonstrates normal activity on a bone scan.
- Sclerotic metastatic disease to the pelvis most commonly originates from prostate and breast carcinoma.
- Paget's disease in the pelvis may demonstrate thickening of the iliopectineal and ilioischial lines.

■ Suggested Readings

Greenspan A. Orthopedic Imaging: A Practical Approach. 5th ed. Lippincott Williams and Wilkins; 2011

Ihde LL, Forrester DM, Gottsegen CJ, et al. Sclerosing bone dysplasias: review and differentiation from other causes of osteosclerosis. Radiographics. 2011; 31(7): 1865–1882

Resnick D, Kransdorf MJ. Bone and joint imaging. 3rd ed. Philadelphia, PA: Elsevier Saunders; 2005

Theodorou DJ, Theodorou SJ, Kakitsubata Y. Imaging of Paget disease of bone and its musculoskeletal complications: review. AJR Am J Roentgenol. 2011; 196(6) Suppl:S64–S75

Case 26

Jasjeet Bindra

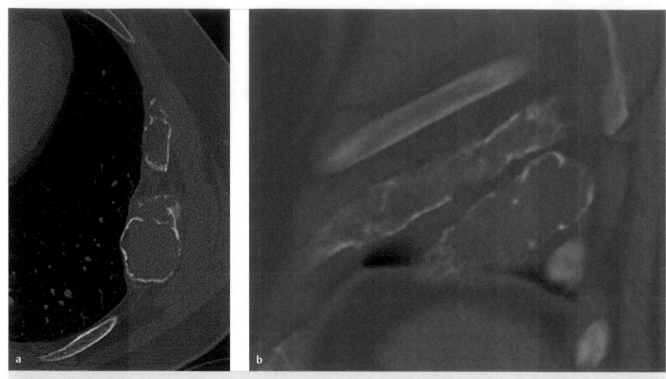

Fig. 26.1 Axial CT image through the midchest **(a)** shows expansile lesions of two consecutive left ribs with thinning of cortices. Sagittal reformatted CT image **(b)** demonstrates that the lesions are relatively long.

■ Clinical History

A 40-year-old male with incidental finding on chest CT (▶ Fig. 26.1).

■ Key Finding

Expansile lytic lesion of rib.

■ Top 3 Differential Diagnoses

- **Fibrous dysplasia:** Fibrous dysplasia is a benign skeletal disorder characterized by replacement of medullary bone with fibrous tissue. The ribs are the most common sites of involvement with monostotic disease. Polyostotic disease can also be seen. Bony lesions are expansile with variable internal matrix; the classic lesion has a ground glass matrix. Any part of the rib may be affected, and involvement of a long segment is common and characteristic.
- **Metastases/Myeloma:** Metastasis is by far the most common cause of malignant involvement of the ribs. A variety of tumors metastasize to the ribs. Expansile metastases are typically seen in renal cell, thyroid and hepatocellular carcinoma, although lytic lesions can be seen with many other types of primary malignancies like breast and lung. Multiple lesions, if present, can help guide the diagnosis. Multiple myeloma rib lesions are often multiple. Plasmacytoma of ribs is less common.
- **Chondroid lesions:** Enchondroma is the second most common benign primary rib lesion after fibrous dysplasia. Chondroid tumors tend to arise near the anterior ends of ribs. Enchondroma is usually a lytic, expansile lesion less than 4 cm in size which may show characteristic chondroid calcifications. Distinguishing from low-grade chondrosarcoma can be challenging on imaging alone. Chondrosarcoma is the commonest primary malignant rib tumor. It presents in relatively older patients and rarely found in patients less than 20 years of age. Chondroid matrix may be seen but the lesions commonly have an associated soft-tissue mass.

■ Diagnosis

Fibrous dysplasia.

✓ Pearls

- Fibrous dysplasia may have "groundglass" matrix with involvement of a long segment.
- Presence of multiple lesions and a known primary malignancy can help guide the diagnosis in metastases.
- Chondroid lesions tend to present near the anterior end and may have "rings and arcs" calcifications.

■ Suggested Readings

Guttentag AR, Salwen JK. Keep your eyes on the ribs: the spectrum of normal variants and diseases that involve the ribs. Radiographics. 1999; 19(5):1125–1142

Zarqane H, Viala P, Dallaudière B, Vernhet H, Cyteval C, Larbi A. Tumors of the rib. Diagn Interv Imaging. 2013; 94(11):1095–1108

Case 27

Eva Escobedo

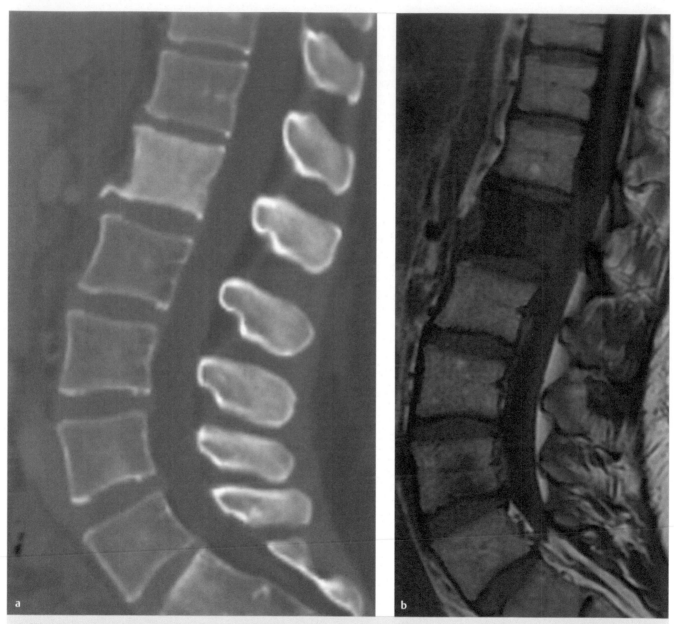

Fig. 27.1 Sagittal reformatted CT image of lumbar spine **(a)** shows diffusely dense L1 vertebral body. Sagittal T1-weighted MR image **(b)** shows diffuse hypointensity of the vertebral body by infiltrative process.

■ **Clinical History**

A 60-year-old female with back pain (► Fig. 27.1).

■ Key Finding

Ivory vertebral body.

■ Top 3 Differential Diagnoses

- **Osteoblastic metastasis:** Increased density is due to abnormal stimulation of osteoblasts. Prostate and breast carcinoma are the most common sources of osteoblastic metastases. Less common sources include lymphoma (see below), bladder, colon, lung, and carcinoid. In most cases, there is involvement of multiple vertebral levels. In children, sclerotic vertebral metastasis can be seen with neuroblastoma and medulloblastoma.
- **Paget's disease:** Paget's disease, which is most common after age 40, is characterized by excessive, abnormal remodeling of bone. The ivory vertebral body is seen in the inactive, sclerotic phase, and can either involve a single level or more than one level. The most common appearance with Paget's in the vertebral body is trabecular thickening with enlargement of the vertebral body. Cortical thickening around the periphery of the body results in a "picture frame" appearance. Because of the common finding of expansion, Paget's does not fully meet the original criteria of an ivory vertebral body, which is "increased density with retained size and shape," but is commonly included in the differential.
- **Lymphoma:** Skeletal involvement is common in both Hodgkin and nonHodgkin lymphomas. Osteosclerosis is rare and more commonly seen in Hodgkin lymphoma. Spinal involvement in patients with Hodgkin disease may result in osteolysis, osteosclerosis, or a combination of the two. Destructive lytic lesions are more common than osteosclerosis. Lymphoma of the vertebral body is characteristically associated with a paraspinal soft-tissue mass. Margins of the vertebral body may show erosions caused by the surrounding mass.

■ Additional Diagnostic Considerations

- **Mastocytosis:** A rare disorder of mast cell proliferation, mastocytosis may present with either osteopenia and lytic lesions, or osteosclerosis, and may be focal or diffuse. In the spine, it commonly involves multiple levels. Multiple organ systems may be affected.
- **Myeloma:** Rarely, myeloma may present with osteosclerotic lesions. Sclerotic bone lesions may be seen with POEMS syndrome, a disease comprising multiple entities. POEMS is an acronym for the most common features of the syndrome: polyneuropathy, organomegaly, endocrinopathy, monoclonal gammopathy, and skin changes.

■ Diagnosis

Hodgkin's lymphoma.

✓ Pearls

- Enlargement of the vertebral body helps differentiate Paget's from other causes of ivory vertebral body.
- The "picture frame" appearance is also a characteristic sign in Paget's disease.
- Prostate and breast carcinoma are the most common sources of osteoblastic metastases.
- Osteosclerosis is rare in lymphoma, more often seen with Hodgkin than with non Hodgkin lymphomas.
- Myeloma can rarely present with sclerotic lesions, which may be a component of POEMS syndrome.

■ Suggested Readings

Graham TS. The ivory vertebra sign. Radiology. 2005; 235(2):614–615

Mulligan ME. Myeloma and lymphoma. Semin Musculoskelet Radiol. 2000; 4(1): 127–135

Resnick D. Diagnosis of bone and joint disorders. 4th ed. Philadelphia, PA: Saunders; 2002

Case 28

Jasjeet Bindra

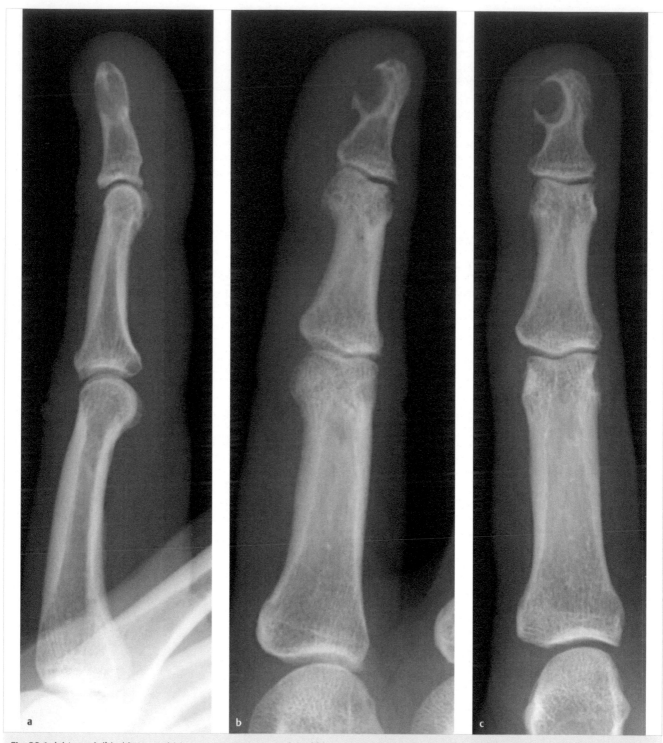

Fig. 28.1 **(a)** Lateral, **(b)** oblique, and **(c)** posteroanterior views of the fifth digit of the hand show a well-defined lucent lesion with sclerotic margins in the terminal phalanx.

■ Clinical History

A 46-year-old male with mass at the fingertip. Patient with history of remote crush injury to the fingers (▶ Fig. 28.1).

■ Key Finding

Lytic lesion of distal phalanx.

■ Top 3 Differential Diagnoses

- **Glomus tumor:** Glomus tumor is a benign hamartomatous tumor with the vast majority occurring at fingertips. Patients present with excruciating pain and temperature sensitivity. Radiographically, the tumor can demonstrate pressure erosion in the terminal phalanx. Typical clinical presentation and MR imaging showing T1 hypointense, T2 hyperintense, and avidly enhancing mass help to make the diagnosis.
- **Epidermal inclusion cyst:** Epidermal inclusion cysts are benign cystic lesions thought to result from prior trauma, with proliferation of implanted epidermal elements, causing the cyst. They can manifest with swelling and pain of the fingertip. Lucency in the terminal phalanx may be seen from erosion of the adjacent soft-tissue inclusion cyst into the bone. They have intermediate signal intensity on T1- and T2-weighted images on MR, and show peripheral enhancement on postcontrast images.
- **Enchondroma:** Enchondroma is the most common benign tumor of the hand. It is seen as a lucent lesion in the medullary cavity of short tubular bones of the hand. The lesion may cause endosteal scalloping and bone expansion, and can show typical ring-and-arcs chondroid matrix. It is more commonly seen in the proximal and middle phalanges than the distal phalanx.

■ Additional Diagnostic Consideration

- **Metastatic lesion:** Metastatic lesions of tubular bones of hands are extremely rare and associated with poor prognosis. When they do occur, distal phalanx is the most common site of involvement. Primary tumors associated with subungual metastases include lung, genitourinary tract and breast. Of these lesions, more than 90% exhibit osseous involvement.

■ Diagnosis

Epidermal inclusion cyst.

✓ Pearls

- Glomus tumors have a typical clinical history and are usually small at presentation.
- Epidermal inclusion cysts can have prior history of trauma and typically show only peripheral enhancement on postcontrast images.
- Enchondromas are the most common benign tumors of hand which involve terminal phalanx less commonly than other short tubular bones.

■ Suggested Readings

Lee CH, Tandon A. Focal hand lesions: review and radiological approach. Insights Imaging. 2014; 5(3):301–319

Melamud K, Drapé JL, Hayashi D, Roemer FW, Zentner J, Guermazi A. Diagnostic imaging of benign and malignant osseous tumors of the fingers. Radiographics. 2014; 34(7):1954–1967

Case 29

Jasjeet Bindra

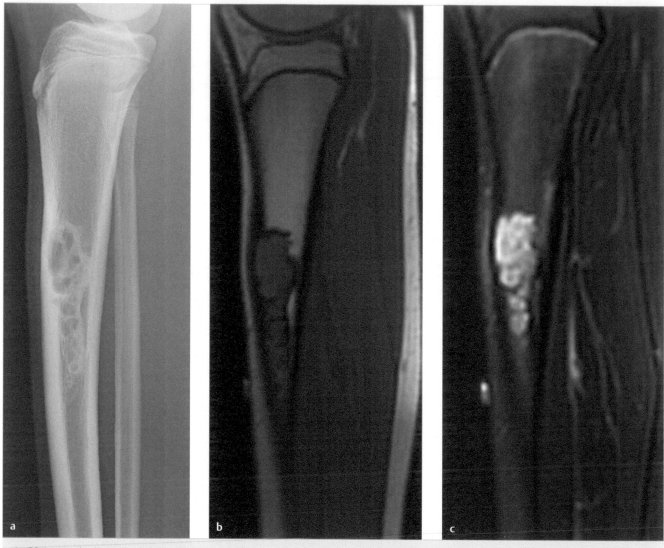

Fig. 29.1 Lateral radiograph of tibia and fibula **(a)** shows a lucent, mildly expansile, bubbly lesion with sclerotic margins along the anterior cortex in the diaphysis of tibia. Sagittal T-weighted **(b)** and fat-suppressed, T2-weighted **(c)** MR images show the lesion to be intermediate signal intensity on T1 and hyperintense on T2-weighted images.

▪ Clinical History

A 13-year-old female with tibial pain (▶ Fig. 29.1).

■ Key Finding

Anterior tibial cystic appearing lesion.

■ Top 3 Differential Diagnoses

- **Osteofibrous dysplasia:** Osteofibrous dysplasia is a benign fibro-osseous lesion, most frequently seen in the first two decades of life. The lesions are usually diaphyseal, involving the anterior cortex of middle to distal third of tibia. The lesions present as intracortical osteolysis with a characteristic sclerotic band, and there is bowing and enlargement of bone. Distinction between this entity, fibrous dysplasia, and adamantinoma on imaging can be difficult but can be made on pathology. Osteofibrous dysplasia has a more favorable prognosis and tends to regress spontaneously without residual deformity.
- **Nonossifying fibroma:** Nonossifying fibroma is usually seen in patients who are less than 20 years of age. Tibia is a common site and the lesions are well-defined, cortical-based lytic lesions with sclerotic margins seen in the metaphyseal or metadiaphyseal regions. They are more likely to involve posterior or medial cortices. With growth, the lesions tend to fill in with fibro-osseous ingrowth and become radiopaque.
- **Adamantinoma:** Adamantinoma is seen usually between 20 to 50 years of age. The lesions are typically seen in the middle third of anterior cortex of tibia, and appear as multilocular or slightly expansile osteolytic lesions that may show local aggressive features. Satellite lesions are not uncommon and can aid in differential diagnosis. Adamantinoma is a low-grade malignancy which has the ability to metastasize.

■ Additional Diagnostic Consideration

- **Fibrous dysplasia:** In fibrous dysplasia, the patient age is typically between 20 to 30 years. Tibial or any long bone involvement tends to be intramedullary and diaphyseal in location. The lesions are well-defined and of variable radiopacity, depending on the proportion of fibrous and osseous tissue in the lesion. Some lesions show characteristic ground glass matrix. With expansile lesions, there can be endosteal scalloping, thinning, and weakening of cortex.

■ Diagnosis

Osteofibrous dysplasia.

✓ Pearls

- Osteofibrous dysplasia shows bowing and enlargement of the bone with intracortical osteolysis.
- Nonossifying fibroma tends to fill in with fibro-osseous in growth over time.
- Adamantinoma may show local aggressive features and satellite lesions.

■ Suggested Readings

Bethapudi S, Ritchie DA, Macduff E, Straiton J. Imaging in osteofibrous dysplasia, osteofibrous dysplasia-like adamantinoma, and classic adamantinoma. Clin Radiol. 2014; 69(2):200–208

Levine SM, Lambiase RE, Petchprapa CN. Cortical lesions of the tibia: characteristic appearances at conventional radiography. Radiographics. 2003; 23(1):157–177

Case 30

Paulomi Kanzaria and Jasjeet Bindra

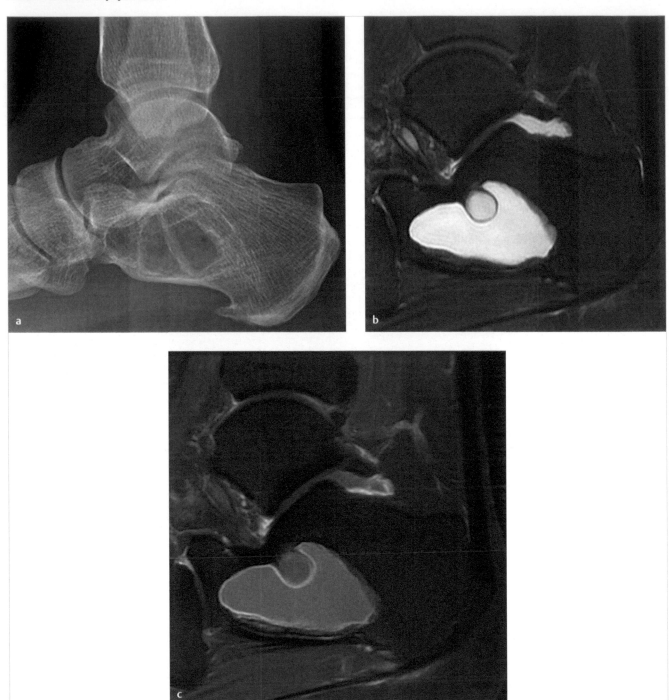

Fig. 30.1 Lateral view of the ankle **(a)** shows a well-marginated lucent lesion with sclerotic margins in the anterior calcaneus. Sagittal, fat-suppressed, T2-weighted MR image **(b)** reveals the lesion to be hyperintense. Sagittal, fat-suppressed, postcontrast, T1-weighted MR image **(c)** shows no significant enhancement or solid components in the lesion.

■ Clinical History

A 40-year-old female with plantar fascial heel pain (▶ Fig. 30.1).

◼ Key Finding

Lucent lesion in calcaneus.

◼ Top 3 Differential Diagnoses

- **Pseudocyst:** Pseudocyst of the calcaneus is a normal variant that appears as an ill-defined triangular area in the anterior to midcalcaneus in which the trabecular network is naturally much sparser. The almost total lack of spongy structure in this area is due to the absence of locally transmitted forces, which pass instead through the thick trabeculae that surround this area. Unlike cysts and lipomas, pseudocysts do not have a peripheral sclerotic rim, sign of expansion or central calcifications, and do show some persistence of sparse spongy bone within.

- **Intraosseous lipoma:** Calcaneal lipomas are benign lesions that are relatively rare. Calcaneus is the most common site for intraosseous lipomas of the skeleton. They are generally seen between 30 to 60 years of age. Many lesions are found incidentally. Typical appearance on radiographs consists of a well-circumscribed lucent lesion that is frequently associated with mild, focal expansile remodeling and may contain central sclerosis or calcification. The fatty tissue contained within lipomas has negative density values on CT (−60 to −130 HU). On MRI, they closely follow the signal of the marrow and subcutaneous fat and are differentiated from marrow fat by a thin margin of low-signal intensity secondary to the capsule or partial ossification. On T1-weighted images, the lesion is of high-signal, with the central sclerosis being of low-signal. On fat suppression sequences, intralesional fat shows corresponding suppression.

- **Simple bone cyst:** A simple bone cyst (SBC) or unicameral bone cyst (UBC) is a benign, fluid-filled lesion that most commonly occurs in the metaphyseal region of proximal humerus or femur. The calcaneal location is relatively rare, but it is the most common tarsal bone affected by UBC. Calcaneal cysts are usually seen in the second or third decades of life. They are generally asymptomatic and found incidentally.

  On radiography, the cyst is a mildly expansile, well-defined lucent lesion with thin sclerotic rim and no central calcification. On CT and MRI imaging, the lesion is fluid-filled, which may, at times, have a fluid level. On MRI, the lesion demonstrates low-T1 signal and high-T2 signal and does not enhance with contrast.

◼ Additional Diagnostic Considerations

- **Aneurysmal bone cyst (ABC):** ABC of calcaneus is a relatively uncommon entity. Most of these lesions occur in patients less than 20 years of age. On radiographs, the lesion appears as a large, expansile, osteolytic process with "eggshell" borders. Fluid levels may be demonstrated within the lesion on CT or MR.

- **Giant cell tumor (GCT):** GCT can also uncommonly involve calcaneus. Most cases are seen in patients between 20 to 40 years of age. Radiographically, the lesion appears osteolytic, expansile, and with well-defined but nonsclerotic margins. On CT or MR, the solid tumor shows enhancement with contrast administration.

◼ Diagnosis

Simple bone cyst of calcaneus.

✓ Pearls

- Calcaneal pseudocyst shows some sparse trabeculae within and does not have a defined sclerotic margin.
- UBC of calcaneus is a well-defined lucent lesion with thin sclerotic rim and without central calcification.

- Fatty contents of calcaneal lipoma can be easily identified with CT or MR imaging.

◼ Suggested Readings

Kumar R, Matasar K, Stansberry S, et al. The calcaneus: normal and abnormal. Radiographics. 1991; 11(3):415–440

Malghem J, Lecouvet F, Vande Berg B. Calcaneal cysts and lipomas: a common pathogenesis? Skeletal Radiol. 2017; 46(12):1635–1642

Case 31

Jasjeet Bindra

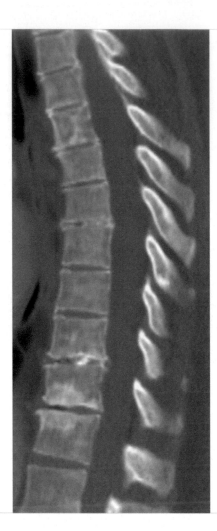

Fig. 31.1 Sagittal reformation CT image of the thoracic spine shows diffusely increased bone density.

■ Clinical History

A 56-year-old male with pancytopenia (▶ Fig. 31.1).

■ Key Finding

Diffusely increased bone density.

■ Top 3 Differential Diagnoses

- **Metabolic disorders:** Renal osteodystrophy, primary hyper-parathyroidism, hypervitaminosis D, and fluorosis are among metabolic disorders that can be associated with increased bone density. Renal osteodystrophy is usually associated with soft-tissue calcifications, osteomalacia, and regions of osteosclerosis especially affecting the ribs, pelvis and spine. Osteosclerosis can produce the classic "rugger-jersey" spine radiographic appearance.
- **Osteoblastic metastases:** Several primary malignancies characteristically produce osteoblastic metastases, including carcinomas of the prostate gland, breast, and pancreas; mucinous adenocarcinoma of the gastrointestinal tract; transitional cell carcinoma; carcinoid tumor; lymphoma; medulloblastoma; and neuroblastoma. Differentiation from other causes of increased bone density can usually be made by considering the entire medical history and invariably patchy nature of metastases.
- **Hematologic disorders:** Myelofibrosis, mastocytosis, and sickle cell anemia are some of the hematologic disorders that can show diffuse osteosclerosis. In myelofibrosis, the bone marrow is replaced by fibrotic tissue, and osteosclerosis is most commonly found in the axial skeleton and proximal portions of long bones, humerus and femur. In sickle cell disease, the abnormal red blood cells increase the incidence of bone infarcts that can ultimately cause a markedly sclerotic appearance, especially in pelvis, spine and ribs.

■ Additional Diagnostic Considerations

- **Paget's disease:** In the blastic phase of the disease, there are areas of sclerosis with cortical thickening, coarse trabeculae and bony enlargement, especially in skull, spine and pelvis.
- **Osteopetrosis:** Osteopetrosis is a rare inherited dysplasia with increased density in the medullary portion of the bone, especially in the long bones, skull and spine. The bones, however, are prone to fractures.

■ Diagnosis

Myelofibrosis.

✓ Pearls

- Osteosclerosis with renal osteodystrophy can be seen as classic "rugger jersey" spine. Soft-tissue calcifications, osteoporosis, and bone resorption are other features.
- Osteoblastic metastases present with patchy areas of increased density much more commonly than diffuse increase in bone density.
- Sickle cell disease patients show multiple other radiologic manifestations like "fish-mouth" vertebrae, areas of avascular necrosis, and extramedullary hematopoiesis.

■ Suggested Readings

Ejindu VC, Hine AL, Mashayekhi M, Shorvon PJ, Misra RR. Musculoskeletal manifestations of sickle cell disease. Radiographics. 2007; 27(4):1005–1021

Ihde LL, Forrester DM, Gottsegen CJ, et al. Sclerosing bone dysplasias: review and differentiation from other causes of osteosclerosis. Radiographics. 2011; 31(7): 1865–1882

Murphey MD, Sartoris DJ, Quale JL, Pathria MN, Martin NL. Musculoskeletal manifestations of chronic renal insufficiency. Radiographics. 1993; 13(2):357–379

Case 32

Robert D. Boutin

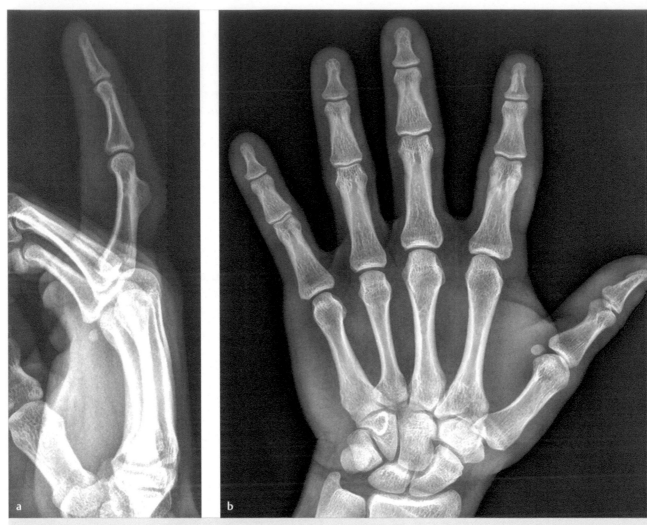

Fig. 32.1 Lateral radiograph **(a)** of the finger demonstrates a well-defined, ossified lesion off the dorsal surface of the proximal phalanx. The underlying cortex shows no full-thickness disruption. The underlying medullary bone is normal. Frontal radiograph **(b)** of the hand appears essentially normal.

■ Clinical History

A 31-year-old man with a finger lump. Radiographs 5 years earlier showed only soft-tissue swelling, but no phalangeal derangement (▶ Fig. 32.1).

■ Key Finding

Well-marginated, ossific mass, projecting off the surface of the bone (without full-thickness cortical disruption or overlying soft-tissue mass).

■ Top 3 Differential Diagnoses

- **Bizarre parosteal osteochondromatous proliferation (BPOP):** BPOP, often referred to as "Nora's lesion" (for the pathologist who described it in 1983), is a well-marginated, mineralized lesion at the cortical surface. BPOP usually is located in the hands and feet (≥75%). A classic target site is the phalanges of the hand. BPOP has a spectrum of appearances that varies from soft-tissue swelling superficial to bone (with or without mineralization) to an osteochondroma-like osseous excrescence.

  BPOP may or may not be associated with a known history of trauma. BPOP is often regarded as a proliferative response to periosteal injury, representing a reactive process that can evolve over time (e.g., from a first-stage of florid reactive periostitis to a final-stage of turret exostosis). BPOP also has been hypothesized to represent a benign neoplasm, and local recurrences may occur after surgical excision.

  Pertinent negatives on imaging generally include: no overlying soft-tissue mass, no aggressive cortical destruction, and no underlying derangement in the medullary bone on radiography. Furthermore, BPOP characteristically does not show trabecular continuity merging the lesion with the underlying cancellous bone (unlike an osteochondroma).
- **Osteochondroma:** An osteochondroma is an osseous excrescence that develops with a cartilage cap. The hallmark of an osteochondroma is continuity of the lesion (both the cortex

  and marrow) with the cortex and marrow of the underlying bone.

  Most symptomatic osteochondromas are diagnosed in patients by the age of 20 years (~80%). Osteochondroma growth is usually proportional to overall patient growth, and lesion growth typically ceases at skeletal maturity. Long bones are affected most commonly, especially the metaphysis/metadiaphysis of the femur, tibia and humerus. Much less commonly, osteochondromas may occur in the hand, classically in the setting of multiple hereditary exostoses (osteochondromatosis).

  The general risk of malignant transformation of a solitary osteochondroma to chondrosarcoma is 1%, but it may occur in up to 5% of patients with multiple hereditary exostoses. The diagnosis of a secondary chondrosarcoma is suggested when the cartilage cap thickness measures ≥2 cm in an adult long bone.
- **Periosteal chondroma:** Periosteal (juxtacortical) chondroma is a benign surface bone lesion. These benign chondroid tumors spare the medullary bone, unlike enchondromas (which are more common benign chondroid tumors).

  Periosteal chondromas most commonly occur in the proximal humerus (metaphysis or metadiaphysis), but they may also occur in the short tubular bones of the hand. Like BPOP, periosteal chondromas are mineralized juxtacortical lesions and are treated with surgical excision.

■ Diagnosis

Bizarre parosteal osteochondromatous proliferation (BPOP).

✓ Pearls

- BPOP is classically seen as a well-marginated, mineralized mass at the surface of bone, which most commonly occurs in the hand.
- BPOP typically does not have an overlying soft-tissue mass, does not violate the underlying cortex, and does not have corticomedullary continuity.

- The hallmark of an osteochondroma is continuity of the lesion (both the cortex and marrow) with the cortex and marrow of the underlying bone.

■ Suggested Readings

Dhondt E, Oudenhoven L, Khan S, et al. Nora's lesion, a distinct radiological entity? Skeletal Radiol. 2006; 35(7):497–502

Fenerty S, Ling S, Wang C, Awan O, Ali S. Test yourself: painless hand mass. Bizarre parosteal osteochondromatous proliferation (Nora lesion) of the metacarpal. Skeletal Radiol. 2017; 46(3):359–360, 405–407

Flint JH, McKay PL. Bizarre parosteal osteochondromatous proliferation and periosteal chondroma: a comparative report and review of the literature. J Hand Surg Am. 2007; 32(6):893–898

Michelsen H, Abramovici L, Steiner G, Posner MA. Bizarre parosteal osteochondromatous proliferation (Nora's lesion) in the hand. J Hand Surg Am. 2004; 29(3):520–525

Rabarin F, Laulan J, Saint Cast Y, Césari B, Fouque PA, Raimbeau G. Focal periosteal chondroma of the hand: a review of 24 cases. Orthop Traumatol Surg Res. 2014; 100(6):617–620

Salna I, Solanki N, Proudman T. Appearances and evolution of a recurrent Nora's lesion of the hand. Eplasty. 2019; 19:ic5

Case 33

Jasjeet Bindra

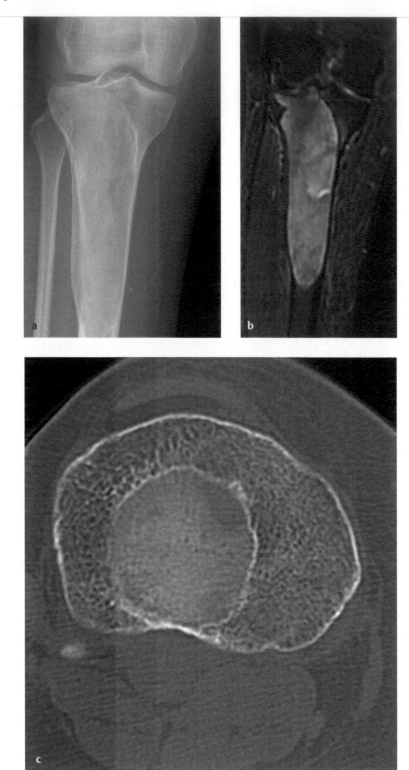

Fig. 33.1 Frontal radiograph of the knee **(a)** shows a long, mildly expansile lesion with ground glass matrix in the proximal tibia. Coronal, fat-suppressed, T2-weighted MR image **(b)** demonstrates the well-defined lesion with internal hyperintensity. Ground glass matrix is seen well on axial CT image **(c)**.

■ Clinical History

A 25-year-old male with pain in the leg (▶ Fig. 33.1).

■ Key Finding

Long lesion in a long bone with ground glass matrix–Roentgen classic.

■ Diagnosis

Fibrous Dysplasia: Fibrous dysplasia is a noninherited bone disease that is characterized by replacement of normal lamellar cancellous bone by abnormal fibrous tissue. It is categorized as monostotic or polyostotic and may occur as a component of McCune–Albright syndrome or the rare Mazabraud syndrome. Classically, the lesions are intramedullary, expansile, and well-defined. There may be endosteal scalloping but a smooth cortical contour is always maintained. Lesions show varying degrees of hazy density. Some lesions may appear completely radiolucent or sclerotic. A well-defined long lesion in a long bone with ground glass matrix is a classic appearance. The most common sites of involvement include rib, femur, tibia, mandible, skull, and humerus. The lesions may show increased uptake of radiotracer on bone scans. CT and MRI are useful for evaluating the extent of the disease. MRI appearance is variable with intermediate–to low-signal intensity on T1-weighted images and intermediate- to high-signal on T2-weighted images. There may be heterogeneous enhancement after administration of gadolinium. Polyostotic form may involve a few or many bones, most commonly skull, facial bones, pelvis and spine. Polyostotic forms tend to involve larger segments of bone, and deformities like shepherd's crook are common. McCune–Albright syndrome consists of a triad of precocious puberty, café' au lait spots, and polyostotic fibrous dysplasia. The cafe au lait spots in this syndrome have characteristically irregular ragged borders (commonly called "coast of Maine" borders) as opposed to the smoothly marginated ("coast of California") borders of the spots seen in neurofibromatosis. Mazabraud syndrome is the rare combination of fibrous dysplasia and soft-tissue myxomas.

Complications that can be associated with fibrous dysplasia are pathologic fractures and, rarely, malignant transformation.

✓ Pearls

- Fibrous dysplasia lesions are intramedullary, expansile, and well-defined.
- Lesions may have varying degrees of density with ground glass appearance being classic.
- Involvement of long segments of bone is more common in polyostotic forms.

■ Suggested Readings

Fitzpatrick KA, Taljanovic MS, Speer DP, et al. Imaging findings of fibrous dysplasia with histopathologic and intraoperative correlation. AJR Am J Roentgenol. 2004; 182(6):1389–1398

Kransdorf MJ, Moser RP, Jr, Gilkey FW. Fibrous dysplasia. Radiographics. 1990; 10(3): 519–537

Case 34

Jasjeet Bindra

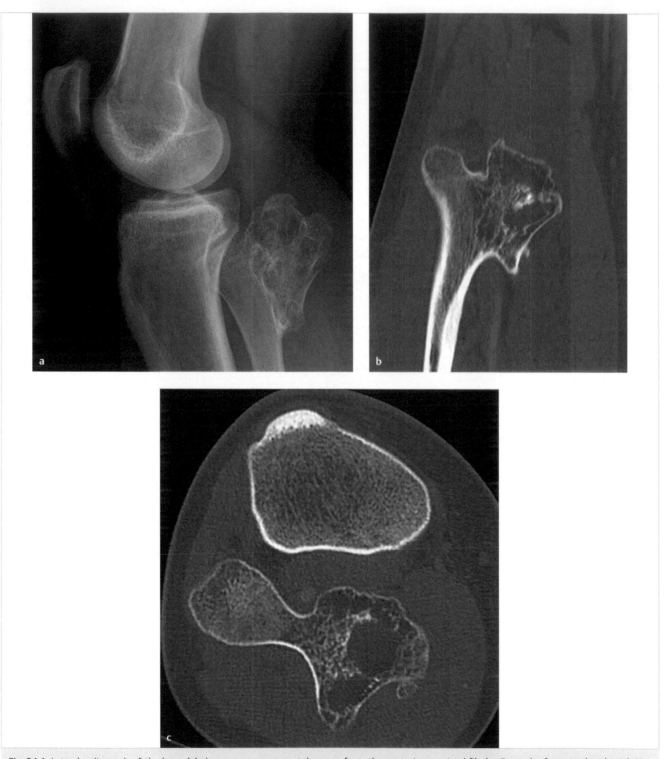

Fig. 34.1 Lateral radiograph of the knee **(a)** shows an osseous protuberance from the posterior proximal fibula. Coronal reformatted and axial CT images **(b, c)** demonstrate the lesion well, showing continuity of the cortex and medullary canal of the lesion with that of the host bone.

■ Clinical History

A 32-year-old female with posterior knee pain (▶ Fig. 34.1).

■ Key Finding

Bony projection with continuation of cortex and medullary cavity of host bone–Roentgen classic.

■ Diagnosis

Osteochondroma: Osteochondroma is the most common benign tumor or tumor-like lesion of bone. The radiographic appearance is often diagnostic and reflective of pathology, that is, a lesion composed of cortical and medullary bone with an overlying hyaline cartilage cap. It is the continuity of this lesion with underlying host bone's cortex and medullary canal that is pathognomonic of osteochondroma. Any bone that forms from preformed cartilage (enchondral ossification) can develop an osteochondroma. The most commonly involved bones are femur, tibia, and humerus. Other more unusual locations are small bones of hand and feet, scapula, pelvis, and spine. The area of osseous continuity with the parent bone may be broad in sessile osteochondromas or narrow in pedunculated lesions. Hyaline cap may have chondroid calcifications on radiography. The thickness of hyaline cartilage cap is variable and best measured by MR although CT is also helpful. CT and MR are best for depicting the pathognomonic marrow and cortical continuity with underlying bone, especially in areas of complex anatomy and in sessile osteochondromas. The cartilage cap in benign osteochondromas averages about 6 to 8 mm with a maximum of 2.5 cm. Cartilage cap thickness also depends on skeletal maturity, and increased thickness of the cartilage cap is a recognized feature in skeletally immature patients.

Hereditary multiple exostoses (HMEs) are characterized by multiple osteochondromas and show an autosomal dominant inheritance pattern. The lesions are similar to solitary osteochondromas. Various complications associated with osteochondromas include osseous deformity, fracture, vascular or neurologic compromise, bursa formation, and malignant transformation. Malignant transformation occurs in 1% of solitary osteochondromas. The prevalence of this complication is higher in HME. Malignant transformation is invariably due to chondrosarcoma arising in the cartilage cap. Features that suggest malignant transformation include growth of a previously stable lesion in a skeletally mature patient, indistinct surface, region of radiolucency in a lesion, erosion or destruction of adjacent bone, and soft-tissue mass. Cartilage cap thickness is another criterion that is helpful. A cartilage cap thickness of greater than 1.5 cm in a skeletally mature patient should be viewed with suspicion of harboring malignant transformation.

✓ Pearls

- Cortical and medullary continuity with underlying bone is pathognomonic of an osteochondroma.
- CT and MR may be more optimal than radiography for depicting the pathognomonic continuity in areas of complex anatomy and in sessile osteochondromas.
- Cartilage cap thickness is best measured on MRI.

■ Suggested Readings

Karasick D, Schweitzer ME, Eschelman DJ. Symptomatic osteochondromas: imaging features. AJR Am J Roentgenol. 1997; 168(6):1507–1512

Murphey MD, Choi JJ, Kransdorf MJ, Flemming DJ, Gannon FH. Imaging of osteochondroma: variants and complications with radiologic-pathologic correlation. Radiographics. 2000; 20(5):1407–1434

Case 35

Jasjeet Bindra

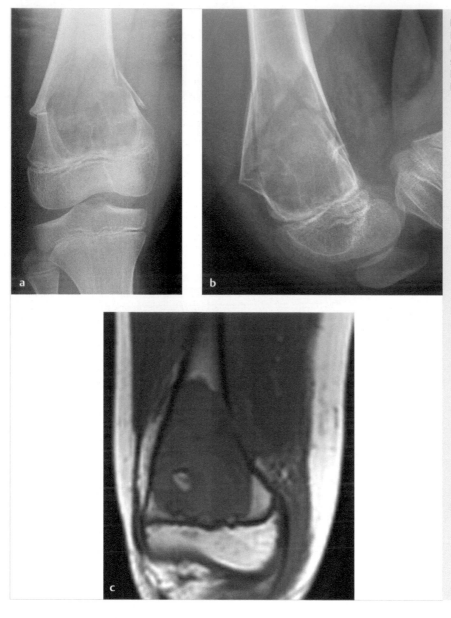

Fig. 35.1 Frontal and lateral radiographs of the knee (**a, b**) show a pathologic fracture through a lytic lesion of metadiaphysis of distal femur in this skeletally immature patient. Coronal T1-weighted image through the lesion (**c**) demonstrates a bony fragment fallen within the lesion.

▪ Clinical History

A 10-year-old male with acute knee pain (▶ Fig. 35.1).

■ Key Finding

Fractured lytic lesion with a fallen fragment–Roentgen classic.

■ Diagnosis

Simple bone cyst: Solitary bone cyst (SBC), also termed simple or unicameral bone cyst, is a very common tumor-like lesion of childhood. It is often found incidentally or as a pathologic fracture. It is most commonly seen in the first and second decades and uncommonly in adults. Proximal humerus and proximal femur are the most common locations. Radiographically, it appears as a well-circumscribed, central, radiolucent metaphyseal or diaphyseal lesion that is mildly expansile, with a narrow zone of transition, and a thin sclerotic rim. The "fallen fragment" sign is considered nearly pathognomonic for SBC with a pathologic fracture. Gravitational settling of a bony fragment within a fractured lucent osseous lesion implies it is hollow or fluid-filled and, therefore, most likely a unicameral bone cyst. This sign helps in differentiation of a bone cyst from other radiographically similar lesions containing solid tissue like fibrous dysplasia. Fractures through other cystic lesions such as hemophiliac pseudotumors, or cystic fibrous dysplasia could conceivably allow for a "fallen fragment" sign to be observed. However, these entities are much less common and typically associated with other characteristic findings that can point toward the correct diagnosis.

MRI is rarely required for these lesions. However, the MRI appearance is typical of a cyst with low-signal intensity on T1-weighted, and high-signal on T2-weighted images and occasional fluid levels. CT and MRI can help to confirm location of bone fragment within the lesion. The lesion may occasionally heal spontaneously following fracture. Otherwise, it is treated with curettage and bone grafting. There is a high recurrence rate with higher likelihood of recurrence in younger patients.

✓ Pearls

- SBC is usually a lucent, mildly expansile lesion with a narrow zone of transition in a child.
- Most common sites of involvement are proximal humerus and proximal femur.
- "Fallen fragment" sign within a lucent osseous lesion is nearly pathognomonic for SBC.

■ Suggested Readings

Killeen KL. The fallen fragment sign. Radiology. 1998; 207(1):261 262

Manaster BJ, May DA, Disler DG. Musculoskeletal Imaging, The Requisites. 4th ed. Philadelphia: Mosby Elsevier; 2013

Part 3

Upper Extremity

Case 36

Cyrus Bateni

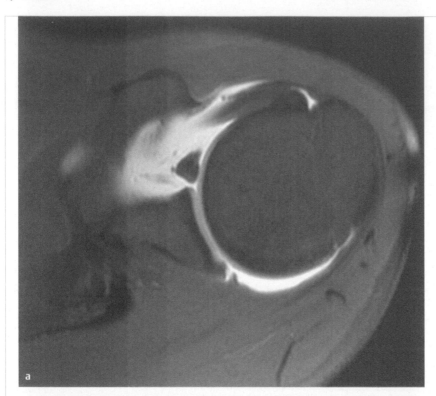

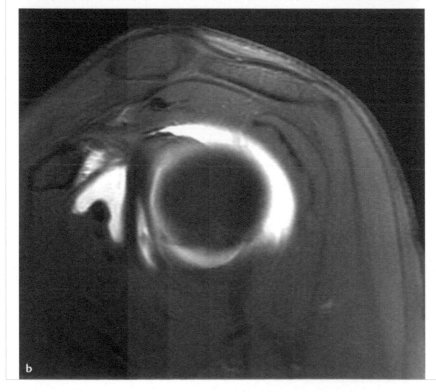

Fig. 36.1 Axial, fat-saturated, T1-weighted MR arthrogram image (a) of the shoulder shows a thickened middle glenohumeral ligament (MGHL) with absence of the anterior superior glenoid labrum. Sagittal, fat-saturated, T1-weighted MR arthrogram image (b) shows the thickened MGHL to a better advantage.

▪ Clinical History

A 21-year-old female with pain at the shoulder with overhead movements (▶ Fig. 36.1).

■ Key Finding

Abnormal/variant appearance of anterosuperior labrum.

■ Top 3 Differential Diagnoses

- **Sublabral sulcus:** A sublabral sulcus or recess is the most common normal variant of glenoid labrum. If one utilizes a clock face description for the glenoid (such that when looking at it en face on sagittal imaging, the biceps tendon attachment upon the labrum is defined as the 12 o'clock position while anterior at the level of the equator is termed the 3 o'clock position), it is usually present between 11 o'clock and 3 o'clock positions. A normal sulcus is identified as a small linear fluid-filled gap between the labrum and the glenoid articular cartilage. This small cleft has smooth margins, parallels the glenoid articular cartilage, and is usually anterior to the biceps anchor. This can be typically identified on conventional MRI but is best depicted on coronal MR arthrographic imaging, with linear fluid signal following the contour of the medial glenoid articular cartilage, and a triangular appearance of the labrum just lateral to the fluid signal cleft.
- **Sublabral foramen:** A sublabral foramen or hole is a focal detachment of the labrum from the glenoid rim in the anterosuperior quadrant, usually located between 12 o'clock to 3 o'clock positions. It is found in about 10% of individuals. Similar to a sublabral sulcus, there will be smooth margins, and there should be no extension into the long head biceps tendon or glenohumeral ligaments.
- **Buford complex:** In a Buford complex, the middle glenohumeral ligament is thickened, and the anterior–superior glenoid labrum is absent. This occurs in about 1% of individuals and can be differentiated from a tear of the labrum by its lack of involvement of the labrum at the biceps tendon attachment. While both a sublabral foramen and a Buford complex are normal variants, individuals with these anatomic variants have an increased risk of a labral tear, which is felt to be due to increased laxity and tension placed upon the remainder of the labrum. It is important to recognize these anatomic variants, as attempts to repair a normal labrum in these cases may lead to decreased range of motion and pain.

■ Additional Diagnostic Consideration

- **SLAP tear:** A tear of the superior glenoid labrum extending anterior to posterior is termed a SLAP tear. This tear can sometimes be challenging to differentiate from normal variants. Key imaging features that can aid the radiologist in making the diagnosis of a SLAP lesion include the presence of fluid signal extending laterally into the labrum, irregular margins, extension into and posterior to the attachment of the long head biceps tendon upon the labrum, more than 2 to 2.5 mm width of signal abnormality, and presence of paralabral cysts.

■ Diagnosis

Buford complex.

✓ Pearls

- Anatomic variants are commonly seen in the anterosuperior and superior labrum.
- Presence of intralabral signal, irregular margins, nonparallel orientation to glenoid margin, and extension of signal posterior to biceps anchor are some features that aid in the diagnosis of a SLAP lesion.

■ Suggested Readings

De Coninck T, Ngai SS, Tafur M, Chung CB. Imaging the glenoid labrum and labral tears. Radiographics. 2016; 36(6):1628–1647

De Maeseneer M, Van Roy F, Lenchik L, et al. CT and MR arthrography of the normal and pathologic anterosuperior labrum and labral-bicipital complex. Radiographics. 2000; 20(Spec No):S67–S81

Case 37

Cyrus Bateni

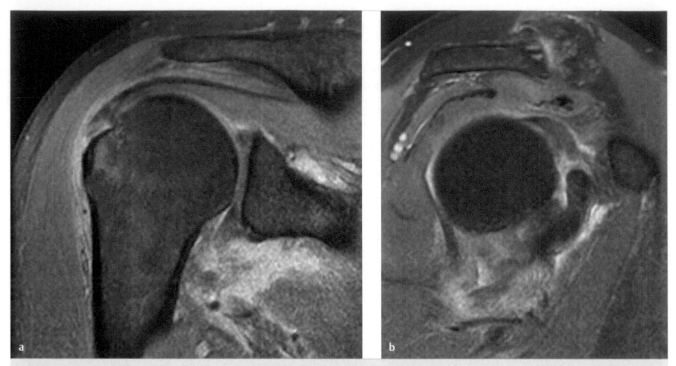

Fig. 37.1 Coronal **(a)** and sagittal **(b)** fat-saturated proton density MR images of the shoulder show significant edema in the right axilla with disruption of the inferior glenohumeral ligament. There is edema in the posterior fibers of the supraspinatus tendon at the attachment upon the greater tuberosity related to the greater tuberosity fracture.

■ Clinical History

A 52-year-old male with recent fall and acute right shoulder pain (▶ Fig. 37.1).

■ Key Finding

Abnormality of inferior glenohumeral ligament.

■ Top 3 Differential Diagnoses

- **Capsular avulsion:** The inferior glenohumeral ligament (IGHL) extends from the inferior labrum to the surgical neck of the humerus and consists of anterior and posterior bands, with an intervening axillary recess of capsule. IGHL can avulse at its humeral or glenoid attachments as a result of acute traumatic glenohumeral subluxation or dislocation. These injuries are termed humeral avulsion of the glenohumeral ligament (HAGL) and glenoid avulsion of the glenohumeral ligament (GAGL), respectively. On MRI, the IGHL is best visualized on oblique coronal sequences as a hypointense "U" shaped band, serving as the inferior portion of the glenohumeral joint capsule, which is also termed the axillary pouch. Both HAGL and GAGL are best identified on MRI as either change in configuration of the IGHL to a "J" shape and extravasation of fluid or injected contrast, extending inferiorly into the axilla. In a subset of patients, there may also be an avulsion fracture at the humeral attachment. The HAGL lesion is an important cause of anterior instability of the glenohumeral joint.

- **Midsubstance tear:** Midsubstance tears represent about a third of IGHL injuries. When the IGHL fails at this location, the fluid within the glenohumeral joint may escape inferiorly into the axilla, or the inferior joint capsule may no longer be its typical "U" shape on oblique coronal MRI sequences.

- **Adhesive capsulitis:** Adhesive capsulitis is a clinically diagnosed condition characterized by painful limitation of motion of shoulder. Multiple imaging findings have been described in this entity, including thickening and intermediate- to high-signal of the inferior glenohumeral ligament. This can be differentiated from IGHL injury primarily by clinical presentation, but also by the lack of other imaging findings that may be found in a shoulder dislocation (Hill–Sachs impaction fracture and anterior inferior labral injury) that led to injury of IGHL. Similar to IGHL injury, the thickening and intermediate/edema signal of the IGHL in adhesive capsulitis is best identified on oblique coronal, fat-suppressed fluid-sensitive sequences. Other findings described on MRI in adhesive capsulitis include edema and soft-tissue thickening within the rotator interval, and thickening of the coracohumeral ligament.

■ Diagnosis

Midsubstance tear of the IGHL related to a shoulder dislocation.

✓ Pearls

- IGHL tears can result from shoulder dislocations. Injuries are best identified in the acute setting as extravasation of fluid, contrast from axillary recess, or abnormal J shape of the inferior joint capsule.

- Thickening and intermediate signal of the IGHL can be seen in adhesive capsulitis.

■ Suggested Readings

Omoumi P, Teixeira P, Lecouvet F, Chung CB. Glenohumeral joint instability. J Magn Reson Imaging. 2011; 33(1):2–16

Walz DM, Burge AJ, Steinbach L. Imaging of shoulder instability. Semin Musculoskelet Radiol. 2015; 19(3):254–268

Case 38

Cyrus Bateni and Jasjeet Bindra

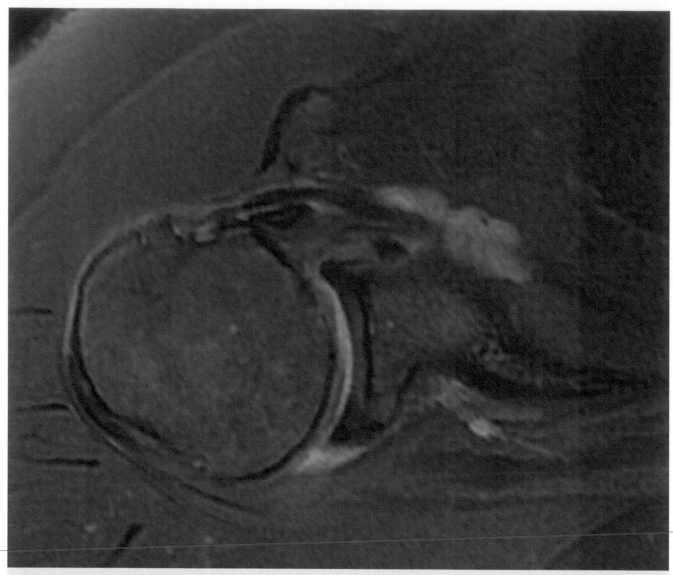

Fig. 38.1 Axial, fat-saturated proton density MR image of the shoulder shows an empty bicipital groove with abnormal position of long head of biceps tendon.

■ Clinical History

A 64-year-old female with chronic shoulder pain (▶ Fig. 38.1).

■ Key Finding

Abnormality of proximal long head of biceps tendon.

■ Top 3 Differential Diagnoses

- **Dislocation or subluxation:** The coracohumeral ligament, superior glenohumeral ligament, subscapularis tendon, and supraspinatus tendon are all important in maintaining the stability of the long head biceps tendon (LHBT) within the bicipital groove. On ultrasound or MRI, if the long head biceps tendon is not identified within the bicipital groove, there should be close inspection for medial displacement or tear of the biceps tendon. Displacement of the LHBT can occurs due to injury of any of the four aforementioned stabilizers, although, most frequently, this is due to a tear of the subscapularis tendon. The dislocated tendon may be anterior to subscapularis tendon, within an intratendinous tear of subscapularis tendon, or deep to the subscapularis tendon in an intra-articular location.
- **Tendon tear:** Partial and complete tears of LHBT are usually associated with underlying tendon pathology like degeneration. Complete rupture occurs most commonly in the bicipital groove or just proximal to the groove. It is commonly accompanied by "popeye" deformity, a bulge that occurs over the anterior arm from retraction of the torn tendon and muscle. Partial tears are seen as sudden reduction in caliber and irregularity of the tendon contour. Complete tears are indicated by absence of the tendon in the groove, and careful inspection confirms that the tendon is not dislocated. In acute ruptures, ventral edema and retracted tendon stump may also be seen. LHBT tears are very common in individuals with rotator cuff abnormalities, occurring in approximately 75% of individuals with rotator cuff tears.
- **Tendinitis:** Biceps tendinitis is not an uncommon finding on MR imaging, especially in the presence of abnormalities of supraspinatus and subscapularis. Tendinitis can occur in both diffuse and segmental form. The imaging findings of tendinitis are increased signal in the tendon on all pulse sequences, and thickening and inhomogeneity of the tendon.

■ Additional Diagnostic Consideration

- **Variant anatomy:** A wide range of anatomic variations has been reported for LHBT and proximal biceps, including aberrant intra-articular and extra-articular origin, congenital absence, and accessory heads. In individuals with a congenitally absent tendon, the bicipital groove will be either hypoplastic or absent. Other common variations about the long head biceps tendon that may mimic an injury include a duplication or bifurcation of the long head biceps tendon. On MRI, an accessory tendon is seen as an additional hypointense structure in the bicipital groove which is flattened and can be misinterpreted as a longitudinal tear of LHBT without carefully tracing the tendon to its origin.

■ Diagnosis

Medial dislocation of the long head biceps tendon into an interstitial tear of subscapularis.

✓ Pearls

- Tears of the subscapularis tendon are the most common cause of medial dislocation of the LHBT.
- There is a very high association of injuries of the LHBT with rotator cuff tears.
- An accessory LHBT tendon can be misinterpreted as a longitudinal tear without carefully tracing it to its origin.

■ Suggested Readings

Beltran J, Jbara M, Maimon R. Shoulder: labrum and bicipital tendon. Top Magn Reson Imaging. 2003; 14(1):35–49

Petchprapa CN, Beltran LS, Jazrawi LM, Kwon YW, Babb JS, Recht MP. The rotator interval: a review of anatomy, function, and normal and abnormal MRI appearance. AJR Am J Roentgenol. 2010; 195(3):567–576

Case 39

Cyrus Bateni and Jasjeet Bindra

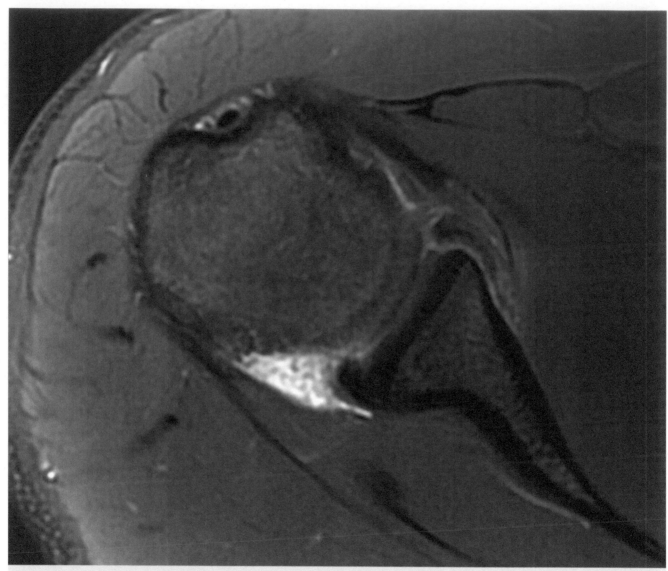

Fig. 39.1 Axial, fat-saturated proton density MRI image of the shoulder demonstrates a fluid signal cleft between the anterior–inferior labrum and glenoid. The nondisplaced labrum remains attached to the periosteum.

■ Clinical History

An 18-year-old male with prior anterior shoulder dislocation (▶ Fig. 39.1).

Key Finding

Tear of the anteroinferior labrum.

Top 3 Differential Diagnoses

- **Bankart lesion:** A Bankart lesion is an injury to the anteroinferior labrum, which may involve the labrum or both the labrum and adjacent bony glenoid. The labrum (and potentially the glenoid) will be displaced due to a tear of the adjacent periosteum. This injury to the labrum is most commonly associated with an anterior shoulder dislocation. It commonly coexists with a Hill–Sachs lesion, which is a compression fracture of posterolateral humeral head. The detached labrum can remain in situ or migrate distal to its attachment site. MR imaging demonstrates a disrupted medial scapular periosteum, irregular fluid, or contrast extending into or deep to the labrum, but the labrum stays continuous to the anterior inferior glenohumeral ligament.
- **Perthes lesion:** When the anteroinferior labrum is detached from the glenoid surface but the labrum is still partially attached by the periosteum and not displaced, the injury is called a Perthes lesion. This can be difficult to see both by imaging and arthroscopy, as the labrum may appear to be in normal position, unlike a Bankart lesion. The pressure placed upon the labrum by distension of the joint with fluid in an MR arthrogram can better depict a Perthes lesion. In addition, placing the arm in the abducted and externally rotated (ABER) position as part of an MR arthrogram can best identify a Perthes lesion due to stress placed upon the anterior labrum by a taut inferior glenohumeral ligament in this position. The Perthes injury can be found both due to an acute traumatic event or repetitive stress.
- **Anterior labroligamentous periosteal sleeve avulsion (ALPSA):** An ALPSA lesion is often the result of a chronic injury rather than acute dislocation. This entity is similar to a Perthes lesion in that the anteroinferior labrum is separated from the glenoid surface, and the labrum will be partially attached to the periosteum. However, unlike in a Perthes lesion, the labrum is displaced medially along the anterior aspect of the scapular neck in an ALPSA lesion. As the labrum is not in its normal position, this is easier to diagnose on MR than its similar correlate, the Perthes lesion.

Additional Diagnostic Consideration

- **Glenoid labral articular disruption (GLAD):** In a GLAD lesion, the anteroinferior labrum and a portion of the adjacent articular cartilage are torn, and these may be either minimally displaced or displaced medially. Unlike the other above-mentioned entities, this more commonly occurs as a direct acute traumatic impaction injury rather than a dislocation injury. MR arthrography can best depict the tear of the glenoid articular cartilage.

Diagnosis

Perthes lesion.

Pearls

- In a Bankart lesion, there is detachment of the labrum and disruption of the scapular periosteum.
- ABER positioning can help in identifying a Perthes lesion on MR.
- In an ALPSA lesion, the labrum is detached, and the scapular periosteum is stripped with medial displacement of labrum.

Suggested Readings

Bencardino JT, Gyftopoulos S, Palmer WE. Imaging in anterior glenohumeral instability. Radiology. 2013; 269(2):323–337

De Coninck T, Ngai SS, Tafur M, Chung CB. Imaging the Glenoid Labrum and Labral Tears. Radiographics. 2016; 36(6):1628–1647

Case 40

Cyrus Bateni and Jasjeet Bindra

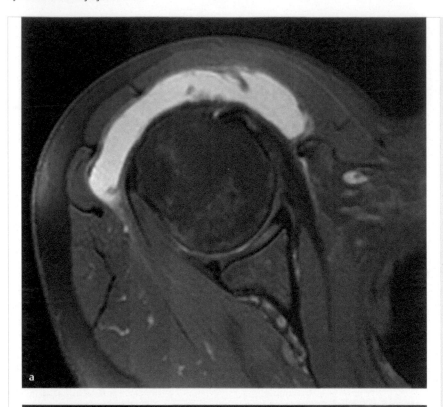

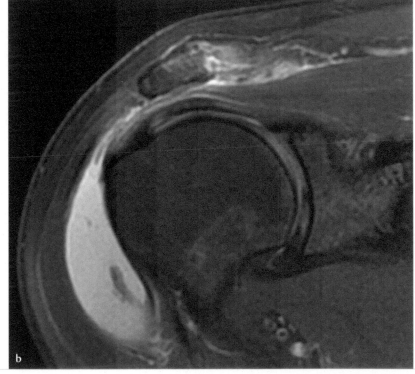

Fig. 40.1 Axial, fat-saturated proton density MR image **(a)** of the shoulder shows a crescentic fluid collection around the shoulder deep to the deltoid. Coronal, fat-saturated proton density image **(b)** of the same shoulder shows the same collection with internal synovitis.

■ **Clinical History**

A 49-year-old female with shoulder swelling (▶ Fig. 40.1).

■ Key Finding

Bursa or cyst around the shoulder.

■ Top 3 Differential Diagnoses

- **Subacromial–subdeltoid bursa:** Subacromial–subdeltoid bursa is superficial to all the rotator cuff tendons. It does not communicate with the glenohumeral joint. If there is a full-thickness tear of rotator cuff, an abnormal communication gets established between the glenohumeral joint and the subacromial–subdeltoid bursa, allowing fluid to escape from the joint into the bursa. Inflammation and distension of this bursa can also occur in infectious or inflammatory conditions, such as calcium hydroxyapatite deposition without a rotator cuff tear. It can be normal to have a trace amount of fluid within this bursa.
- **Geyser sign:** In a full-thickness rotator cuff tear, fluid can escape from the glenohumeral joint into the subacromial–subdeltoid bursa and then into the acromioclavicular (AC) joint. If considerable pressure and fluid are present, a fluid-filled mass called geyser sign can develop above the AC joint. The geyser sign on shoulder arthrography is characterized by extension of contrast from the glenohumeral joint to subacromial–subdeltoid bursa and then into the AC joint space. It usually indicates full-thickness tear of the rotator cuff of long duration, with erosion of the inferior capsule of AC joint. Sometimes, this mass can get large and simulate a tumor clinically.
- **Subcoracoid bursa:** Subcoracoid bursa is located anterior to the subscapularis and inferior to coracoid and subscapularis recess. It does not communicate with glenohumeral joint but does communicate with subacromial–subdeltoid bursa. Distension of this bursa occurs with bursitis or full-thickness rotator cuff tears. The subcoracoid bursa can be differentiated from the subscapularis recess by its further inferior extent anterior to the subscapularis muscle, and its location purely anterior to the subscapularis muscle.

■ Additional Diagnostic Considerations

- **Paralabral cyst:** A paralabral cyst usually shows close relationship with the labrum and is frequently found in association with a labral tear. MRI appearance may vary from a small unilocular to a large multilocular cystic lesion. Paralabral cyst of suprascapular or spinoglenoid notch can cause entrapment of suprascapular nerve.
- **Long head of biceps tendon sheath fluid:** The synovial sheath of long head of biceps tendon communicates with the glenohumeral joint. Fluid in the biceps tendon sheath should not be considered abnormal unless the tendon is completely surrounded by it or there are morphological alterations in the biceps tendon.

■ Diagnosis

Subacromial–subdeltoid bursitis.

✓ Pearls

- If there is more than a trace fluid within the subacromial–subdeltoid bursa, the rotator cuff should be closely evaluated for a tear.
- Geyser sign usually indicates full-thickness tear of rotator cuff of long duration.
- Subcoracoid bursa is differentiated from subscapularis recess by its further inferior extent and entirely anterior location to subscapularis.

■ Suggested Readings

Mellado JM, Salvadó E, Camins A, et al. Fluid collections and juxta-articular cystic lesions of the shoulder: spectrum of MRI findings. Eur Radiol. 2002; 12(3): 650–659

Motamedi D, Everist BM, Mahanty SR, Steinbach LS. Pitfalls in shoulder MRI: part 2– biceps tendon, bursae and cysts, incidental and postsurgical findings, and artifacts. AJR Am J Roentgenol. 2014; 203(3):508–515

Case 41

Cyrus Bateni and Jasjeet Bindra

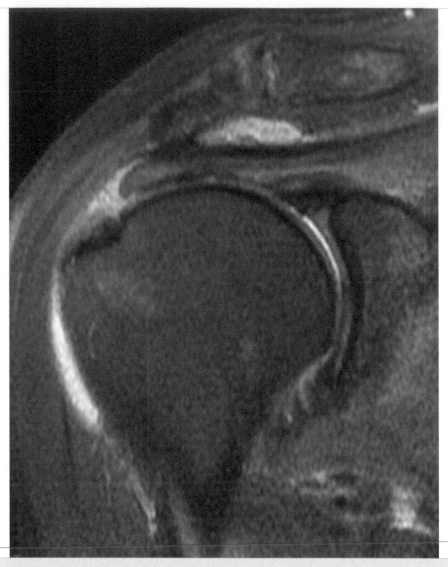

Fig. 41.1 Coronal, fat-suppressed proton density MR image of the shoulder demonstrates a full-thickness tear of the supraspinatus tendon with mild retraction. There is a moderate amount of fluid in subacromial–subdeltoid bursa.

■ Clinical History

A 52-year-old male with recent worsening of shoulder pain (▶ Fig. 41.1).

■ Key Finding

Rotator cuff abnormality.

■ Top 3 Differential Diagnoses

- **Partial thickness tear:** Partial-thickness rotator cuff tears can be described according to the surface of the tendon involved as well as the percentage of tendon involved. Tears may involve the articular surface, bursal surface, or intrasubstance. Articular surface tears are the most common type. They are seen as the focal region of tendon discontinuity which is filled with fluid on T2-weighted imaging. Fat-suppressed, T2-weighted imaging increases lesion conspicuity. Additional findings may include surface fraying or changes in tendon caliber such as attenuation or thickening. Tendon retraction may occasionally be seen in high-grade, partial-thickness tears. Intrasubstance tears are characterized by intratendinous T2 fluid signal without extension to either articular or bursal surface. Bursal-sided tears involve the superior or bursal surface of the tendon with an extra-articular, fluid-filled gap. Partial-thickness tears are classified arthroscopically according to the degree of tendon involvement. Grade 1 lesions involve less than 25% (less than 3 mm) of tendon thickness; grade 2 lesions involve 25 to 50% (3–6 mm); and grade 3 lesions involve greater than 50% of the tendon (greater than 6 mm).
- **Full-thickness tear:** In full-thickness tears, the discontinuity of the tendon extends from the articular surface to the bursal surface. Of the four rotator cuff tendons (supraspinatus, infraspinatus, subscapularis, and teres minor), a full-thickness tear most commonly involves the supraspinatus, and this most often is at its insertion upon the greater tuberosity. Full-thickness tears can be classified based on the size of the tears —small (less than 1 cm), medium (1–3 cm), large (3–5 cm), and massive (greater than 5 cm). The tear does not need to involve the entire tendon in an AP dimension to be considered a full-thickness tear. The most characteristic sign of a full-thickness tear is tendon discontinuity with a fluid-filled gap. Secondary signs include presence of fluid in subacromial–subdeltoid bursa, tendon retraction, and muscle atrophy. Muscle atrophy usually indicates chronicity, although there can be other causes of muscle atrophy even in the presence of an intact cuff.
- **Rotator cuff tendinosis:** Classically, rotator cuff tears occur in cuff tendons with preexisting tendinosis. On MRI, there is increased signal in the tendon on proton density and T2-weighted images, but signal intensity will not reach that of fluid, and the area of abnormality is more globular in appearance than linear as would be found with a tear. Differentiation between tendinosis and a partial-thickness tear can sometimes be challenging. One pitfall of assessing the tendons on short TE images is that magic angle phenomenon can result in artificially increased signal in regions where the tendon courses at a 55-degree angle in relation to the main magnetic field. Magic angle artifact should resolve on T2-weighted (long TE) sequences.

■ Diagnosis

Full thickness tear of the supraspinatus tendon.

✓ Pearls

- The supraspinatus is the most commonly torn tendon of the rotator cuff.
- Rotator cuff tears should be described by thickness as well as width (anterior to posterior dimension).
- Differentiation between a partial-thickness tear and tendinosis of rotator cuff can sometimes be challenging; in tendinosis, the increased T2 signal of the tendon tends to be globular rather than linear and not reach fluid intensity.

■ Suggested Readings

Kassarjian A, Bencardino JT, Palmer WE. MR imaging of the rotator cuff. Radiol Clin North Am. 2006; 44(4):503–523

Morag Y, Jacobson JA, Miller B, De Maeseneer M, Girish G, Jamadar D. MR imaging of rotator cuff injury: what the clinician needs to know. Radiographics. 2006; 26(4): 1045–1065

Case 42

Jasjeet Bindra

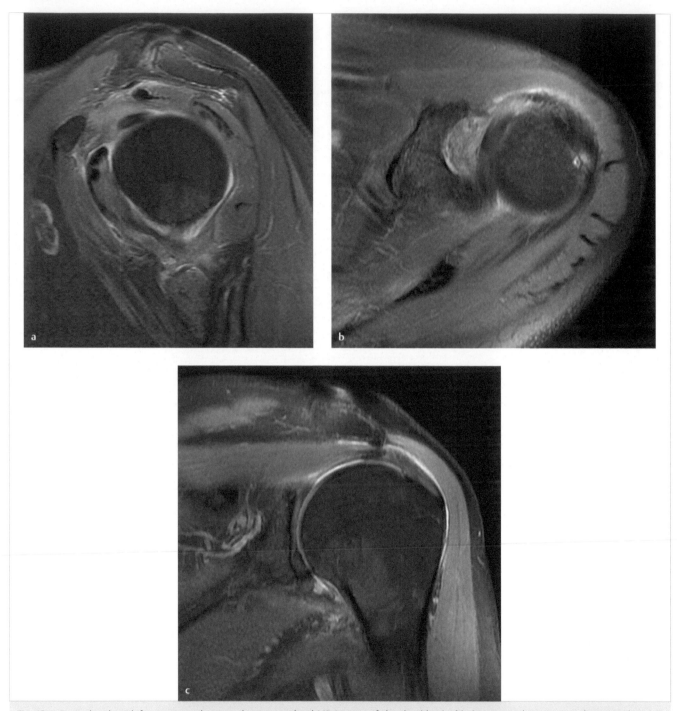

Fig. 42.1 Sagittal and axial, fat-suppressed proton density-weighted MR images of the shoulder **(a, b)** show amorphous intermediate signal in the rotator interval. Coronal, fat-suppressed proton density-weighted image of the same shoulder **(c)** shows edema signal and thickening of inferior glenohumeral ligament.

■ Clinical History

A 53-year-old female with shoulder pain and restricted range of motion (▶ Fig. 42.1).

Key Finding

Rotator interval abnormality.

Top 3 Differential Diagnoses

- **Biceps pulley abnormality:** The coracohumeral ligament (CHL) and superior glenohumeral ligament (SGHL) form a sling-like structure surrounding the long head of biceps tendon proximal to the bicipital groove, and this reflection pulley plays an important role in the stability of intraarticular biceps tendon. The reflection pulley can be injured by acute trauma, repetitive overhead activity, or degenerative change, or injury may be secondary to anterosuperior rotator cuff tears. Because of intimate insertion patterns, tears of the far anterior supraspinatus and superior subscapularis footprint (known as anterosuperior rotator cuff tears) can dissect to involve CHL and SGHL, respectively. On MRI, when the biceps tendon is perched on the lesser tuberosity, medially subluxed or dislocated, injury to the biceps pulley can be inferred. Identifying abnormality of the component structures may not be possible at MRI. Abnormalities of the superior border of subscapularis tendon have high-sensitivity and specificity in diagnosing abnormalities of the pulley.

- **Adhesive capsulitis:** Adhesive capsulitis is a relatively common clinically diagnosed condition characterized by painful limitation of motion, usually in middle aged women. The pathology is felt to be a cascade of events, leading to thickening and contraction of joint capsule and synovium. On MRI, there can be replacement of normal rotator interval fat by granulation or fibrous tissue, thickening of rotator interval capsule, thickening of SGHL and CHL in rotator interval, and thickening of axillary recess capsule. Rotator interval abnormalities of adhesive capsulitis are best seen on oblique sagittal images.

- **Lax rotator interval:** Rotator interval capsular lesions are believed to result in posterior and inferior instability of the shoulder joint. Tears of the rotator interval capsule may manifest as thinning or focal discontinuity of the capsule. Extra-articular contrast may be seen in this region on MR arthrography, and the dimensions and volume of rotator interval may appear larger than routine on MR arthrography.

Diagnosis

Adhesive capsulitis.

Pearls

- Biceps pulley lesions may be inferred from nonanatomic position of long head of biceps tendon.
- Adhesive capsulitis can present with replacement of rotator interval fat by granulation or fibrous tissue.

- Thinning, focal irregularity, and patulous appearance of rotator interval capsule can be associated with shoulder instability.

Suggested Readings

Nakata W, Katou S, Fujita A, Nakata M, Lefor AT, Sugimoto H. Biceps pulley: normal anatomy and associated lesions at MR arthrography. Radiographics. 2011; 31(3): 791–810

Petchprapa CN, Beltran LS, Jazrawi LM, Kwon YW, Babb JS, Recht MP. The rotator interval: a review of anatomy, function, and normal and abnormal MRI appearance. AJR Am J Roentgenol. 2010; 195(3):567–576

Case 43

Paulomi Kanzaria and Jasjeet Bindra

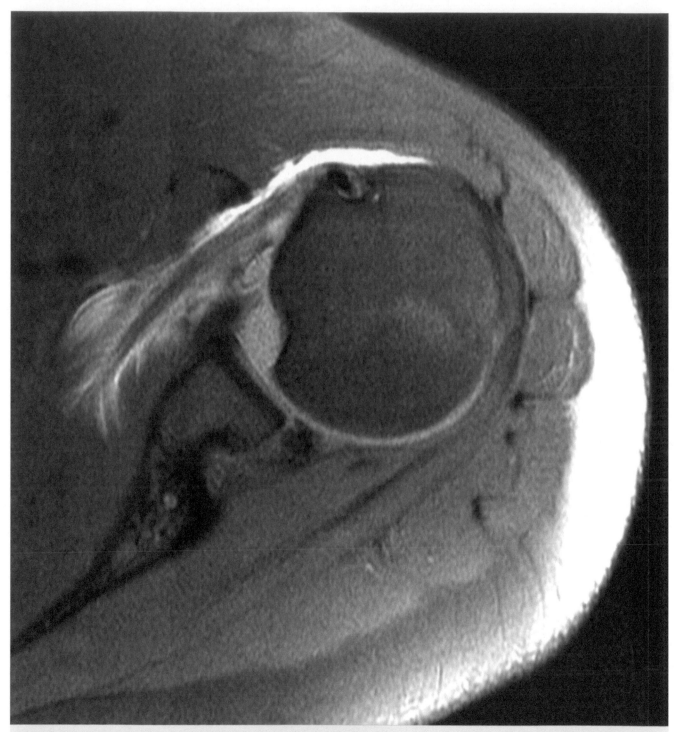

Fig. 43.1 Axial, fat-suppressed, T1-weighted MR arthrogram image of the shoulder shows a posteroinferior labral tear, posterior scapular periosteal tear, and impaction deformity of the anterior aspect of the humeral head.

■ Clinical History

A 45-year-old female with acute shoulder pain after a seizure
(▶ Fig. 43.1).

■ Key Finding

Posterior glenoid labral abnormality.

■ Top 3 Differential Diagnoses

- **Posterior glenoid labral tear:** A tear of the posterior labrum is less common than an anterior labral tear. It can be associated with posterior instability. The spectrum can include a nondetached tear, detached tear, or frayed or crushed labrum. A paralabral cyst may also be seen in association with a labral tear, and when large, it can cause muscle denervation from compressive neuropathy.
- **Reverse Bankart lesion:** A reverse Bankart lesion occurs secondary to posterior dislocation of the shoulder and commonly coexists with a reverse Hill–Sachs lesion. In this type of injury, there is detachment of the posterior inferior labrum from its glenoid attachment in combination with an avulsive tear of the posterior scapular periosteum. This results in increased laxity of the posterior band of the inferior glenohumeral ligament and posterior capsule, which results in abnormal posterior translation of the humeral head. An associated reverse osseous Bankart lesion may be seen and can range from avulsion fracture of the posterior inferior glenoid rim to a large comminuted fracture.
- **POLPSA lesion:** A posterior labrocapsular periosteal sleeve avulsion (POLPSA) lesion occurs secondary to impingement of the humeral head on the posterior labrocapsular complex during posterior shoulder dislocation or recurrent subluxation. It is characterized by stripping of the posterior inferior labrum and intact posterior scapular periosteum from the glenoid. This results in a redundant recess that communicates with the joint space. There occurs fibrous tissue proliferation underneath the periosteal sleeve on arthroscopy.

■ Additional Diagnostic Considerations

- **Posterior GLAD Lesion:** A posterior GLAD lesion is similar to its anterior counterpart. MR imaging demonstrates a focal cartilage defect involving the posteroinferior glenoid, which is associated with subtle tearing of the labrum.
- **Kim's Lesion:** A Kim's lesion occurs secondary to repetitive posterior subluxations of the humeral head, with posteroinferiorly directed force on the labrum. There is a superficial tear between the posterior inferior labrum and the glenoid articular cartilage (marginal crack), and a separate deep and/or intrasubstance incomplete detachment of the posteroinferior labrum from the glenoid. At MR arthrography, flattening of the posteroinferior labrum, increased glenoid retroversion, and a preserved relationship between the glenoid cartilage and posterior labrum may be seen.

■ Diagnosis

Reverse Bankart with reverse Hill–Sachs lesion from posterior dislocation.

✓ Pearls

- Paralabral cysts associated with posterior labral tears can cause muscle denervation from compressive neuropathy.
- A reverse Bankart lesion is characterized by detachment of the posterior inferior labrum from glenoid in combination with an avulsive tear of the posterior scapular periosteum.
- POLPSA lesion is seen as stripping of the posterior inferior labrum and intact posterior scapular periosteum from the glenoid.

■ Suggested Readings

De Coninck T, Ngai SS, Tafur M, Chung CB. Imaging the glenoid labrum and labral tears. Radiographics. 2016; 36(6):1628–1647

Shah N, Tung GA. Imaging signs of posterior glenohumeral instability. AJR Am J Roentgenol. 2009; 192(3):730–735

Case 44

Cyrus Bateni

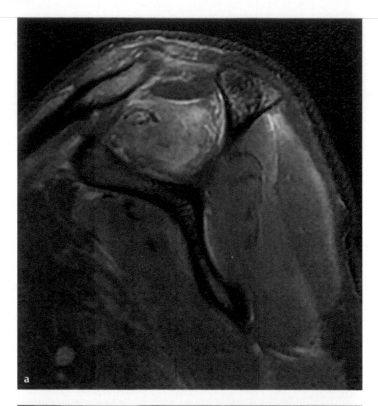

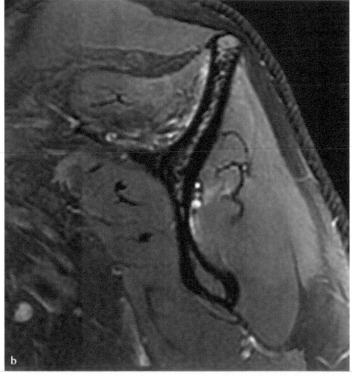

Fig. 44.1 Sagittal, fat-saturated proton density MR image **(a)** of the shoulder shows edema within the supraspinatus, infraspinatus, teres minor, and deltoid muscles. A second sagittal image **(b)** performed 6 months later demonstrates improvement of the muscular edema, although with mild residual edema within the supraspinatus and infraspinatus muscles. There is atrophy of the supraspinatus muscle.

▪ Clinical History

A 19-year-old male with shoulder pain and weakness after a motor vehicle accident (▶ Fig. 44.1).

■ Key Finding

Nerve entrapment at shoulder.

■ Top 3 Differential Diagnoses

- **Suprascapular nerve:** The suprascapular nerve courses through the suprascapular foramen medial to the coracoid, enters the supraspinatus fossa, and then supplies the supraspinatus muscle. Finally, it curves around the spinoglenoid notch and supplies the infraspinatus muscle. If the nerve is affected at the suprascapular foramen, both the supraspinatus and infraspinatus muscles will be involved. Isolated infraspinatus denervation suggests compression at the spinoglenoid notch. Evidence for suprascapular nerve entrapment may be best visualized on sagittal, fluid-sensitive sequences as edema of both muscles. Chronic compression presents with reduction in muscle bulk and fatty infiltration of the involved muscles. Common causes of suprascapular nerve injury or entrapment are trauma, hypertrophy of the transverse scapular ligaments, or extrinsic compression due to space-occupying lesions, most commonly paralabral cysts or ganglia.
- **Brachial plexus:** The brachial plexus may be affected in impingement at the thoracic outlet or may be injured in cervical spine injuries. Motorcycle accidents and falls are common etiologies for direct brachial plexus injuries. Common causes of impingement may include fractures of the clavicle or fibrosis of the scalene muscles. Parsonage–Turner syndrome, also known as acute idiopathic brachial neuritis, can have similar manifestations. The most commonly affected muscles in Parsonage–Turner syndrome are the supraspinatus and infraspinatus muscles, which are similar to suprascapular nerve entrapment. However, it may have other muscle involvement, including deltoid, teres minor, and subscapularis.
- **Axillary nerve:** The axillary nerve originates from the brachial plexus, descends inferolaterally, anterior to subscapularis, before passing through the quadrilateral space, accompanied by the posterior circumflex artery. It innervates the teres minor and deltoid muscles. The axillary nerve may be affected by glenohumeral dislocation, humeral fractures, inferior labral cysts, ganglia, or fibrosis at the level of the inferior glenohumeral joint and the quadrilateral space. Similar to other nerve entrapments, MRI will demonstrate muscular edema, and in chronic cases, loss of muscle bulk and fatty infiltration.

■ Additional Diagnostic Considerations

- **Myositis:** In inflammation of muscles with connective tissue disorders, infections, and drugs, the imaging manifestations of edema and muscle atrophy are similar to nerve entrapment, so clinical history is key. Additionally, muscular involvement without specific nerve distribution can indicate a myositis.
- **Rotator cuff tear:** Tears of the rotator cuff can show muscle edema and loss of muscle bulk on MRI. Close inspection of the tendons will best reveal tendon injury as the etiology for muscular abnormalities.

■ Diagnosis

Brachial plexus injury.

✓ Pearls

- The supraspinatus and infraspinatus muscles are most commonly involved in suprascapular nerve entrapment and Parsonage–Turner syndrome.
- If there is edema and loss of muscle bulk of the supraspinatus and infraspinatus muscles, the most common cause is rotator cuff tearing, not nerve injury or entrapment.
- Sagittal, fat-saturated, T2-weighted sequences of the shoulder can best evaluate edema and muscle bulk.

■ Suggested Readings

Linda DD, Harish S, Stewart BG, Finlay K, Parasu N, Rebello RP. Multimodality imaging of peripheral neuropathies of the upper limb and brachial plexus. Radiographics. 2010; 30(5):1373–1400

Yanny S, Toms AP. MR patterns of denervation around the shoulder. AJR Am J Roentgenol. 2010; 195(2):W157:63

Case 45

Jasjeet Bindra

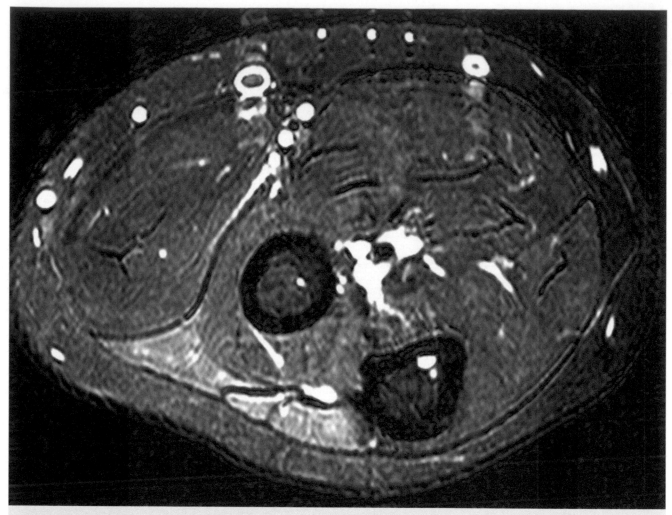

Fig. 45.1 Axial, fat-suppressed, T2-weighted MR image of the proximal forearm shows signal hyperintensity in several extensor muscles, including extensor digitorum, extensor carpi ulnaris, and anconeus.

■ Clinical History

A 23-year-old female with weakness of finger extension (► Fig. 45.1).

■ Key Finding

Nerve entrapment at elbow.

■ Top 3 Differential Diagnoses

- **Ulnar nerve:** Ulnar nerve compression at the elbow is the second most common nerve entrapment of the upper extremity after carpal tunnel syndrome. Patients with ulnar neuropathy complain of pain, paresthesias, weakness in the fifth finger and ulnar side of fourth finger, and they may develop claw deformities of these digits over time. The most common location of ulnar nerve compression is the cubital tunnel, and its most common structural abnormality is anconeusepitrochlearis, an anomalous muscle. MRI of the symptomatic nerve may show signal hyperintensity on T2-weighted images and nerve swelling. Signal hyperintensity can be seen in asymptomatic nerves also. Nerve enlargement can also be seen with ultrasound, which has the added advantage of being able to draw comparison with the contralateral asymptomatic side at the time of examination.
- **Radial nerve:** At the level of the elbow joint, the radial nerve divides into a superficial sensory branch and a deep motor branch. The deep branch pierces the supinator muscle and exits its posterior aspect as posterior interosseous nerve (PIN). Radial nerve compression can lead to either radial tunnel syndrome or posterior interosseous nerve syndrome. Patients with radial tunnel syndrome have a burning sensation along the lateral aspect of the forearm, whereas patients with PIN syndrome present with weakness of the extensor muscles of the forearm. In PIN syndrome, on MRI, the most common abnormality is denervation edema or atrophy of the supinator and extensor muscles of the forearm. Less commonly, mass effect on the nerve may be seen due to anatomic variation, which is a mass or bicipitoradial bursa.
- **Median nerve:** Median nerve courses alongside the brachial artery anterior to the elbow. The nerve passes between the superficial and deep heads of the pronator teres muscle at the elbow and then enters the anterior compartment of the forearm. Compression of median nerve has two presentations—pronator syndrome in which patients have pain and paresthesias, mimicking carpal tunnel syndrome, and the anterior interosseous nerve (AIN) syndrome in which patients have muscle weakness. The anterior interosseous nerve, a purely motor nerve, arises from the median nerve at the distal margin of pronator teres, and supplies pronator quadratus, flexor pollicis longus and flexor digitorum profundus muscle for the index and middle fingers. Patients with AIN syndrome or Kiloh–Nevin syndrome typically have inability to pinch thumb with index finger. The most frequent causes of AIN syndrome are direct trauma and external compression from surgery, venous punctures, and cast pressure. On MRI, there may be denervation edema and fatty atrophy of the muscles supplied by the nerve. Pronator quadratus is always involved, followed by flexor digitorum profundus, and then flexor pollicis longus muscle.

■ Diagnosis

Posterior interosseous nerve compression.

✓ Pearls

- Most common structural abnormality of cubital tunnel is anconeus epitrochlearis, an anomalous muscle.
- In PIN syndrome, denervation edema or atrophy of supinator and extensor muscles of the forearm is seen.
- In AIN syndrome, pronator quadratus muscle is always involved.

■ Suggested Readings

Linda DD, Harish S, Stewart BG, Finlay K, Parasu N, Rebello RP. Multimodality imaging of peripheral neuropathies of the upper limb and brachial plexus. Radiographics. 2010; 30(5):1373–1400

Miller TT, Reinus WR. Nerve entrapment syndromes of the elbow, forearm, and wrist. AJR Am J Roentgenol. 2010; 195(3):585–594

Case 46

Jasjeet Bindra

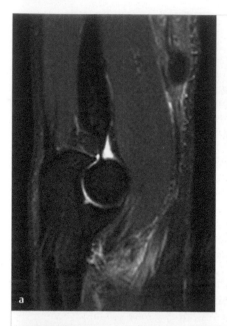
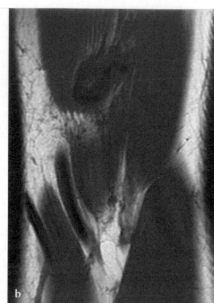
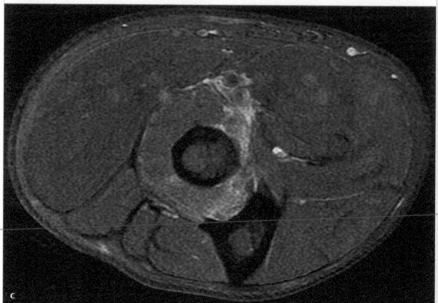

Fig. 46.1 Sagittal STIR MR image of the elbow **(a)** shows an ovoid low-signal intensity mass-like structure in the anterior distal arm. Coronal, T1-weighted image **(b)** reveals the same structure to be U-shaped. Axial, fat-suppressed, proton density-weighted image **(c)** shows edema near the radial tuberosity without any tendon attaching to the tuberosity.

■ Clinical History

A 48-year-old male with acute pain over the elbow (▶ Fig. 46.1).

■ Key Finding

Distal biceps tendon abnormality.

■ Top 3 Differential Diagnoses

- **Complete tear:** The distal biceps brachii tendon courses through the antecubital fossa to insert on the bicipital tuberosity of radius. The superficial fibers form bicipital aponeurosis or lacertus fibrosis, which sweeps from the distal tendon to anchor it to the fascia of flexor pronator mass. Complete tears of distal biceps tendon are usually associated with a single traumatic event, often involving a fairly large force acting against a flexed elbow. Amongst various sports, it is most frequently seen in weightlifters, particularly those using anabolic steroids. Most tears occur 1 to 2 cm above radial tuberosity where there is relative hypovascularity. In complete tears of the tendon, if the bicipital aponeurosis is intact, the myotendinous junction retracts only minimally, and it is difficult to distinguish complete tears from partial tears clinically. Biceps tendon is best evaluated on sagittal and axial images. Additionally, a FABS position (flexion, abduction and supination) can be used as an adjunct to evaluate the distal insertion. For this position, the patient is placed prone in the MRI scanner with shoulder abducted, elbow flexed 90 degrees, and forearm supinated. MRI findings include discontinuity of tendon with a fluid-filled gap with edema and hemorrhage in the surrounding tissues. Variably retracted tendon stump also shows increased signal and irregularity.

- **Partial tear:** Partial tears are precipitated by minor trauma or not even associated with a traumatic event in cases where there is preexisting degeneration in the tendon. Findings usually include a change in caliber, abnormal contour of the tendon, and abnormal intratendinous signal. Peritendinous fluid, edema, and bursitis may also be visible.

- **Bicipitoradial bursitis:** Bicipitoradial or cubital bursa lies between the distal biceps tendon and anterior part of the radial tuberosity. As the forearm moves from supination to pronation, the biceps tendon curls around the radius and compresses the interposed bursa. There is another bursa in close medial vicinity called the interosseous bursa. Communication may occur between these two bursae. Repetitive mechanical trauma from recurrent supination and pronation is the most common cause of cubital bursitis. Inflammatory arthropathies, infection, and synovial chondromatosis may also result in cubital bursitis. Bursal distension can be seen as a cystic lesion on ultrasound or MRI.

■ Diagnosis

Complete tear of distal biceps tendon with retraction of the tendon stump.

✓ Pearls

- FABS position provides a detailed view of the distal biceps insertion and is helpful in differentiating partial from complete tears on MRI.

- Partial tears can be sometimes difficult to distinguish from tendinosis.
- Distension of cubital bursa by simple or complex fluid is readily demonstrated by ultrasound or MRI.

■ Suggested Readings

Bucknor MD, Stevens KJ, Steinbach LS. Elbow imaging in sport: sports imaging series. Radiology. 2016; 279(1):12–28

Chew ML, Giuffrè BM. Disorders of the distal biceps brachii tendon. Radiographics. 2005; 25(5):1227–1237

Case 47

Cyrus Bateni and Jasjeet Bindra

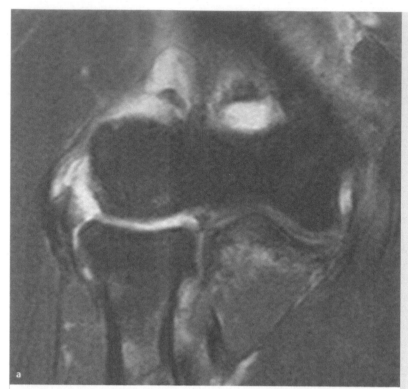

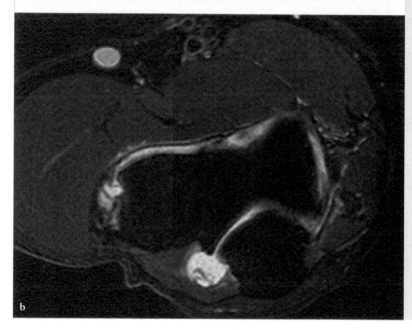

Fig. 47.1 Coronal (**a**) and axial (**b**), fat-saturated proton density MR images of the elbow show discontinuity of the proximal fibers of the radial collateral ligament. There is abnormal fluid signal and thinning of the proximal fibers of the common extensor tendon.

■ Clinical History

A 56-year-old male with chronic elbow pain and recent trauma (▶ Fig. 47.1).

■ Key Finding

Radial-sided, soft-tissue injury at elbow on MRI.

■ Top 3 Differential Diagnoses

- **Lateral epicondylitis:** Lateral epicondylitis or tennis elbow is a pathologic condition of the common extensor tendon at its origin from the lateral epicondyle of humerus. It is thought to be due to repeated contraction of the forearm extensor muscles, with microtears, degeneration, and poor repair at the common extensor tendon. Typically, this is diagnosed clinically, but MRI can help to determine the extent of the disease and exclude other causes of lateral elbow pain. On MRI, tendinosis is seen as thickening and intermediate or increased T2 signal of the common extensor tendon. Radiographs commonly will show no significant findings, but there may be calcium hydroxyapatite deposition adjacent to the lateral humeral epicondyle. Partial-thickness tears are seen as fluid signal intensity, partway extending across the tendon. A full-thickness tear appears as fluid signal intensity gap across the substance of the tendon.

- **Lateral collateral ligament complex injury:** Lateral collateral ligament complex consists of the radial collateral ligament (RCL), lateral ulnar collateral ligament (LUCL), and annular ligament. The LUCL is the most important stabilizer against varus and rotatory stress. It arises from the posterior aspect of the lateral epicondyle, slings around the posterolateral margin of the radial head, and inserts on the supinator crest of the ulna. RCL runs from the lateral epicondyle inferiorly to blend with annular ligament. The RCL and LUCL are best assessed on coronal MRI. Injury to the LUCL is unusual but may occur after an acute varus extension injury or an elbow dislocation. Occasionally, overaggressive release of common extensor tendon for lateral epicondylitis may lead to disruption of the LUCL. Tears of the LUCL lead to a condition called posterolateral rotatory instability (PLRI) of elbow. Most tears of LUCL occur at the humeral origin. On MRI, there is signal hyperintensity with discontinuity of fibers. Posterior subluxation of the radial head relative to capitellum may be observed on sagittal images. Isolated tears of the RCL are uncommon. As RCL shares a common origin with the common extensor tendon, injuries at the lateral elbow commonly involve both the RCL and common extensor tendon. Portions of the LUCL and annular ligament are also inseparable from the radial collateral ligament and may be injured.

- **Humeroradial plica syndrome:** At elbow, symptomatic plicae are seen most frequently within the lateral and posterosuperior elbow, insinuating in the radiocapitellar joint. Young adult athletes tend to be most frequently affected, particularly those involved in sports requiring repetitive flexion and extension. On MRI, plicae are seen as low-signal intensity bands outlined by fluid or intra-articular contrast. A cutoff of 3 mm thickness or greater than one-third coverage of the radial head can be used to accurately suggest the diagnosis. Focal adjacent synovitis and chondrosis of the anterolateral aspect of radial head may also be seen.

■ Diagnosis

Complete tear of the radial collateral ligament.

✓ Pearls

- A tear of the common extensor tendon will be identified on MRI by thinning of the fibers with a fluid-filled gap. Enlargement and intermediate signal of the tendon indicate tendinosis.

- Injury to the RCL most commonly occurs in conjunction with injuries to the common extensor tendon due to their intimate relationship.
- LUCL is best seen on coronal images. In PLRI, subluxation of the radial head with respect to capitellum is best seen on sagittal images.

■ Suggested Readings

Bucknor MD, Stevens KJ, Steinbach LS. Elbow imaging in sport: sports imaging series. Radiology. 2016; 280(1):328

Walz DM, Newman JS, Konin GP, Ross G. Epicondylitis: pathogenesis, imaging, and treatment. Radiographics. 2010; 30(1):167–184

Case 48

Cyrus Bateni and Jasjeet Bindra

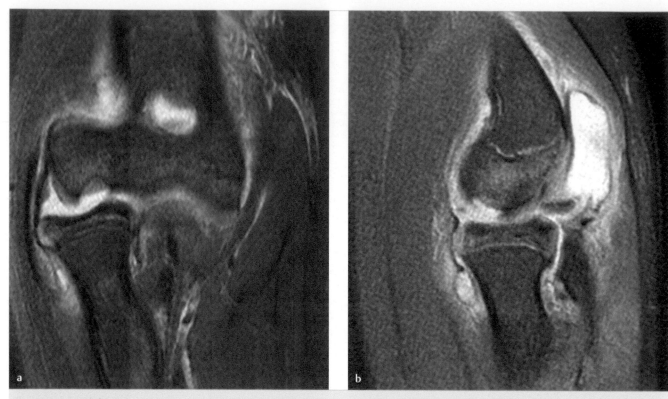

Fig. 48.1 Coronal, fat-saturated proton density MR image (**a**) of the elbow shows an osteochondral crater at the capitellum. Sagittal, fat-saturated proton density image (**b**) in the same patient shows the osteochondral defect at the anterior capitellum with a displaced fragment more posteriorly. A moderate elbow joint effusion is present.

■ Clinical History

A 12-year-old male with acute pain at the elbow after injury (► Fig. 48.1).

■ Key Finding

Osteochondral lesion of elbow.

■ Top 3 Differential Diagnoses

- **Osteochondritis dissecans (OCD) of the capitellum:** An osteochondral lesion is defined as a site of injury to the articular cartilage and subchondral bone. Although the mechanism of injury is unclear, OCD is thought to result from repetitive microtrauma. In the elbow, the most common location is at the capitellum, although lesions of the trochlea, radial head, olecranon, and olecranon fossa have been described. OCD primarily affects young males between 12 and 15 years of age. Radiographs are relatively insensitive in the detection of osteochondral injuries at the elbow, but they may be suggested by a flattened contour to the capitellum, lucent lesion within the capitellum, and intra-articular bodies. MRI best evaluates an OCD lesion, demonstrating whether the defect is stable, and it is the lack of stability that indicates surgical management may be appropriate. The lesion may be unstable if there is a tear of the articular cartilage, thin fluid bright fracture line, rim of fluid surrounding the lesion, multiple cysts around the lesion, or single cyst exceeding 5 mm in size.

- **Panner disease:** Panner disease is a benign and self-limited condition of elbow that involves the entire capitellum. It presents in childhood, primarily in boys less than 10 years of age. It is unclear if this is a separate entity or exists on a spectrum with OCD. Radiographs show a demineralized capitellum with ill-defined margins. There may also be sclerosis, fragmentation, or cortical fissuring. MRI is more sensitive and shows diffuse capitellar edema without damage to the overlying cartilage or intra-articular loose bodies.

- **Pseudodefect of the capitellum:** Pseudodefect of capitellum is an abrupt trough-like undermining at the junction of capitellum and lateral epicondyle. This is a normal finding seen in a large number of patients undergoing elbow MRI. It is significant as it can be mistaken for an osteochondral lesion or an impaction fracture. This can be differentiated from an osteochondral defect or arthritis by the complete lack of cartilage at this site and lack of subchondral marrow edema. Typically, pseudodefects occur in a more posterior location than OCD.

■ Additional Diagnostic Consideration

- **Osteoarthritis.** The elbow is not a commonly affected site of osteoarthritis; when it does occur, it is often secondary due to other conditions such as preceding trauma, including a prior osteochondral injury. Imaging findings of osteoarthritis include osteophytes, joint space narrowing, sclerosis, and subchondral cysts. On MRI, there may be accompanying subchondral marrow edema. Whereas OCD of the elbow most commonly involves the capitellum, osteoarthritis of the elbow is predominantly at the ulnohumeral articulation. If findings of arthritis are noted at the elbow, other causes including rheumatoid arthritis, septic arthritis, and hemophilic arthropathy should also be considered.

■ Diagnosis

Osteochondral lesion of the capitellum.

✓ Pearls

- MRI findings of an unstable osteochondral lesion include a T2 hyperintense cartilage fracture line, fluid signal rim surrounding a bony fragment, and surrounding cyst formation of at least 5 mm.

- Panner disease affects the entire capitellum without damage to the overlying cartilage.
- Pseudodefect of capitellum occurs in a more posterior location and there is no subchondral edema.

■ Suggested Readings

Binaghi D. MR imaging of the elbow. Magn Reson Imaging Clin N Am. 2015; 23 (3):427–440

Wong TT, Lin DJ, Ayyala RS, Kazam JK. Elbow injuries in pediatric overhead athletes. AJR Am J Roentgenol. 2017; 209(4):849–859

Case 49

Cyrus Bateni and Jasjeet Bindra

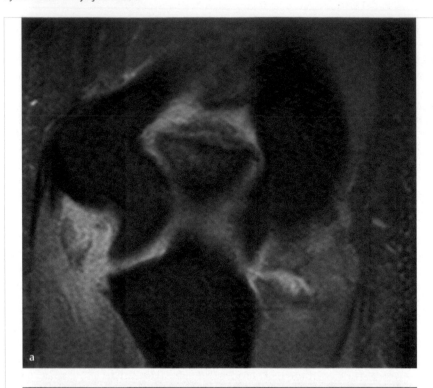

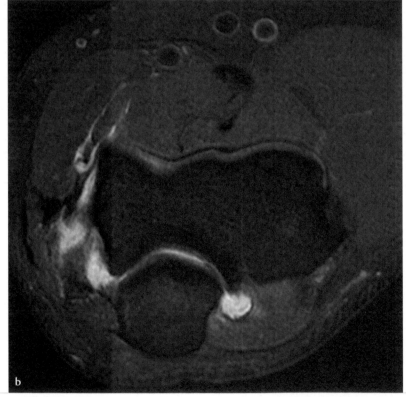

Fig. 49.1 Coronal **(a)** and axial **(b)**, fat-saturated proton density MR images of the elbow demonstrate discontinuity of the ulnar collateral ligament (UCL), adjacent edema, and a moderate joint effusion.

■ Clinical History

A 37-year-old male baseball pitcher with acute medial elbow pain (▶ Fig. 49.1).

■ Key Finding

Ulnar-sided, stabilizer injury at elbow on MRI.

■ Top 3 Differential Diagnoses

- **Partial tear of the ulnar collateral ligament:** The ulnar collateral ligament (UCL) at the elbow is composed of three bundles—anterior, posterior, and transverse. The anterior bundle is the primary restraint to valgus stress and is best evaluated on coronal MRI images. On T1-weighted images, the anterior bundle of the UCL may be purely hypointense, or there may be interspersed linear bands of fat signal within the broad proximal (humeral) attachment, with the ligament tapering distally. On fat-suppressed, T2-weighted images, there should be low-signal to the UCL, and the presence of edema within the fibers, partial disruption of the fibers, and adjacent soft tissue edema indicate a partial tear of the UCL. Partial tears of the distal attachment at the sublime tubercle can show the "T sign" with fluid or contrast material insinuating below the ligament along the margin of the bone. Amongst athletes, injury to the UCL is highly associated with baseball pitching due to the valgus stress placed by the throwing motion. Partial tears are very common within this group, even in asymptomatic individuals. While typical MRI sequences can evaluate for tears of the UCL, MR or CT arthrography have improved sensitivity and specificity for partial tears relative to routine MRI of the elbow.
- **Complete tear of the ulnar collateral ligament:** Complete tears of the UCL are often associated with significant physical examination findings of valgus instability. Most tears occur in the midsubstance of anterior bundle, although avulsions of proximal and distal attachments also occur. Similar to partial tears, coronal MRI fluid-sensitive, fat-suppressed sequences can best demonstrate a complete tear of the UCL. MRI findings consistent with a complete tear include complete disruption of the UCL fibers, laxity, and adjacent soft-tissue edema.
- **Medial epicondylitis:** The flexor pronator mass comprises the pronator teres, flexor carpiradialis, palmaris longus, flexor digitorum superficialis, and flexor carpi ulnaris muscles. The common flexor pronator tendon is a dynamic stabilizer to valgus instability. Degeneration of the origin of the common flexor tendon at the elbow is a common source of pain at the medial elbow. Common flexor tendon injuries at the attachment upon the medial humeral epicondyle may also be associated with overhead throwing sports and UCL injuries. The common flexor tendon can be differentiated from the UCL best on coronal MRI sequences by the more proximal and medial origin of the common flexor tendon relative to the UCL. Additionally, the proximal anterior bundle of the UCL will normally have a broad attachment, while the common flexor tendon origin is of smaller caliber. On MRI, tendinosis can be seen as enlargement of the tendon, intermediate to hyperintense T2 signal within the tendon, and paratendinous soft-tissue edema. Partial-thickness or full-thickness tears can also occur.

■ Diagnosis

Complete tear of the UCL.

✓ Pearls

- UCL tears are best demonstrated on coronal T2-weighted sequences.
- MR or CT arthrography are more sensitive relative to routine MRI for detection of partial tears of the UCL.
- Common flexor tendinosis may show an enlarged tendon, intermediate to hyperintense T2 signal within the tendon, and adjacent soft-tissue edema.

■ Suggested Readings

Bucknor MD, Stevens KJ, Steinbach LS. Elbow imaging in sport: sports imaging series. Radiology. 2016; 280(1):328

Wong TT, Lin DJ, Ayyala RS, Kazam JK. Elbow injuries in adult overhead athletes. AJR Am J Roentgenol. 2017; 208(3):W110–W120

Case 50

Robert D. Boutin

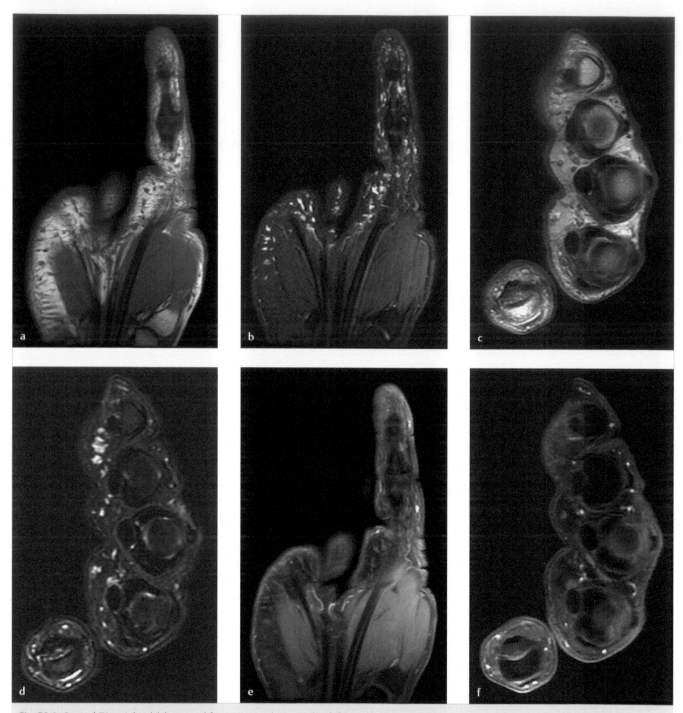

Fig. 50.1 Coronal T1-weighted **(a)**, coronal fat-suppressed T2-weighted **(b)**, axial proton density-weighted **(c)**, and axial fat-suppressed T2-weighted **(d)** images of the hand show tiny nodular foci in the palmar subcutaneous fat layer that are T1-isointense and T2-hyperintense. After contrast administration, coronal, fat-suppressed, T1-weighted **(e)** and axial fat-suppressed T1-weighted **(f)** images show no enhancement of these nodular foci in the palmar subcutis.

■ Clinical History

A 39-year-old man with workers' compensation claim related to repetitive work (▶ Fig. 50.1).

■ Key Finding

Numerous tiny T2-hyperintense subcutaneous nodules.

■ Top 3 Differential Diagnoses

- **Pacinian corpuscles:** Pacinian corpuscles are sensory receptors for vibration and deep pressure, particularly in the palms of the hands and the soles of the feet. Pacinian corpuscles are most commonly regarded as incidental findings, although there are reports describing symptomatic presentations that may be related to a history of trauma or repetitive microtrauma. Normal Pacinian corpuscles are rounded foci that usually measure <2 mm (range, 1–5 mm).

  With MRI, the typical appearance is that of tiny nodules that are T1-isointense and T2-hyperintense compared to muscle, without any contrast enhancement because of a tight blood–nerve barrier. A subtle, thread-like connection to a neighboring digital nerve also may be seen. With high-resolution ultrasound, Pacinian corpuscles may be seen as echolucent dots, particularly adjacent to digital nerves and vessels in the palmar subcutis.
- **Neurofibromatosis:** Neurofibromatosis is characterized by tumors involving the nerves and skin, and may present with multiple soft-tissue nodules. In addition to neurofibromas

  (localized, diffuse, and plexiform), classic features of neurofibromatosis type 1 include cutaneous lesions (e.g., café-au-lait spots, axillary/groin freckling) and distinctive osseous lesions (e.g., kyphoscoliosis, pseudoarthrosis, posterior vertebral body scalloping). Compared to Pacinian corpuscles, however, it is important to note that neurofibromas are usually larger, show contrast enhancement on MRI, and have higher echogenicity on sonography.
- **Angiomatous lesions:** Angiomatous lesions in the musculoskeletal and cutaneous tissues most commonly present in relatively young patients, often infants and children. The two competing classification systems used for vascular soft-tissue masses are published by the World Health Organization (WHO) and the International Society for the Study of Vascular Anomalies (ISSVA). Although the 2013 WHO classification system remains in use in many clinical practices with adult patients, the 2018 ISSVA classification system is generally favored in multidisciplinary centers treating affected children and young adults.

■ Diagnosis

Pacinian corpuscles.

✓ Pearls

- Pacinian corpuscles are mechanoreceptors that are commonly seen as incidental, tiny T2 hyperintense nodules in the subcutaneous fat layer.
- Pacinian corpuscles do *not* enhance after contrast administration, but neurogenic and angiomatous lesions *do* enhance.

- The vast majority of soft-tissue tumors are solitary. When *multiple* soft-tissue masses are present, the differential diagnosis becomes limited, with considerations that most often include neurofibromatosis, angiomatous lesions, fibromatosis, and metastases.

■ Suggested Readings

Fletcher CDM, Bridge JA, Hogendoorn PCW, et al, eds. World Health Organization Classification of Tumours of Soft Tissue and Bone. 5th ed. Lyon: IARC Press; 2020

International Society for the Study of Vascular Anomalies. ISSVA Classification of Vascular Anomalies. Available at: issva.org/classification. Accessed May 1, 2020

Rhodes NG, Murthy NS, Lachman N, Rubin DA. Normal Pacinian corpuscles in the hand: radiology-pathology correlation in a cadaver study. Skeletal Radiol. 2019; 48(10):1591–1597

Riegler G, Brugger PC, Gruber GM, Pivec C, Jengojan S, Bodner G. High-resolution ultrasound visualization of Pacinian corpuscles. Ultrasound Med Biol. 2018; 44(12): 2596–2601

Wildgruber M, Sadick M, Müller-Wille R, Wohlgemuth WA. Vascular tumors in infants and adolescents. Insights Imaging. 2019; 10(1):30

Part 4

Lower Extremity

Case 51

Robert D. Boutin

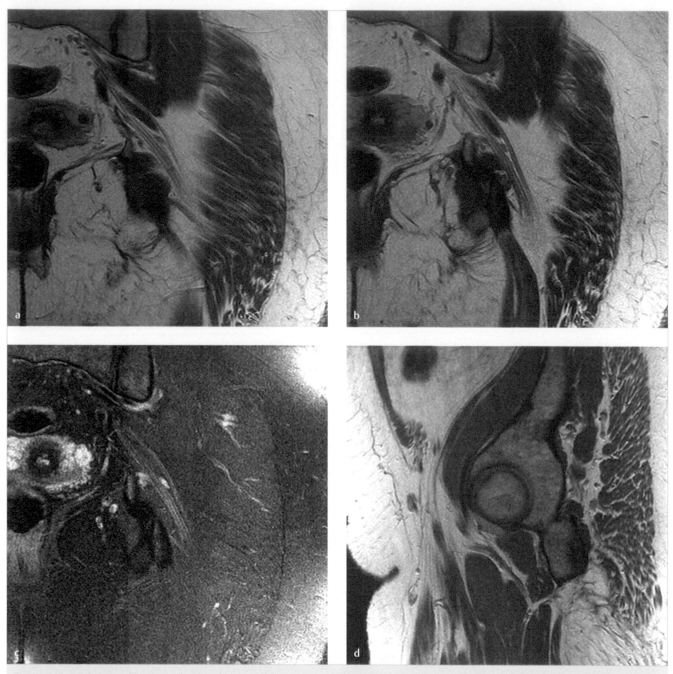

Fig. 51.1 Coronal proton density-weighted (**a, b**), coronal fat-suppressed T2-weighted (**c**) and sagittal proton density-weighted (**d**) images of the pelvis show that the sciatic nerve is divided by the piriformis muscle. One division of the sciatic nerve (tibial component) courses normally along the inferior margin of the piriformis, but another division (common peroneal component) pierces the piriformis.

■ Clinical History

A 39-year-old woman with a history of buttock pain, aggravated by sitting, and "sciatic-like" symptoms (► Fig. 51.1).

■ Key Finding

Variant sciatic nerve anatomy.

■ Top 3 Differential Diagnoses

- **Piriformis syndrome:** Piriformis syndrome refers to entrapment of the sciatic nerve at the level of the piriformis muscle. Two general categories are described: primary (i.e., anatomical cause such as sciatic nerve splitting) and secondary (i.e., due to a precipitating case such as a mass or trauma).

    Clinical features of piriformis syndrome reported most commonly include tenderness near the greater sciatic notch, buttock pain, pain aggravated on sitting or any maneuver that increases piriformis muscle tension, and limitation in straight leg raising.

    On MRI, sciatic nerve variations are relatively common (≤20%). Such variant sciatic nerve anatomy is not necessarily associated with piriformis syndrome. Abnormal caliber and T2 hyperintensity in the sciatic nerve may be associated with sciatica. MR neurography and diffusion tensor imaging are increasingly used to evaluate the sciatic nerve.

    In patients undergoing cross-sectional imaging for clinically suspected piriformis syndrome, derangements at the level of the piriformis muscle (e.g., tumors) can be identified as important etiologies that drastically alter patient management (e.g., with percutaneous injection, surgery, antibiotics, and radiation therapy).

- **Incidental anatomic variation:** Anatomically, an undivided sciatic nerve most commonly emerges inferior to the piriformis muscle (~80%).

    The most common anatomic variation involves the sciatic nerve splitting into two divisions, with one division of the sciatic nerve passing *through* the piriformis and the other passing *inferior* to the piriformis. Other variations are also possible (e.g., the sciatic nerve splitting, with one division *above* and one division *below* the piriformis).

- **Double crush syndrome:** Multifocal neuropathy, commonly referred to as double crush syndrome, refers to multiple simultaneous nerve insults (e.g., nerve entrapment and diabetes) that results in nerve dysfunction. Double crush syndrome specifically refers to multiple sites of physical compression along a single nerve (e.g., at the level of the piriformis and lumbar spine). Currently, the concept has been expanded to recognize that nonmechanical etiologies (e.g., systemic, pharmacological) may also contribute to neuropathic symptoms. Imaging is most helpful in identifying anatomic sites of nerve entrapment that may be amenable to surgical decompression. In order to avoid suboptimal outcomes after nerve decompression at a single site, successful management focuses on treating *all* contributing factors (e.g., decompression of both proximal and distal sites of nerve entrapment).

■ Diagnosis

Piriformis syndrome.

✓ Pearls

- Piriformis syndrome may be related to anatomic variations in some cases but, importantly, extraspinal sciatica may be secondary to focal derangements, such as a space-occupying mass.

- Anatomic variations in the relationship of the piriformis muscle and sciatic nerve are relatively common, and they may not have a significant association with clinically diagnosed piriformis syndrome.

- Double crush syndrome (multifocal neuropathy) occurs when multiple etiologies are responsible for a neuropathy. Recognition of this concept helps physicians avoid "satisfaction of search" errors that can result in suboptimal outcomes.

■ Suggested Readings

Bartret AL, Beaulieu CF, Lutz AM. Is it painful to be different? Sciatic nerve anatomical variants on MRI and their relationship to piriformis syndrome. Eur Radiol. 2018; 28(11):4681–4686

Hopayian K, Danielyan A. Four symptoms define the piriformis syndrome: an updated systematic review of its clinical features. Eur J Orthop Surg Traumatol. 2018; 28(2):155–164

Kane PM, Daniels AH, Akelman E. Double crush syndrome. J Am Acad Orthop Surg. 2015; 23(9):558–562

Probst D, Stout A, Hunt D. Piriformis Syndrome: a narrative review of the anatomy, diagnosis, and treatment. PM R. 2019; 11 Suppl 1:S54–S63

Shah SS, Consuegra JM, Subhawong TK, Urakov TM, Manzano GR. Epidemiology and etiology of secondary piriformis syndrome: A single-institution retrospective study. J Clin Neurosci. 2019; 59:209–212

Vassalou EE, Katonis P, Karantanas AH. Piriformis muscle syndrome: a cross-sectional imaging study in 116 patients and evaluation of therapeutic outcome. Eur Radiol. 2018; 28(2):447–458

Wada K, Goto T, Takasago T, Hamada D, Sairyo K. Piriformis muscle syndrome with assessment of sciatic nerve using diffusion tensor imaging and tractography: a case report. Skeletal Radiol. 2017; 46(10):1399–1404

Case 52

Robert D. Boutin and Geoffrey M. Riley

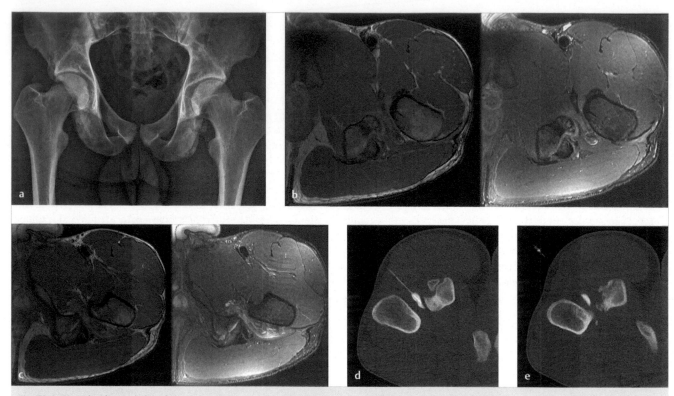

Fig. 52.1 Frontal radiograph **(a)** of the pelvis shows asymmetric osteosclerosis at the left ischial tuberosity, with osseous irregularity indicative of chronic avulsive injury. In addition to the nonacute avulsion injury at the origins of the hamstring tendons, axial proton density-weighted and fat-suppressed T2-weighted **(b, c)** images demonstrate narrowing of the ischiofemoral space and edema in the quadratus femoris muscle. With the patient positioned prone, axial CT images **(d, e)** of the left hip show percutaneous injection of the ischiofemoral interval, confirmed by the presence of contrast material.

■ **Clinical History**

A 21-year-old man with a history of buttock pain associated with elite collegiate athletics (▶ Fig. 52.1).

■ Key Finding

Ischiofemoral space narrowing and quadratus femoris muscle edema in a patient with chronic ischial tuberosity avulsion (nonunion).

■ Top 3 Differential Diagnoses

- **Ischiofemoral impingement:** Ischiofemoral impingement is generally defined by a triad of findings: (1) pain in the hip or buttock region, (2) narrowing of the space between the ischial tuberosity and lesser trochanter, and (3) quadratus muscle abnormality on MRI (edema or atrophy). Ischiofemoral impingement is more common in women, and it may be related to increased ischial and femoral neck angles compared with controls.

  Radiographs may show chronic osseous changes associated with narrowing between the ischium and lesser trochanter. Although the ischiofemoral space may change with patient positioning, narrowing to ≤15 mm has an optimal diagnostic sensitivity and specificity (~80%). Imaging also may show associated derangements in the hamstring and iliopsoas tendons.

  Management may include image-guided percutaneous treatment (e.g., corticosteroid injection of the quadratus femoris muscle) and, occasionally, surgery (endoscopic or open).
- **Hamstring disorders:** Acute and chronic osseous avulsion injuries at the ischial tuberosity (origin of the hamstring tendons) are commonly observed on radiography, MRI, and CT.

When nonunion or malunion occurs at an ischial avulsion fracture, there is often narrowing of the ischiofemoral space that predisposes patients to ischiofemoral impingement. Other disorders involving the proximal hamstring tendons are also associated with ischiofemoral impingement, including hamstring enthesopathy, tendon tearing, and peritendinitis.

- **Deep gluteal syndrome:** Deep gluteal syndrome is a recently popularized entity that describes the presence of pain in the buttock region and extraspinal entrapment of the sciatic nerve. Disorders involving the deep gluteal space may include a broad array of disorders, including ischiofemoral impingement, piriformis syndrome, obturator internus/gemellus syndrome, and fibrous bands causing sciatic nerve entrapment. Although the term "deep gluteal syndrome" is controversial, proponents suggest it is a unifying concept that should promote improved awareness for diagnosis (e.g., with MR neurography) and treatment (e.g., with percutaneous and endoscopic procedures).

■ Diagnosis

Ischiofemoral impingement, which is associated with chronic hamstring avulsion injury.

✓ Pearls

- Ischiofemoral impingement is a syndrome defined by hip/buttock pain, ischiofemoral space narrowing, and quadratus femoris muscle edema/atrophy.
- Hamstring disorders may be primary pain generators, in addition to predisposing patients to ischiofemoral impingement.

- Deep gluteal syndrome is an overarching term, encompassing a wide variety of extraspinal disorders that cause sciatica.

■ Suggested Readings

Backer MW, Lee KS, Blankenbaker DG, Kijowski R, Keene JS. Correlation of ultrasound-guided corticosteroid injection of the quadratus femoris with MRI findings of ischiofemoral impingement. AJR Am J Roentgenol. 2014; 203(3):589–593

Balius R, Susín A, Morros C, Pujol M, Pérez-Cuenca D, Sala-Blanch X. Gemelli-obturator complex in the deep gluteal space: an anatomic and dynamic study. Skeletal Radiol. 2018; 47(6):763–770

Hernando MF, Cerezal L, Pérez-Carro L, Abascal F, Canga A. Deep gluteal syndrome: anatomy, imaging, and management of sciatic nerve entrapments in the subgluteal space. Skeletal Radiol. 2015; 44(7):919–934

Hernando MF, Cerezal L, Pérez-Carro L, Canga A, González RP. Evaluation and management of ischiofemoral impingement: a pathophysiologic, radiologic, and therapeutic approach to a complex diagnosis. Skeletal Radiol. 2016; 45(6):771–787

Singer AD, Subhawong TK, Jose J, Tresley J, Clifford PD. Ischiofemoral impingement syndrome: a meta-analysis. Skeletal Radiol. 2015; 44(6):831–837

Taneja AK, Bredella MA, Torriani M. Ischiofemoral impingement. Magn Reson Imaging Clin N Am. 2013; 21(1):65–73

Case 53

Robert D. Boutin

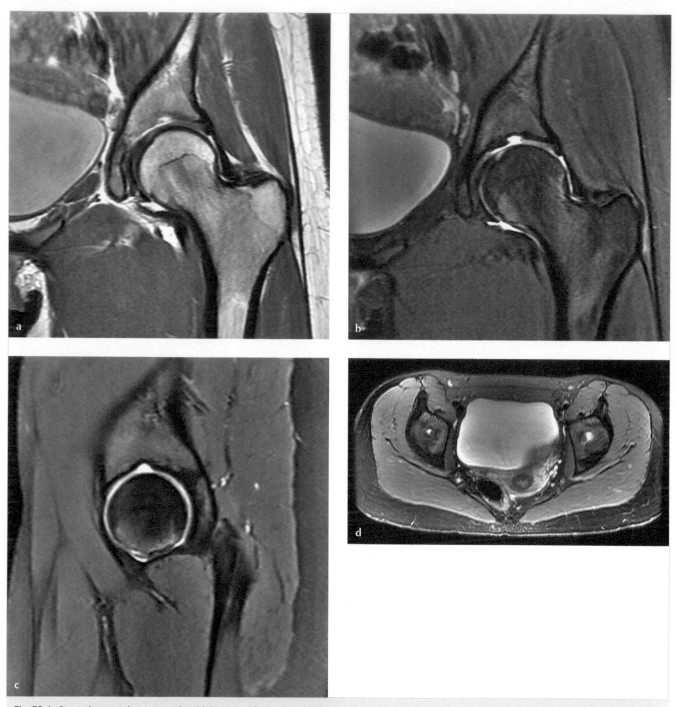

Fig. 53.1 Coronal proton density-weighted (**a**), coronal fat-suppressed T2-weighted (**b**), and sagittal fat-suppressed T2-weighted (**c**) images of the left hip show a focal morphologic concavity involving the subchondral bone at the superior aspect of the acetabulum. On the axial fat-suppressed T2-weighted (**d**) image of the pelvis, similar foci of high signal intensity at the acetabular roof are present bilaterally (left greater than right).

■ Clinical History

A 14-year-old girl with a history of low back and hip pain (▶ Fig. 53.1).

Key Finding

Small smoothly marginated depression ("fossa") at the mid-acetabular roof.

Top 3 Differential Diagnoses

- **Supraacetabular fossa:** The supraacetabular fossa (pseudodefect of acetabular cartilage) is a focal concavity located in the acetabular roof at the 12 o'clock position (both on coronal and sagittal images). This apparent depression in the articular surface is smoothly marginated and small (generally measures approximately 3 mm in depth and 5 mm in transaxial diameter).

  The supraacetabular fossa is considered an incidental anatomic variation. It is observed in approximately 10% of hip MRI examinations (often in adolescents and young adults).

  On MRI, the supraacetabular fossa may be filled with articular cartilage or fluid. Unlike a typical chondral/osteochondral defect, there is no adjacent bone edema or loose body.
- **Superior acetabular notch:** The superior acetabular notch is also considered an anatomic variant. This notch is located in the acetabular roof superomedially (superior to the acetabular fossa and medial the chondral surface).

  The "superior acetabular notch," like the "supraacetabular fossa," is an incidental anatomic variant and is seen in only a minority of patients. These two terms for anatomic variants are easy to confuse with "acetabular fossa" and "acetabular notch," which are both constant anatomic features. (The "acetabular fossa" is at the medial aspect of the acetabulum; it is occupied by the ligamentum teres and fibrofatty tissue. At the inferior margin of the acetabular fossa, there is an "acetabular notch," which is the attachment site for the transverse acetabular ligament).
- **Chondral/osteochondral defect:** A chondral or osteochondral lesion must be differentiated from normal anatomic variants in the acetabular roof. Chondral lesions most commonly occur at the anterosuperior or superolateral rim of the acetabulum. In addition to having different locations than anatomic variants, chondral or osteochondral lesions are typically associated with subchondral bone edema/reaction, adjacent chondrosis, or loose bodies.

Diagnosis

Supraacetabular fossa.

✓ Pearls

- The supraacetabular fossa and the superior acetabular notch are incidental anatomic variants that occur at specific locations in the roof of the acetabulum.
- Anatomic variations in the roof of the acetabulum, especially the supraacetabular fossa, can be mistaken for a chondral/osteochondral defect.
- A chondral/osteochondral defect is typically associated with subchondral bone edema, adjacent chondrosis, or loose bodies.

Suggested Readings

Boutris N, Gardner SL, Yetter TR, Delgado DA, Pulido L, Harris JD. MRI prevalence and characteristics of supraacetabular fossae in patients with hip pain. Hip Int. 2018; 28(5):542–547

Dallich AA, Rath E, Atzmon R, et al. Chondral lesions in the hip: a review of relevant anatomy, imaging and treatment modalities. J Hip Preserv Surg. 2019; 6(1):3–15

Dietrich TJ, Suter A, Pfirrmann CW, Dora C, Fucentese SF, Zanetti M. Supraacetabular fossa (pseudodefect of acetabular cartilage): frequency at MR arthrography and comparison of findings at MR arthrography and arthroscopy. Radiology. 2012; 263(2):484–491

Omoumi P, Vande Berg B. Hip Imaging: normal variants and asymptomatic findings. Semin Musculoskelet Radiol. 2017; 21(5):507–517

Sampatchalit S, Chen L, Haghighi P, Trudell D, Resnick DL. Changes in the acetabular fossa of the hip: MR arthrographic findings correlated with anatomic and histologic analysis using cadaveric specimens. AJR Am J Roentgenol. 2009; 193(2):W127–W133

Case 54

Robert D. Boutin

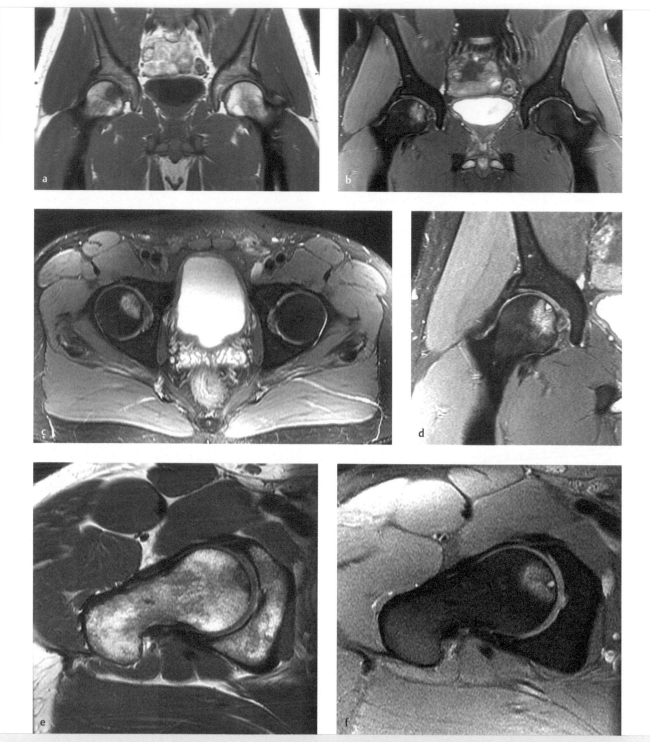

Fig. 54.1 Coronal T1-weighted **(a)**, coronal fat-suppressed T2-weighted **(b)** and axial fat-suppressed T2-weighted **(c)** images of the pelvis show a unilateral focus of nonspecific edema-like signal in the anteromedial aspect of the right femoral head. Small field-of-view, coronal fat-suppressed T2-weighted **(d)**, oblique–axial proton density-weighted **(e)** and oblique–axial fat-suppressed T2-weighted **(f)** images of right hip show better anatomic detail, including a tiny subchondral cyst and slight overlying chondral signal heterogeneity. At arthroscopy, chondrosis was present at this site, with an adjacent tear in the middle-third of the ligamentum teres (visible on **b** and **d**).

▪ Clinical History

A 38-year-old man with a history of right hip pain (▶ Fig. 54.1).

■ Key Finding

Focal subchondral bone edema in the femoral head.

■ Top 3 Differential Diagnoses

- **Subchondral stress fracture:** Stress fractures may occur at numerous characteristic locations in the skeleton, including the subchondral bone of the femoral head.

  Two types of stress fractures may occur: (1) fatigue fractures and (2) insufficiency fractures. *Fatigue-type stress fractures* occur in normal bone with chronic repetitive microtrauma (e.g., endurance athletes and military recruits during intensive training). *Insufficiency-type stress fractures* generally occur when normal stress is exerted on weakened bones. In the femoral head, subchondral insufficiency fractures are diagnosed most commonly in elderly female patients with osteopenia and acute onset severe hip pain. There is an association with insufficiency fractures elsewhere (e.g., vertebral body compression fracture).

  Both types of femoral head subchondral fractures cause hip pain, are relatively small, and are subtle (or occult) with radiography. Both types of fractures can benefit from early diagnosis with a high-spatial resolution MRI, which enables appropriate early management (e.g., non-weight bearing) and improves the likelihood of preventing progression to subchondral collapse, secondary osteonecrosis, and early onset osteoarthritis.

  At MRI, both subchondral stress fractures and avascular necrosis (AVN) have some overlapping features that can make evaluation difficult, including potentially a "crescent sign," a low-signal intensity band of demarcation (corresponding to osteosclerosis on CT), and adjacent bone edema.

  Two MRI findings can help differentiate a femoral head subchondral stress fracture versus AVN. With a subchondral stress fracture, there is typically (1) a serpentine, hypointense fracture line that parallels the articular surface and (2) hyperintense signal between the fracture line and the subchondral bone plate on fat-saturated T2 and postcontrast images (in other words, bone edema and enhancement occur *on both sides* of the fracture line).

  By comparison, with AVN, there is often (1) a continuous, rounded hypointense line that is concave superiorly, and (2) hypointense, necrotic bone completely fills the zone between the hypointense line and the subchondral bone on fat-saturated T2 and postcontrast images (in other words, bone edema and enhancement occur only *outside* the necrotic bone).

  With follow-up MRI of subchondral stress fractures, improvement is characterized by fracture healing and decreased bone edema, while worsening is characterized by progression to secondary AVN with femoral head collapse.

- **Osteonecrosis:** With femoral head AVN, bone marrow edema is associated with hip pain and radiographically-occult subchondral fracture/femoral head collapse (the last case discusses femoral head AVN in detail).

- **Reactive subchondral bone edema:** A bone marrow edema pattern on MRI is a nonspecific finding seen in association with a wide spectrum of pathological conditions, including posttraumatic contusions, subchondral fractures, AVN, osteochondral lesions, and articular cartilage degeneration (histologically, true edema may not be the predominant finding in the bone marrow, and therefore some purists prefer terms such as "bone marrow edema-like pattern" or "bone marrow lesion").

  The term "reactive bone edema" is sometimes used to indicate that the edema-like pattern of signal in the subchondral bone is secondary to a process such as overlying chondrosis. With MRI, articular cartilage degeneration in the hip may be difficult to visualize, but reactive bone edema and degenerative subchondral cysts are often recognizable.

  Notably, the term "idiopathic transient bone marrow edema syndrome" has largely fallen out of favor, because clinical correlation or high-resolution MRI often reveal an underlying etiology for the bone edema pattern, such as stress reaction, stress fracture, or overlying chondrosis.

■ Diagnosis

Reactive subchondral bone edema.

✓ Pearls

- Focal signal alteration in the subchondral bone of the femoral head is not always due to AVN.
- Subchondral fracture and AVN can occur at similar anatomical locations, but they often have different imaging appearances and different treatment algorithms.

- Reactive subchondral bone edema and subchondral cysts are commonly associated with overlying chondrosis in the hip.

■ Suggested Readings

Ando W, Yamamoto K, Koyama T, Hashimoto Y, Tsujimoto T, Ohzono K. Radiologic and clinical features of misdiagnosed idiopathic osteonecrosis of the femoral head. Orthopedics. 2017; 40(1):e117–e123

Gonzalez-Espino P, Van Cauter M, Gossing L, Galant CC, Acid S, Lecouvet FE. Uncommon observation of bifocal giant subchondral cysts in the hip: diagnostic role of CT arthrography and MRI, with pathological correlation. Skeletal Radiol. 2018; 47(4):587–592

Hatanaka H, Motomura G, Ikemura S, et al. Differences in magnetic resonance findings between symptomatic and asymptomatic pre-collapse osteonecrosis of the femoral head. Eur J Radiol. 2019; 112:1–6

Kim SM, Oh SM, Cho CH, et al. Fate of subchondral fatigue fractures of femoral head in young adults differs from general outcome of fracture healing. Injury. 2016; 47(12):2789–2794

Lee S, Saifuddin A. Magnetic resonance imaging of subchondral insufficiency fractures of the lower limb. Skeletal Radiol. 2019; 48(7):1011–1021

Leydet-Quilici H, Le Corroller T, Bouvier C, et al. Advanced hip osteoarthritis: magnetic resonance imaging aspects and histopathology correlations. Osteoarthritis Cartilage. 2010; 18(11):1429–1435

Case 55

Robert D. Boutin

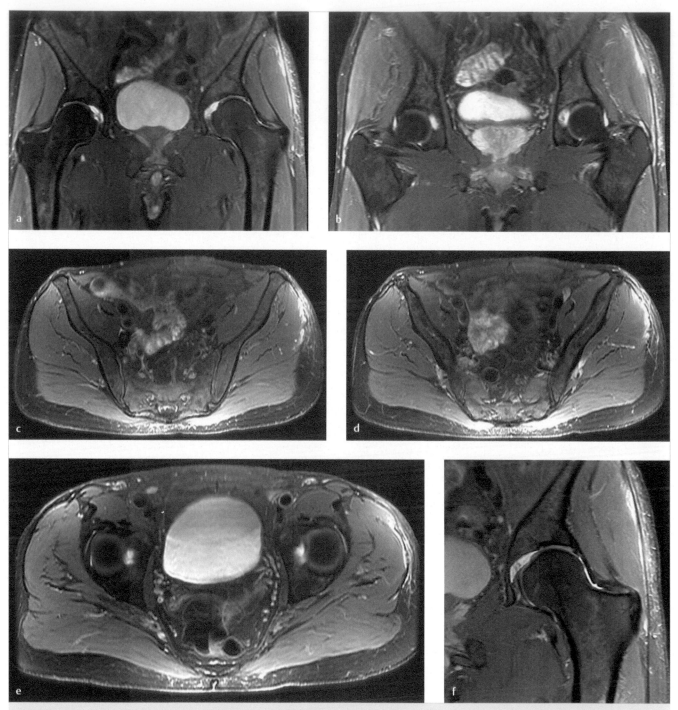

Fig. 55.1 Coronal fat-suppressed T2-weighted (**a, b**) and axial fat-suppressed T2-weighted (**c–e**) images of the pelvis demonstrate soft-tissue edema tracking along the deep and superficial surfaces of the left iliotibial band (ITB). At the superolateral aspect of the left hip, the ITB fibers are ill-defined. Coronal fat-suppressed T2-weighted (**f**) image of the left hip confirms the distribution of the soft-tissue edema.

■ Clinical History

A 64-year-old athletic man with persistent pain at the lateral aspect of the hip, presenting for an MRI to "rule out stress fracture, trochanteric bursitis, and abductor tendon tear" (▶ Fig. 55.1).

■ **Key Finding**

Low-grade tearing of the iliotibial band (ITB), with soft-tissue edema along the fascia.

■ **Top 3 Differential Diagnoses**

- **Proximal iliotibial band syndrome:** Anatomically, the ITB is a longitudinally-oriented band of fascial tissue that is best seen on coronal images originating from an origin at the iliac tubercle (at the superior–lateral lip of the iliac crest, approximately 5 cm posterior to the anterior superior iliac spine). The ITB extends distally along the superficial aspect of the gluteus medius/minimus and greater trochanter. The ITB continues distally beyond the hip region along the entire lateral thigh and knee, inserting distally at the anterolateral tibia (Gerdy's tubercle).

  Distally, ITB syndrome at the lateral aspect of the knee is a well-known overuse injury in athletes such as runners and cyclists. However, a *proximal* ITB syndrome is increasingly recognized as an important cause of pain at the lateral aspect of the hip, which can be associated with repetitive use/microtrauma and low-grade inflammation. Proximal ITB syndrome may occur as an overuse injury in athletes as well as in older (predominantly female) nonathletes.

  On MRI, proximal ITB syndrome is characterized by the presence of soft-tissue edema along the ITB, typically at the proximal attachment or more distally at the lateral aspect of the hip (without other causes of edema such as contusion). At the iliac tubercle enthesis, edema may be seen in the bone marrow and overlying soft tissue. Regardless of the location in the hip region, soft-tissue edema may be accompanied by subtle thickening or partial tearing.

- **Greater trochanteric pain syndrome:** With the given clinical history, the differential diagnosis could include numerous potential pain generators located at the lateral aspect of the hip.

  Regardless of the pain generator, the accuracy of MRI and sonography is enhanced by detailed anatomic knowledge and high-resolution imaging. Causes of greater trochanteric pain syndrome may or may not be well-demonstrated with imaging, and therefore some humility on the part of imagers is appropriate.

  The term "greater trochanteric pain syndrome" is important to recognize, however, because it has largely replaced the clinical diagnosis of "trochanteric bursitis." There is now a more nuanced understanding of pain at the lateral aspect of the hip. In addition to bursitis, pain generators are now known to commonly involve one or more other sites. Examples of conditions include abductor tendinopathy (with or without tears), abductor peritendinitis, calcific tendinitis, and snapping hip (external coxa saltans). Proximal ITB syndrome could also be included under this umbrella term.

  Greater trochanteric pain syndrome is often diagnosed in middle-aged women, but it is also reported in other demographic groups such as athletes and patients after hip arthroplasty.

  Treatment of greater trochanteric pain syndrome varies with the source, severity, and duration of symptoms. In most cases, nonoperative management suffices (e.g., physical therapy, percutaneous injection). In a minority of cases failing conservative management, surgical interventions may be performed (e.g., tendon repair, tendon release, and bursectomy).

- **Referred pain:** With the given clinical history, the clinical differential diagnosis includes pain referred to the lateral aspect of the hip. For many of these diagnoses, radiologists are extremely helpful with imaging and/or image-guided injections, including the diagnosis of hip osteoarthritis, stress fracture, myopathy/myositis, sacroiliitis, and lumbar spine degeneration.

■ **Diagnosis**

Proximal ITB syndrome.

✓ **Pearls**

- The term "greater trochanteric pain syndrome" is a clinical diagnosis. In addition to trochanteric bursitis, there are numerous other potential pain generators located at the lateral aspect of the hip.
- Proximal ITB syndrome refers to low-grade edema/inflammation involving the ITB at the ischial enthesis or at the lateral aspect of the hip, often related to overuse (degenerative or athletic). Partial tearing of the ITB may or may not be present.
- Proximal ITB syndrome is easily overlooked if one is not aware of the characteristic appearance on MRI.

■ **Suggested Readings**

Flato R, Passanante GJ, Skalski MR, Patel DB, White EA, Matcuk GR, Jr. The iliotibial tract: imaging, anatomy, injuries, and other pathology. Skeletal Radiol. 2017; 46(5):605–622

Hirschmann A, Falkowski AL, Kovacs B. Greater trochanteric pain syndrome: abductors, external rotators. Semin Musculoskelet Radiol. 2017; 21(5):539–546

Huang BK, Campos JC, Michael Peschka PG, et al. Injury of the gluteal aponeurotic fascia and proximal iliotibial band: anatomy, pathologic conditions, and MR imaging. Radiographics. 2013; 33(5):1437–1452

Khoury AN, Brooke K, Helal A, et al. Proximal iliotibial band thickness as a cause for recalcitrant greater trochanteric pain syndrome. J Hip Preserv Surg. 2018; 5(3):296–300

Redmond JM, Chen AW, Domb BG. Greater trochanteric pain syndrome. J Am Acad Orthop Surg. 2016; 24(4):231–240

Sher I, Umans H, Downie SA, Tobin K, Arora R, Olson TR. Proximal iliotibial band syndrome: what is it and where is it? Skeletal Radiol. 2011; 40(12):1553–1556

Case 56

Robert D. Boutin

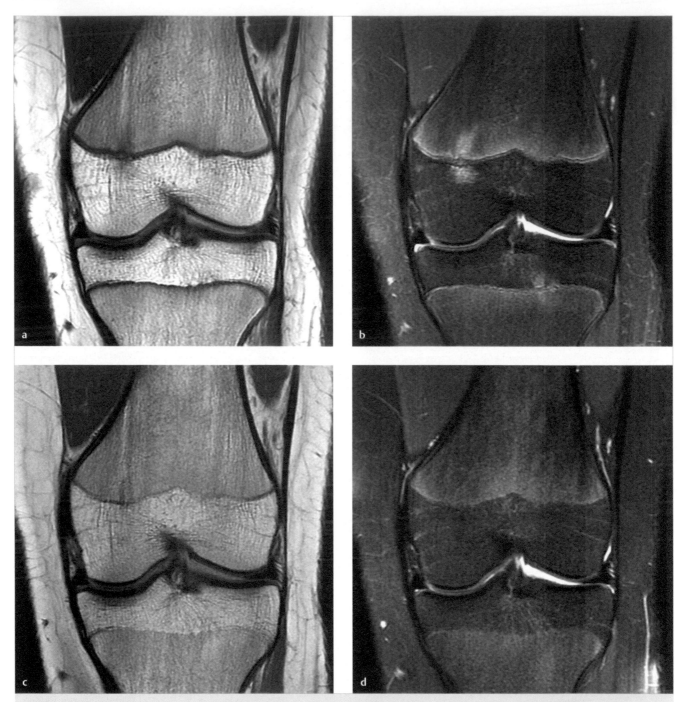

Fig. 56.1 Coronal proton density-weighted **(a)** and fat-suppressed T2-weighted **(b)** images of knee demonstrate a focal, patchy area of T2 hyperintensity on both sides of the medial femoral physis. There is also a smaller, more faint patchy focus of bone marrow edema on both sides of the lateral tibial physis on the T2 image. After 10 months, a follow-up MRI examination with coronal proton density-weighted **(c)** and fat-suppressed T2-weighted **(d)** images show interval closing of the physes (most prominently centrally) and resolution of the focal periphyseal edema in the femur and tibia.

■ Clinical History

A 12-year-old athletic girl with a history of knee pain and negative radiographs (▶ Fig. 56.1).

■ Key Finding

Focal periphyseal edema.

■ Top 3 Differential Diagnoses

- **Focal periphyseal edema (FOPE) zone:** Focal periphyseal edema (FOPE) refers to a focal zone of bone edema centered around a physis. It can be seen in adolescents with pain in the early stages of physiologic physeal closure.

  FOPE zones are most commonly observed at the knee, but can occur elsewhere (e.g., in the hip at the greater trochanter apophysis). In the knee, FOPE zones generally occur in patients with bone ages ranging from 11 to 14 years. FOPE zones are characteristically seen in an eccentric central location at sites of early physeal closure and resolve within one year. FOPE zones are managed conservatively and do not need follow-up imaging.
- **Physeal stress reaction (repetitive microtrauma):** Children and adolescents participating in organized sports are vulnerable to stress injury. In addition to bone edema, physeal widening and reactive sclerosis may occur.

  Although stress injury is usually reversible with conservative management, there is occasionally, premature bone bridging across the physis and subsequent deformity.
- **Contusion/fracture:** Injuries can involve the physis, such as a contusion or fracture. Imaging findings of physeal injury can include physeal widening, bone edema, fracture lines, and periosteal injury (elevation or disruption).

  At the knee, the most common physeal fracture pattern targets the lateral distal femoral metaphysis, with fracture extension through the medial physis (Salter–Harris type II fracture). Subsequent premature physeal fusion with leg length inequality may then occur.

■ Diagnosis

Focal periphyseal edema (FOPE) zone.

✓ Pearls

- FOPE zones are observed on MRI examinations of adolescents during early physiologic physeal closure.
- On knee MRI, a FOPE zone is generally seen as a patchy focus of bone edema, abutting the proximal and distal margins of the physis; this bone edema resolves in less than 1 year with conservative management.
- Bone edema on MRI is a nonspecific finding and may be caused by stress reaction or fracture, depending on the clinical context.

■ Suggested Readings

Giles E, Nicholson A, Sharkey MS, Carter CW. Focal periphyseal edema: are we over-treating physiologic adolescent knee pain? J Am Acad Orthop Surg Glob Res Rev. 2018; 2(4):e047

Jaimes C, Jimenez M, Shabshin N, Laor T, Jaramillo D. Taking the stress out of evaluating stress injuries in children. Radiographics. 2012; 32(2):537–555

Leschied JR, Udager KG. Imaging of the pediatric knee. Semin Musculoskelet Radiol. 2017; 21(2):137–146

Sakamoto A, Matsuda S. Focal periphyseal edema zone on magnetic resonance imaging in the greater trochanter apophysis: a case report. J Orthop Case Rep. 2017; 7(4):29–31

Ueyama H, Kitano T, Nakagawa K, Aono M. Clinical experiences of focal periphyseal edema zones in adolescent knees: case reports. J Pediatr Orthop B. 2018; 27(1): 26–30

Zbojniewicz AM, Laor T. Focal periphyseal edema (FOPE) zone on MRI of the adolescent knee: a potentially painful manifestation of physiologic physeal fusion? AJR Am J Roentgenol. 2011; 197(4):998–1004

Case 57

Robert D. Boutin

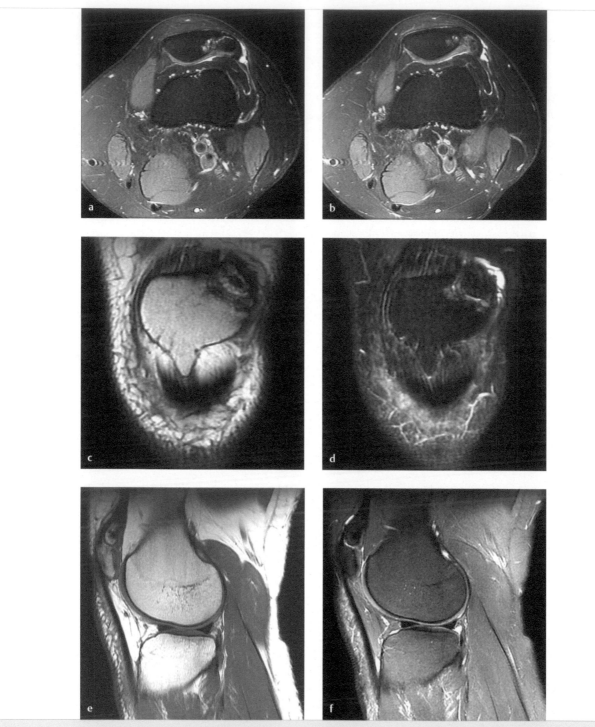

Fig. 57.1 Axial fat-suppressed T2-weighted (**a, b**), coronal proton density-weighted (**c**), coronal fat-suppressed T2 weighted (**d**), sagittal proton density-weighted (**e**) and sagittal fat-suppressed T2-weighted (**f**) images of the knee show a corticated ossific fragment at the superolateral aspect of the patella. T2 hyperintensity is seen between the fragment and the remainder of the patella, with mild adjacent reactive edema and sclerosis.

■ Clinical History

A 35-year-old woman with anterior knee pain (► Fig. 57.1).

■ Key Finding

Curvilinear signal separating the patella into two fragments.

■ Top 3 Differential Diagnoses

- **Bipartite patella:** The patella begins to ossify at 3 to 5 years of age, with secondary ossification centers that develop and usually fuse during adolescence. When one (or more) of these ossification centers fail to fuse, a bipartite (or multipartite) patella occurs. The prevalence is approximately 1 to 2% (9 times more common in males than females; bilateral in >25 %).

  A bipartite patella may be discovered as an asymptomatic incidental finding, or it may be associated with symptoms. With MRI of an asymptomatic bipartite patella, bone edema is not present. Conversely, in most symptomatic patients, bone edema abuts the interface (fibrocartilaginous synchondrosis or pseudarthrosis) between the fragment and the adjacent patella.

  With imaging, the bipartite patella is seen as a well-corticated fragment that is located at the superolateral patella in the vast majority of cases (i.e., insertion site for the vastus lateralis and lateral retinaculum in ≥75% of cases). Less commonly, a bipartite patella has a longitudinal orientation along the lateral patellar facet. A small fragment at the distal margin was originally described as a "type I" bipartite patella, but many investigators now categorize this finding as Sinding–Larsen–Johansson (SLJ) syndrome.

  Imaging features that favor a bipartite patella (rather than fracture) include bilateral distribution, superolateral location, curvilinear orientation, and smooth, sclerotic, corticated margins.

- **Patellar fracture:** Fractures of the patella are commonly due to a traumatic event involving a direct blow or excessive tension through the extensor mechanism. Osteochondral fractures are commonly seen after a transient lateral patellar dislocation.

  Other patellar fractures are often described by their orientation as transverse (~80% occur in the mid to lower third of the patella, typically from indirect trauma), vertical (~20% of patellar fractures), or stellate (comminuted, typically from direct trauma).

  Patellar stress fractures are rare, but they may occur in athletes (runners, jumpers, and kickers). These fractures are typically located either in the distal third of the patella (transversely) or in the lateral patella facet (longitudinally).

- **Patellar calcar:** A calcar is a normal condensation of bone trabeculae. In the subchondral bone of the lateral patellar facet, a calcar can be observed in most knees, particularly in adolescents and young adults (~80%).

  The patellar calcar is displayed as curvilinear low-signal with anterior convexity, which is generally best seen on two to three contiguous, nonfat-suppressed images. The patellar calcar is often inconspicuous and is not normally associated with any bone edema, but it rarely may mimic a patellar stress fracture or an osteochondral lesion.

■ Diagnosis

Bipartite patella.

✓ Pearls

- A bipartite patella is a developmental anomaly caused by failed fusion of an accessory ossification center with the remainder of the patella, usually superolaterally.
- A bipartite patella is commonly an incidental finding; these patients do not have bone edema along the synchondrosis between fragments. In most symptomatic patients with a bipartite patella, MRI shows bone edema.

- In the lateral patellar facet, a patellar calcar is a normal incidental finding seen as curvilinear low signal, without bone edema. The patellar calcar should not be confused with a fracture or osteochondral lesion.

■ Suggested Readings

Brown GA, Stringer MR, Arendt EA. Stress fractures of the patella. In: Miller TL, Kaeding CC (eds). Stress Fractures in Athletes. Cham, Switzerland: Springer; 2015:125–135

Collins MS, Tiegs-Heiden CA, Stuart MJ. Patellar calcar: MRI appearance of a previously undescribed anatomical entity. Skeletal Radiol. 2014; 43(2):219–225

Jarraya M, Diaz LE, Arndt WF, Roemer FW, Guermazi A. Imaging of patellar fractures. Insights Imaging. 2017; 8(1):49–57

Kavanagh EC, Zoga A, Omar I, Ford S, Schweitzer M, Eustace S. MRI findings in bipartite patella. Skeletal Radiol. 2007; 36(3):209–214

O'Brien J, Murphy C, Halpenny D, McNeill G, Torreggiani WC. Magnetic resonance imaging features of asymptomatic bipartite patella. Eur J Radiol. 2011; 78(3):425–429

Oohashi Y. Developmental anomaly of ossification type patella partita. Knee Surg Sports Traumatol Arthrosc. 2015; 23(4):1071–1076

Case 58

Robert D. Boutin

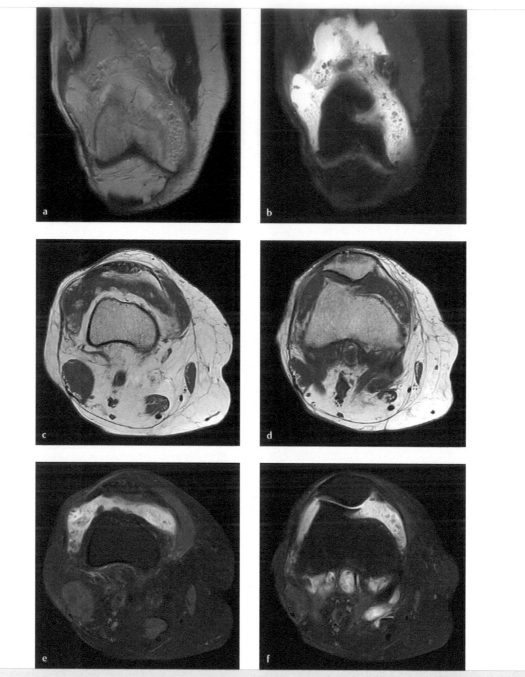

Fig. 58.1 Coronal proton density-weighted **(a)** coronal fat-suppressed T2-weighted **(b)** images of the knee show a joint effusion outlining frond-like tissue in the joint. Axial T1-weighted **(c, d)** and axial fat-suppressed T2-weighted images **(e, f)** demonstrate the frond-like lobules of tissue are isointense with fat on all pulse sequences.

■ Clinical History

A 62-year-old woman with a history of chronic knee osteo-arthritis and "swelling" (▶ Fig. 58.1).

■ Key Finding

Frond-like lobules of fatty tissue in the suprapatellar recess, with effusion.

■ Top 3 Differential Diagnoses

- **Lipoma arborescens:** Lipoma arborescens is a non-neoplastic lipomatous proliferation of the subsynovial connective tissue. Although an idiopathic (primary) type is described in younger patients, the vast majority of cases are in older patients, secondary to chronic synovial irritation in the setting of osteoarthritis or (much less commonly) rheumatoid arthritis. Affected joints have a chronic or recurring effusion.

  Lipoma arborescens is generally a monoarticular process. The most common location for lipoma arborescens is the knee, particularly in the suprapatellar recess. With knee MRI, the frequency of this finding is approximately 0.3%. Lipoma arborescens may also be seen in other synovial-lined locations (e.g., glenohumeral joint in the setting of chronic osteoarthritis). More rarely, bursae or tendon sheaths may be affected.

  Diagnosis can be made on MRI examinations showing hypertrophic lipomatous tissue with a lobular or villous morphology projecting into an effusion. Unlike pigmented villonodular synovitis (PVNS), there is no low-T2 signal or susceptibility artifact to suggest hemosiderin.

  Arthroscopic synovectomy is an accepted treatment to address the proliferative process itself, although management of any underlying cause (e.g., osteoarthritis) is also an important consideration.

- **Intraarticular (loose) bodies:** Multiple intraarticular (loose) bodies are associated with internal derangements of joints, most commonly osteoarthritis. These fragments vary in signal intensity, depending on whether they are cartilaginous (chondral), osteochondral, or osseous.

  Fragments containing fatty marrow, such as osseous loose bodies, are commonly seen in joints with substantial osteoarthritis. This condition is sometimes referred to as secondary osteochondromatosis to differentiate it from primary synovial chondromatosis.

  Osseous loose bodies contain fatty signal (like lipoma arborescens), but typically have a thin sclerotic rim and are not confined to the suprapatellar recess. Unlike lipoma arborescens, osseous loose bodies are mineralized (radio dense) on radiography and CT.

- **Rice bodies:** Rice bodies are fibrinoid fragments that grossly resemble grains of rice. They are thought to occur when hypertrophic synovium undergoes fibrinoid necrosis and is shed into a joint, bursa, or tendon sheath.

  Rice body formation is typically seen in patients with chronic synovitis which is caused by inflammatory arthritis (e.g., rheumatoid arthritis, juvenile chronic arthritis) or mycobacterial infection (e.g., tuberculosis arthritis).

  On MRI, rice bodies are recognized as numerous, very small fragments of uniform caliber outlined by synovial fluid (not fixed to the synovium).

■ Diagnosis

Lipoma arborescens.

✓ Pearls

- Lipoma arborescens is displayed as synovial-based hypertrophic lipomatous tissue projecting into an effusion.
- Lipoma arborescens is typically seen in the suprapatellar recess of older patients with knee osteoarthritis.
- Both lipoma arborescens and osseous loose bodies can be seen as foci of high-T1 signal intensity in arthritic joints.

■ Suggested Readings

Coll JP, Ragsdale BD, Chow B, Daughters TC. Best cases from the AFIP: lipoma arborescens of the knees in a patient with rheumatoid arthritis. Radiographics. 2011; 31(2):333–337

Evenski AJ, Stensby JD, Rosas S, Emory CL. Diagnostic imaging and management of common intra-articular and peri-articular soft tissue tumors and tumor like conditions of the knee. J Knee Surg. 2019; 32(4):322–330

Susa M, Horiuchi K. Rice bodies in a patient with oligoarticular juvenile idiopathic arthritis. J Rheumatol. 2019; 46(9):1157–1158

Wang CK, Alfayez S, Marwan Y, Martineau PA, Burman M. Knee arthroscopy for the treatment of lipoma arborescens: a systematic review of the literature. JBJS Rev. 2019; 7(4):e8

Case 59

Robert D. Boutin

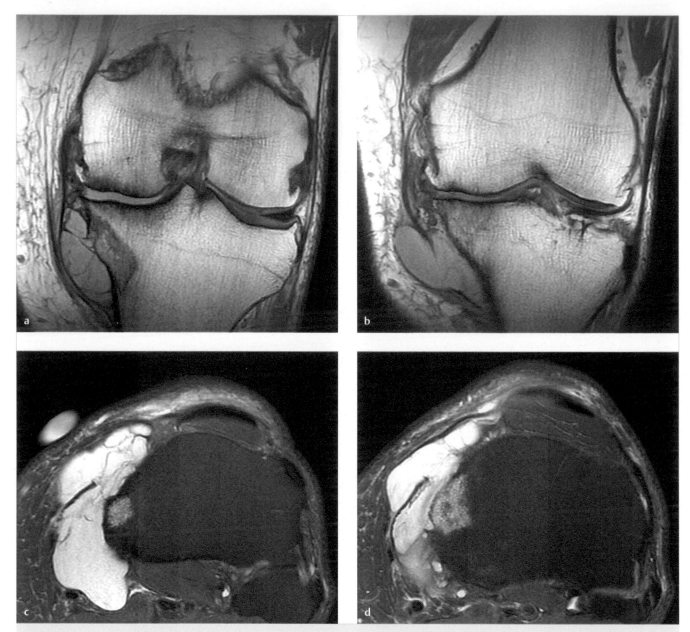

Fig. 59.1 Coronal proton density-weighted (**a, b**) and axial fat-suppressed T2-weighted (**c, d**) images of the knee show an ovoid, well-defined lesion at the medial aspect of the tibia. The lesion is mostly isointense with fluid, has thin septations, and is deep to the pes anserinus and medial collateral ligament. The underlying bone shows slight cortical scalloping and localized reactive bone marrow edema.

■ Clinical History

A 70-year-old man with a palpable mass and pain at the medial aspect of the knee (► Fig. 59.1).

■ Key Finding

Cystic-appearing lesion centered inferior to the medial joint line of the knee.

■ Top 3 Differential Diagnoses

- **Bursitis:** Bursae are sac-like structures lined by synovial tissue which function to mitigate friction in the musculoskeletal system. When inflamed, these bursae characteristically fill with fluid, which is considered the *sine qua non* of bursitis. Classic symptoms can include pain, swelling, and tenderness.

    Bursitis at the medial aspect of the knee is associated most commonly with osteoarthritis and overuse (e.g., in runners). Fluid may collect in three bursae at the medial aspect of the knee (in order of frequency).

    The *semimembranosus–tibial collateral ligament bursa* is located near the posteromedial joint line, typically along the superficial aspect of the semimembranosus tendon.

    The *pes anserinus bursa* is located between the medial tibial plateau region and the pes anserine tendons (i.e., sartorius, gracilis, and semitendinosus). With imaging, there is a rounded fluid collection with well-defined margins located inferior to the joint line along the medial aspect of the tibia, superficial to the medial collateral ligament. These fluid collections do not communicate with the knee joint or with popliteal bursal fluid collections. However, in rare cases of pes anserine bursitis (<2%), there are underlying bone changes (e.g., cortical scalloping, subcortical sclerosis, reactive bone marrow edema, and even intramedullary extension at the medial tibial surface), which may mimic a neoplasm.

    The *medial collateral ligament (MCL) bursa* is located between the superficial and deep MCL fibers (at the central third of the medial knee). Fluid can collect proximal to the joint line, distal to the joint line, or both.
- **Parameniscal cyst:** Parameniscal cysts are well-defined, rounded collections that are typically in continuity with a horizontal or complex tear of the subjacent meniscus.

    Almost all patients going to arthroscopy with parameniscal cysts have meniscus tears at surgery. An important exception to this "rule" is observed at the anterior and anterolateral regions of the lateral meniscus; underlying meniscus tears are not present in approximately one-third of patients with cysts at the anterolateral joint line.
- **Synovial sarcoma:** Solid lesions, such as synovial sarcoma, may have a high-water content and mimic fluid collections on noncontrast MRI. Synovial sarcoma can appear relatively homogeneous when small, but larger lesions usually are seen as heterogeneously hyperintense on T2-weighted images that undergo diffuse heterogeneous contrast enhancement. Dystrophic calcification is present in approximately one-third of synovial sarcomas. Underlying bone erosion is rarely seen. Unlike a periarticular cyst, there is no pedicle connecting to the joint.

■ Diagnosis

Pes anserinus bursitis.

✓ Pearls

- Bursitis at the medial aspect of the knee occurs at characteristic anatomic locations, typically involving one of three bursae: the semimembranosus–tibial collateral ligament bursa, pes anserinus bursa, or MCL bursa.
- Parameniscal cysts are very highly associated with underlying meniscus tears, *except* at the anterolateral joint line.
- Synovial sarcoma may mimic a fluid collection on noncontrast MRI. However, synovial sarcoma typically does *not* occur in the anatomic distribution of bursa and is *not* associated with an underlying meniscus tear.

■ Suggested Readings

Colak C, Ilaslan H, Sundaram M. Bony changes of the tibia secondary to pes anserine bursitis mimicking neoplasm. Skeletal Radiol. 2019; 48(11):1795–1801

Curtis BR, Huang BK, Pathria MN, Resnick DL, S, mitaman E. Pes anserinus: anatomy and pathology of native and harvested tendons. AJR Am J Roentgenol. 2019; 213 (5):1107–1116

De Maeseneer M, Shahabpour M, Van Roy F, et al. MR imaging of the medial collateral ligament bursa: findings in patients and anatomic data derived from cadavers. AJR Am J Roentgenol. 2001; 177(4):911–917

De Smet AA, Graf BK, del Rio AM. Association of parameniscal cysts with underlying meniscal tears as identified on MRI and arthroscopy. AJR Am J Roentgenol. 2011; 196(2):W180–6

Rennie WJ, Saifuddin A. Pes anserine bursitis: incidence in symptomatic knees and clinical presentation. Skeletal Radiol. 2005; 34(7):395–398

Steinbach LS, Stevens KJ. Imaging of cysts and bursae about the knee. Radiol Clin North Am. 2013; 51(3):433–454

Case 60

Paulomi Kanzaria and Jasjeet Bindra

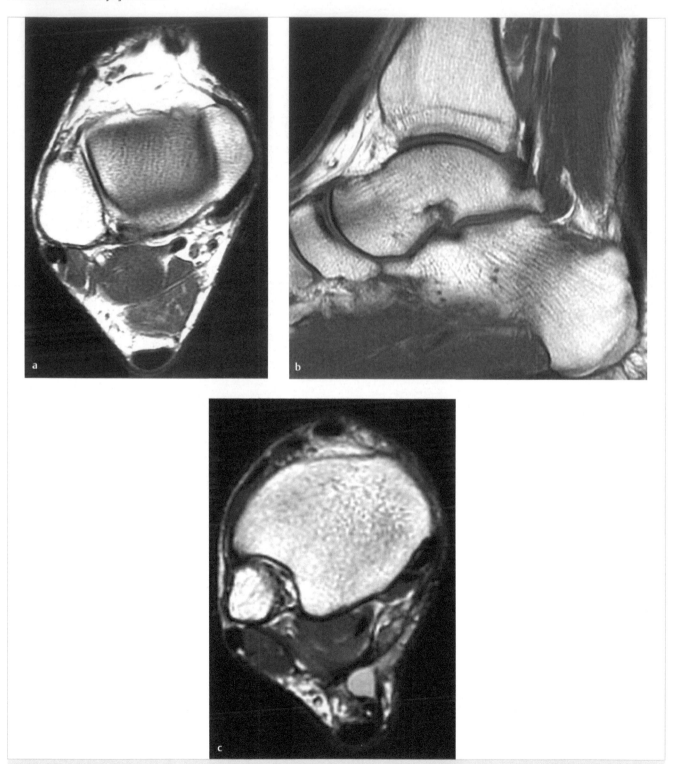

Fig. 60.1 Axial proton density-weighted MR image of the ankle **(a)** shows a triangular accessory muscle in the tarsal tunnel and another accessory muscle anterior to the Achilles tendon. Sagittal T1-weighted image **(b)** reveals the accessory muscles longitudinally. Axial proton density-weighted MR image **(c)** of the same ankle shows postsurgical changes after resection of both accessory muscles.

■ Clinical History

A 38-year-old female with recurrent posterior ankle pain after exercising (▶ Fig. 60.1).

Key Finding

Accessory muscle around ankle.

Top 3 Differential Diagnoses

- **Accessory soleus:** Accessory soleus muscle is typically asymptomatic but can manifest as a soft-tissue mass, and hypertrophy may cause compression of the posterior tibial-nerve. The accessory soleus is more common in males. Radiographs reveal obscuration of the normal triangular appearance of Kager fat pad by a well-defined area of increased soft-tissue density. Cross-sectional imaging is more sensitive and specific for identification. MR imaging demonstrates the accessory muscle anterior to the Achilles tendon and superficial to the flexor retinaculum, typically extending medially to the area between the medial edge of the Achilles tendon and medial malleolus. Five types of accessory soleus have been described based on the insertion characteristics. The insertion points include the Achilles tendon, the superior surface of the calcaneus either with a fleshy muscular insertion or a tendinous insertion, and the medial surface of the calcaneus either with a fleshy muscular insertion or a tendinous insertion.

- **Peroneus quartus:** Peroneus quartus is commonly encountered as an asymptomatic variant but may cause lateral ankle pain or ankle instability in athletes. Peroneus quartus extends medial and posterior to the other peroneal tendons and has a variety of insertion sites, the most common insertion is into the calcaneus. MR imaging delineates the muscle optimally. On axial MR images, a peroneus quartus is visualized posteromedial or medial to the peroneus brevis and is separated from it by a fat plane. The muscle belly of peroneus quartus may vary in size. It can be associated with longitudinal tears of the peroneal tendons secondary to crowding of the peroneal tendons deep to the peroneal retinaculum.

- **Flexor digitorum accessorius longus:** The accessory flexor digitorum originates either from the medial margin of the tibia or from the lateral margin of the fibula, and the origin can vary widely, arising from any structure in the posterior compartment. The tendon descends posterior and superficial to the tibial nerve, courses beneath the flexor retinaculum through the tarsal tunnel, and is intimately related to the posterior tibial artery and tibial nerve. It can be associated with tarsal tunnel syndrome because of its close relationship to the neurovascular bundle in the tarsal tunnel. On axial MR images, the muscle is demonstrated within the tarsal tunnel, typically superficial to the neurovascular bundle.

Diagnosis

Accessory soleus and flexor digitorum accessorius longus.

Pearls

- Accessory soleus is present at the posterior aspect of the ankle and can mimic a mass on radiography.
- Peroneus quartus can be associated with longitudinal tears of the peroneal tendons, secondary to crowding deep to the peroneal retinaculum.

- Flexor digitorum accessorius longus is present medially and can be a cause of tarsal tunnel syndrome.

Suggested Readings

Cheung Y, Rosenberg ZS. MR imaging of the accessory muscles around the ankle. Magn Reson Imaging Clin N Am. 2001; 9(3):465–473, x

Sookur PA, Naraghi AM, Bleakney RR, Jalan R, Chan O, White LM. Accessory muscles: anatomy, symptoms, and radiologic evaluation. Radiographics. 2008; 28(2): 481–499

Case 61

Paulomi Kanzaria and Jasjeet Bindra

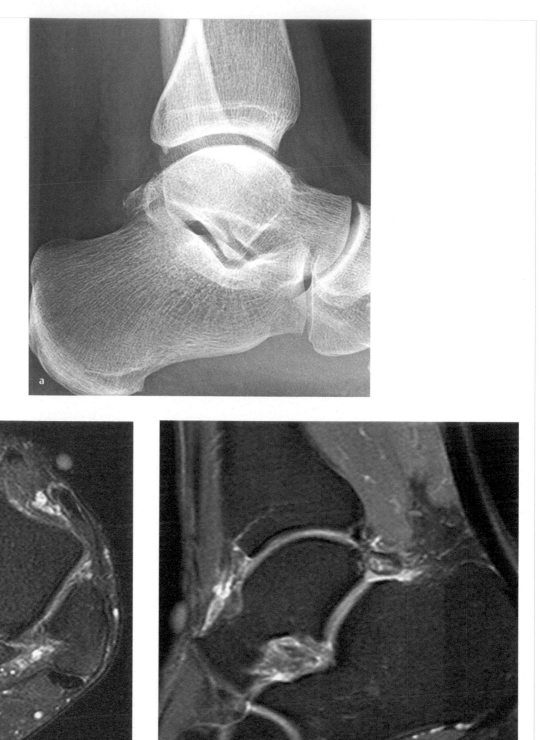

Fig. 61.1 Lateral radiograph of the ankle (**a**) shows an ovoid ossicle posterior to the talus. Axial fat-saturated, proton density-weighted (**b**) and sagittal STIR MR (**c**) images reveal the ossicle and cystic and edematous changes in it and in the posterior talus along the synchondrosis.

■ **Clinical History**

A 28-year-old female with posterior ankle pain (▶ Fig. 61.1).

■ Key Finding

Accessory ossicle around ankle.

■ Top 3 Differential Diagnoses

- **Os trigonum:** An os trigonum is the unfused ossification center posterior to the talus. Normally, this ossification center forms between the ages of 8 and 13 years and fuses with the talus within 1 year. When it remains separate, it is referred to as the os trigonum. On lateral radiographs of the ankle/foot, the os trigonum is round or oval with well-defined corticated margins, and the accessory ossicle articulates with the lateral talar tubercle through a synchondrosis. An os trigonum can be associated with os trigonum syndrome or posterior impingement. This is best evaluated on sagittal and axial MR sequences where bone edema or fragmentation of the os, degenerative changes at the synchondrosis, and adjacent synovitis may be seen.

- **Os peroneum:** An os peroneum is a small sesamoid in the distal peroneus longus tendon near the cuboid. It can be bipartite or multipartite. Painful os peroneum syndrome (POPS) results from a wide spectrum of conditions presenting with pain at the lateral aspect of the cuboid. It can be a consequence of acute trauma or chronic overuse. Acute cases are due to fracture of the os or tear of peroneus longus tendon. Chronic cases may be due to hypertrophic os peroneum or activities that involve repetitive hypersupination.

  On radiographs, a fractured sesamoid will have fragments with sharp margins. Displacement of the os peroneum is an indirect sign of peroneal tendon rupture. MRI, however, is the best imaging modality to evaluate bone marrow changes and abnormalities in adjacent soft tissues and tendon.

- **Os navicularis:** Three types of accessory navicular or os tibiale externum have been described.

  Type I accessory navicular is a round or oval, small sesamoid within the posterior tibial tendon, near the navicular bone, and is rarely associated with symptoms. Type II accessory navicular is the most common type and also most commonly associated with symptoms secondary to dysfunction of the posterior tibial tendon. On radiographs, the ossification center is triangular in shape, located adjacent to the tubercle of the navicular bone, with presence of a fibrocartilaginous-synchondrosis. The entire or majority of the posterior tibial tendon inserts on the type II accessory ossicle, which is best seen on MR imaging. MR imaging can also demonstrate bone marrow reactive change, associated abnormality or tear of the posterior tibial tendon, or fluid in the tendon sheath in symptomatic cases. In type III, the accessory navicular bone is fused with the navicular, resulting in a prominent navicular tuberosity. This type is also known as a cornuate navicular, and these are generally asymptomatic but may be associated with pain secondary to a prominent medial navicular.

■ Diagnosis

Os trigonum with posterior impingement.

✓ Pearls

- An ostrigonum can be associated with posterior impingement, which is best evaluated on MR imaging.
- Displacement of osperoneum is an indirect sign of peroneus longus tendon rupture.

- Among the three types of accessory navicular, Type II is most commonly associated with symptoms.

■ Suggested Readings

Bianchi S, Bortolotto C, Draghi F. Os peroneum imaging: normal appearance and pathological findings. Insights Imaging. 2017; 8(1):59–68

Mellado JM, Ramos A, Salvadó E, Camins A, Danús M, Saurí A. Accessory ossicles and sesamoid bones of the ankle and foot: imaging findings, clinical significance and differential diagnosis. Eur Radiol. 2003; 13 Suppl 4:L164–L177

Case 62

Paulomi Kanzaria and Jasjeet Bindra

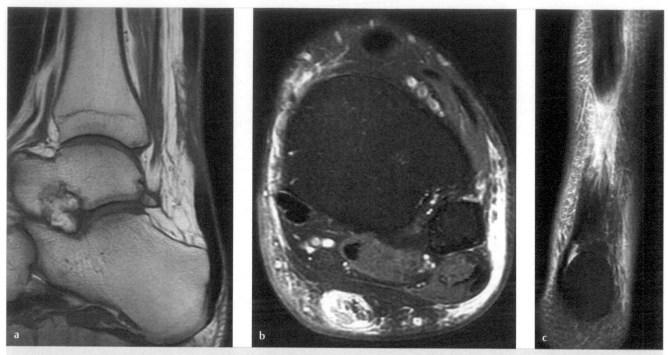

Fig. 62.1 Sagittal T1-weighted, MR image **(a)** of the ankle shows an intermediate signal gap in the Achilles tendon, approximately 5 cm above the insertion. Axial and coronal fat-saturated, proton density-weighted, MR images **(b, c)** show the fluid-filled gap to a better advantage.

■ Clinical History

A 50-year-old male with sudden onset posterior ankle pain while playing badminton (▶ Fig. 62.1).

■ Key Finding

Achilles tendon abnormality.

■ Top 3 Differential Diagnoses

- **Achilles tendinosis:** The Achilles tendon lacks a tendon sheath; however, it has a peritendon. Achilles peritendinosis manifests at MR imaging as linear or irregular areas of altered signal in the pre-Achilles tendon fat pad. Achilles tendinosis manifests on axial MR images as loss of the anterior concave or flat surface of the tendon, and on sagittal images, as fusiform thickening. Focal areas of increased signal intensity within the tendon are also noted.
- **Achilles tendon tear:** Typical tears of Achilles tendon occur at the avascular zone, approximately 2 to 6 cm above the insertion on posterior calcaneus. Atypical tears are more proximal at the myotendinous junction or, rarely, distally at the insertion site. Tears may be partial or complete. In acute cases, the tendon edges are separated by a hematoma. In chronic tears, atrophy of the muscles can be seen. Achilles tendon tears may be detected with ultrasound or MRI and are seen as

discontinuity and focal fluid at the location of the tear, with retraction of the torn edges of the tendon.
- **Haglund's disease:** Haglund's disease is a constellation of osseous and soft-tissue abnormalities that present as posterior heel pain. It is frequently associated with particular footwear such as women's high-heeled shoes and hockey skates, which compress the retro-Achilles bursa against the posterior calcaneal prominence. Haglund deformity is prominence of bony projection along the posterior superior aspect of calcaneal tuberosity. This bony deformity may lead to mechanically induced inflammation of retro-Achilles bursa, Achilles tendinosis, and retrocalcaneal bursitis. MR imaging findings include insertional Achilles tendinosis, calcaneal marrow edema, distended retrocalcaneal and retro-Achilles bursae, and enlarged calcaneal tuberosity.

■ Additional Diagnostic Consideration

- **Achilles tendon xanthoma:** Xanthomas are non-neoplastic lesions that are characterized by local collection of lipid-laden macrophages, giant cells, and other inflammatory cells. Tendinous xanthomas are usually found in familial

hypercholesterolemia and should be suspected in patients with bilateral Achilles tendon abnormalities. MR imaging reveals fusiform thickening of the Achilles tendon associated with intrasubstance heterogeneity and stippling.

■ Diagnosis

Achilles tendon tear.

✓ Pearls

- Achilles tendinosis can present as loss of anterior concave or flat surface of the tendon on axial MR images.
- Typical Achilles tendon tears are seen 2 to 6 cm above the insertion with discontinuity and focal fluid.

- Haglund's disease is a constellation of osseous and soft-tissue findings at the posterior calcaneus.

■ Suggested Readings

Rosenberg ZS, Beltran J, Bencardino JT. From the RSNA refresher courses. Radiological Society of North America. MR imaging of the ankle and foot. Radiographics. 2000; 20(Spec No):S153–S179

Schweitzer ME, Karasick D. MR imaging of disorders of the Achilles tendon. AJR Am J Roentgenol. 2000; 175(3):613–625

Case 63

Paulomi Kanzaria and Jasjeet Bindra

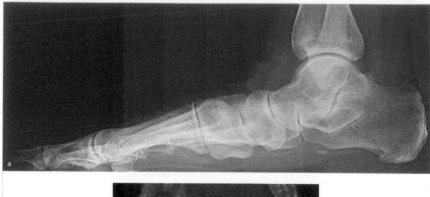

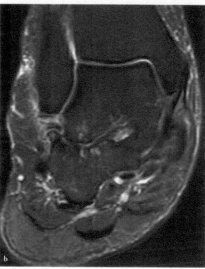

Fig. 63.1 Lateral radiograph of the ankle **(a)** shows considerable pes planus. Coronal fat-suppressed, proton density-weighted, MR image **(b)** reveals extra-articular subcortical cystic changes and mild edema at the lateral process of talus and adjacent calcaneus.

■ Clinical History

A 52-year-old male with chronic posterolateral ankle pain (▶ Fig. 63.1).

■ Key Finding

Impingement syndrome at ankle.

■ Top 3 Differential Diagnoses

- **Anterior impingement:** Anterior impingement is caused by repetitive microtrauma or forced dorsiflexion injuries at ankle. It is a relatively common cause of chronic ankle pain, especially in athletes and particularly soccer players. Radiographs show a beak-like prominence at the anterior rim of the tibial plafond and at the opposing margin of the talus, proximal to the talar neck. MR imaging is useful in visualizing the cartilage damage, synovitis in the anterior capsular recess, and bone marrow edema.
- **Posterior impingement:** Posterior impingement results from repetitive or acute forced plantar flexion of the foot and is most common in classical ballet dancers. The mechanism of injury is compression of the posterior talus and soft tissues between the tibia and the calcaneus during plantar flexion. Osseous causes of impingement are more common and may include a prominent or fragmented ostrigonum, elongated lateral tubercle of the talus (Stieda's process), or loose bodies. Soft tissue causes of impingement include synovitis of the flexor hallucis longus (FHL) tendon sheath and presence of the posterior intermalleolar ligament. MR imaging shows bone marrow edema or occult fractures in the lateral talar tubercle or ostrigonum, synovitis in the posterior recess of the subtalar or tibiotalar joint, as well as FHL tenosynovitis.
- **Anterolateral impingement:** Anterolateral impingement results from minor inversion injuries of the ankle and is relatively uncommon. Repeated microtrauma results in hypertrophied synovial tissue and fibrosis in the anterolateral gutter of the ankle. MR imaging can show abnormal soft-tissue mass in the anterolateral gutter, distinct from the anterior talofibular ligament.

■ Additional Diagnostic Considerations

- **Extra-articular posterolateral hindfoot impingement:** With severe pes planus and hindfoot valgus, there can be talocalcaneal impingement (between the lateral talus and calcaneus) and subfibular impingement (between the calcaneus and fibula). The most common MRI manifestations of talocalcaneal impingement are cystic changes, and sclerosis and edema in the posterior subtalar joint, lateral process of the talus and lateral calcaneus.
- **Medial impingement:** Anteromedial and posteromedial impingements are rare and result from inversion injuries. Scarring, synovitis, and capsular and deltoid ligament thickening may be seen.

■ Diagnosis

Posterolateral hindfoot impingement.

✓ Pearls

- Plain radiographs showing anterior tibiotalar spurring may be the only imaging study necessary in appropriate clinical presentation of anterior impingement.
- In posterior impingement, MR imaging can show edema, fragmentation or occult fracture of Stieda's process, or os trigonum with adjacent synovitis.
- Plain radiography has limited utility in anterolateral impingement as it is a soft-tissue abnormality.

■ Suggested Readings

Cerezal L, Abascal F, Canga A, et al. MR imaging of ankle impingement syndromes. AJR Am J Roentgenol. 2003; 181(2):551–559

Donovan A, Rosenberg ZS. MRI of ankle and lateral hindfoot impingement syndromes. AJR Am J Roentgenol. 2010; 195(3):595–604

Case 64

Jasjeet Bindra

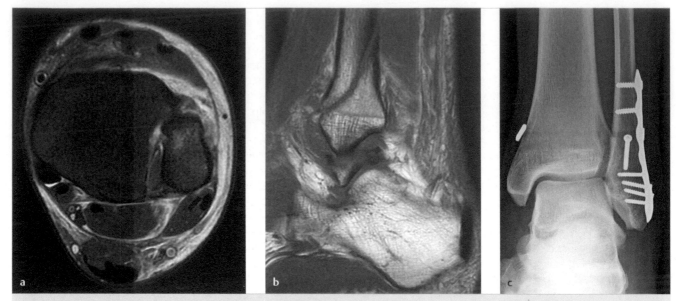

Fig. 64.1 Axial fat-saturated, proton density-weighted, MR image of the ankle **(a)** shows disruption of anteroinferior tibiofibular ligament and edema in posteroinferior tibiofibular ligament. Sagittal T1-weighted, MR image of the same ankle **(b)** reveals a Weber type B fracture of the distal fibula. Postoperative AP radiograph of the ankle **(c)** shows tight rope reconstruction of syndesmotic ligaments and open reduction internal fixation of distal fibular fracture.

■ Clinical History

A 42-year-old female with acute ankle pain after fall (▶ Fig. 64.1).

■ Key Finding

Ankle sprain.

■ Top 3 Differential Diagnoses

- **Syndesmotic injury or high ankle sprain:** Distal tibiofibular syndesmosis consists of three major ligaments: the anterior inferior tibiofibular ligament (AITFL), posterior inferior tibiofibular ligament (PITFL), and interosseous ligament. Most syndesmotic injuries are related to Lauge–Hansen supination external rotation (SER)/Weber B type fractures or pronation external rotation (PER)/Weber C type fractures. These injuries are associated with greater risk of chronic ankle dysfunction and pain. The AITFL and PITFL are usually seen on two or more sequential axial and coronal MR images at the level of the tibial plafond and talar dome. The talar dome is somewhat square at this level, and ligaments insert into fibula above the malleolar fossa, where the cross-section of the fibula is round. This morphology of the talus and fibula can be used to distinguish the syndesmotic ligaments from more inferior talofibular ligaments on axial MRI images. The AITFL is the most commonly torn ligament and is almost always torn before the other syndesmotic ligaments. Injuries usually manifest as attenuation, laxity, or discontinuity of the ligaments on MR imaging.
- **Lateral ankle sprain:** The lateral complex, comprising the anterior talofibular (ATFL), calcaneofibular (CFL), and posterior talofibular (PTFL) ligaments, is the most commonly injured group of ankle ligaments. Injury to the lateral complex typically occurs during forced plantar flexion and inversion. The predictable pattern of injury involves first the ATFL, followed by the CFL, and then the PTFL. The ATFL is best seen on axial T1 or PD MR images as a thin, flat, homogeneous band of low-signal intensity arising from lateral malleolus and coursing anteromedially to the talar neck. The talus is oblong, and fibula has a crescentic configuration from malleolar fossa, serving as a landmark in localization. CFL arises from the deep aspect of inferior tip of lateral malleolus and courses posteroinferiorly to attach to the lateral aspect of the calcaneus. The PTFL is multifascicular, extending inferomedially from the deep aspect of the lateral malleolus to the mid-to-posterior aspect of the talus. A complete tear of any of these ligaments can be seen as discontinuity across the ruptured ligament with retraction of lax fibers. Chronic tears may manifest either as severe attenuation or as thickening.
- **Medial ankle sprain:** Isolated medial collateral or deltoid ligament injuries are infrequent. Acute disruption usually occurs with pronation–eversion or pronation–abduction injuries. The medial collateral ligament complex is further divided into superficial and deep layers. The three components that are most often visualized on MRI include the tibiospring and tibionavicular ligaments in the superficial layer and the posterior tibiotalar ligament in the deep layer. Deep ligament tears are more common than superficial tears, and partial tears are more common than full-thickness tears. Most ligaments are best seen in the coronal plane. In high-grade sprains, high-T2 signal can be seen on fat-saturated PD or T2-weighted MR images, with associated fluid-filled gaps or complete discontinuity of the ligament.

■ Diagnosis

Tibiofibular syndesmotic injury.

✓ Pearls

- Amongst the syndesmotic ligaments, the AITFL is the most commonly torn ligament.
- In lateral ankle sprains, the predictable pattern of injury involves the ATFL first.
- Deltoid ligament components are best seen on coronal MRI images.

■ Suggested Readings

Nazarenko A, Beltran LS, Bencardino JT. Imaging evaluation of traumatic ligamentous injuries of the ankle and foot. Radiol Clin North Am. 2013; 51(3):455–478

Perrich KD, Goodwin DW, Hecht PJ, Cheung Y. Ankle ligaments on MRI: appearance of normal and injured ligaments. AJR Am J Roentgenol. 2009; 193(3):687–695

Case 65

Paulomi Kanzaria and Jasjeet Bindra

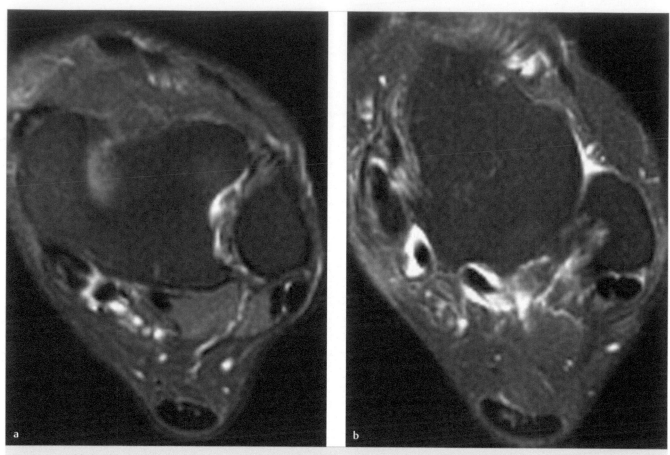

Fig. 65.1 Axial fat-suppressed, proton density-weighted, MR images at the level of medial malleolus and inferior to it **(a, b)** demonstrate two subtendons of posterior tibial tendon resulting from a split tear. There is fluid in the tendon sheaths of all three medial tendons.

■ Clinical History

A 72-year-old woman with progressive flat foot deformity (▶ Fig. 65.1).

■ Key Finding

Medial tendon abnormality at ankle.

■ Top 3 Differential Diagnoses

- **Posterior tibial tendon disease:** Dysfunction of the posterior tibial tendon can be seen with abnormalities ranging from tenosynovitis and tendinosis to partial or complete rupture of the tendon. Acute tenosynovitis is more commonly seen in young athletic individuals, whereas chronic tears are more common in middle-aged and elderly women. On MR imaging, fluid is seen within the tendon sheath with normal signal intensity and morphology of the tendon in tenosynovitis. With tendinosis, there is heterogeneity and thickening of the tendon. Chronic posterior tibial tendon rupture is commonly noted behind the medial malleolus, secondary to friction encountered from the medial malleolus, and is associated with progressive flatfoot deformity. Acute tears are less common and are usually seen at the insertion of the tendon on the navicular bone.
- **Flexor hallucis longus (FHL) tendon injury:** FHL tendon is among the least commonly injured tendons of the foot and ankle. The tendon is susceptible to injuries as it passes through the fibro-osseous tunnel between the lateral and medial talar tubercles. Entrapment may occur from an enlarged ostrigonum, especially in people who engage in activities that involve repetitive weight-bearing with plantar flexion, such as ballet dancing. Repetitive friction may cause chronic or stenosing tenosynovitis, tendinosis, and tears. The tendon is also susceptible to tenosynovitis and tendinosis secondary to its long course, most commonly at the tibiotalar joint, followed by distal disease at the hallux sesamoids, and at the intersection with the flexor digitorum longus in the region of the knot of Henry. The tendon sheath of the FHL can communicate with the ankle joint, so it is important not to mistake a small amount of physiologic fluid in the tendon sheath with an abnormality. Large amount of synovial fluid surrounding an otherwise intact tendon with disproportionately small amount of fluid in the ankle joint is characteristic of chronic synovitis. FHL tendon abnormalities are best seen on axial and sagittal MR images.
- **Flexor digitorum longus (FDL) tendon injury:** Isolated injuries to the FDL tendon are rare but are typically associated with penetrating injuries to the forefoot where the tendon is quite superficial. Spectrum of pathologic conditions also include tendinosis and tendon tear and may clinically mimic plantar fasciitis or tarsal tunnel syndrome. Hammertoe or cross-toe deformities and plantar plate injuries can predispose to tenosynovitis. Other less common causes of FDL disease include overuse, direct trauma, inflammatory arthropathies, and infection. Intersection syndrome may occur at the knot of Henry. On MR, imaging findings of tenosynovitis include peritendinous fluid and edema surrounding the tendon.

■ Diagnosis

Chronic posterior tibial tendon dysfunction with split tear.

✓ Pearls

- The normal posterior tibial tendon at the level of the medial malleolus is about three times larger than the adjacent FDL tendon.
- Sequelae of chronic injury to the posterior tibial tendon include progressive flatfoot deformity and sinus tarsi syndrome.
- Intersection syndrome in the midfoot occurs where the FHL and FDL tendons cross at the knot of Henry.

■ Suggested Readings

Donovan A, Rosenberg ZS, Bencardino JT, et al. Plantar tendons of the foot: MR imaging and US. Radiographics. 2013; 33(7):2065–2085

Rosenberg ZS, Beltran J, Bencardino JT. MD. MR Imaging of the ankle and foot. Radiographics. 2000; 20:S153–S179

Case 66

Jasjeet Bindra

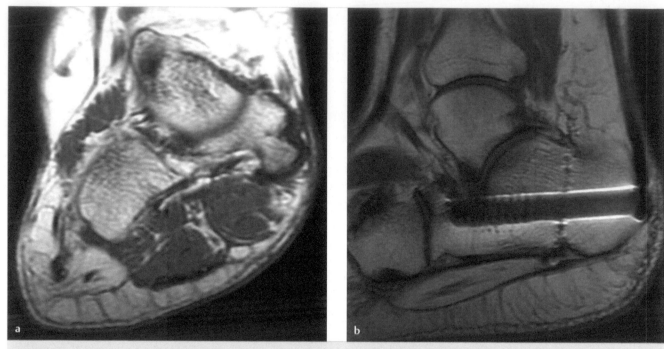

Fig. 66.1 Coronal T1-weighted, MR image of the ankle **(a)** shows atrophy and fatty infiltration of abductor digiti minimi muscle. Sagittal T1-weighted image of the same ankle **(b)** demonstrates calcaneal osteotomy with hardware along with fatty atrophy of abductor digiti minimi muscle.

■ Clinical History

A 55-year-old male with heel pain (▶ Fig. 66.1).

■ Key Finding

Nerve entrapment around ankle and foot.

■ Top 3 Differential Diagnoses

• **Posterior tibial nerve:** Posterior tibial nerve (PTN) and its branches are most commonly entrapped in the tarsal tunnel. The tarsal tunnel is a fibro-osseous space that extends from the posteromedial aspect of the ankle to the plantar aspect of the foot. In the tarsal tunnel, the PTN trifurcates into its terminal branches—medial and lateral plantar nerves and the medial calcaneal nerve. The major mechanisms of neuropathy in tarsal tunnel are compression and tension. Tarsal tunnel syndrome typically results in paresthesia or burning pain at the plantar aspect of the foot and toes. Muscle atrophy is a late outcome. The medial plantar nerve may be compressed adjacent to the master knot of Henry (anatomic crossover of the flexor hallucis longus and flexor digitorum longus tendons). This can be caused by repetitive microtrauma in runners, leading to "jogger's foot" with paresthesias at the medial side of the sole. The inferior calcaneal nerve, a branch of the lateral plantar nerve, provides motor branches to the abductor digitiminimi muscle. Compression of this nerve (Baxter neuropathy) may occur secondary to plantar fasciitis and can manifest as isolated fatty atrophy of the abductor digitiminimi muscle on MRI.

• **Digital nerves:** Morton neuroma is a well-known disorder of the digital nerves. It results from chronic nerve entrapment under the intermetatarsal ligament, typically at second or third web spaces. On coronal MR images, Morton neuroma may be seen as low-to-intermediate signal intensity, teardrop-shaped mass, extending toward the plantar aspect of the web space.

• **Sural nerve:** At the ankle, the sural nerve first runs lateral to the Achilles tendon, and then inferior to the peroneal tendon sheath. It is quite thin and difficult to identify at MR imaging. It can be localized by finding the lesser saphenous vein, as the nerve should lie adjacent to the vein. Nerve entrapment can occur secondary to acute trauma-like fracture of fifth metatarsal base, secondary to callus, or scarring due to trauma or surgery. Sural neuropathy presents with pain and paresthesia of the lateral border of the ankle and foot.

■ Additional Diagnostic Consideration

• **Deep peroneal nerve:** The deep peroneal nerve (DPN) crosses anterior to the ankle, usually adjacent and lateral to the anterior tibial artery. It divides into a medial sensory branch for the first interspace and a lateral motor branch for the extensor digitorum brevis muscle. The nerve may be compressed at the inferior extensor retinaculum, where the extensor hallucis longus tendon crosses it, resulting in anterior tarsal tunnel syndrome.

■ Diagnosis

Baxter neuropathy.

✓ Pearls

• Baxter neuropathy can manifest as isolated atrophy of the abductor digitiminimi.
• Lesser saphenous vein can be used to localize sural nerve lateral to the Achilles tendon.

• Morton neuroma is typically a low-to-intermediate signal intensity mass, extending inferiorly from the webspace.

■ Suggested Readings

De Maeseneer M, Madani H, Lenchik L, et al. Normal anatomy and compression areas of nerves of the foot and ankle: US and MR imaging with anatomic correlation. Radiographics. 2015; 35(5):1469–1482

Delfaut EM, Demondion X, Bieganski A, Thiron MC, Mestdagh H, Cotten A. Imaging of foot and ankle nerve entrapment syndromes: from well-demonstrated to unfamiliar sites. Radiographics. 2003; 23(3):613–623

Case 67

Paulomi Kanzaria and Jasjeet Bindra

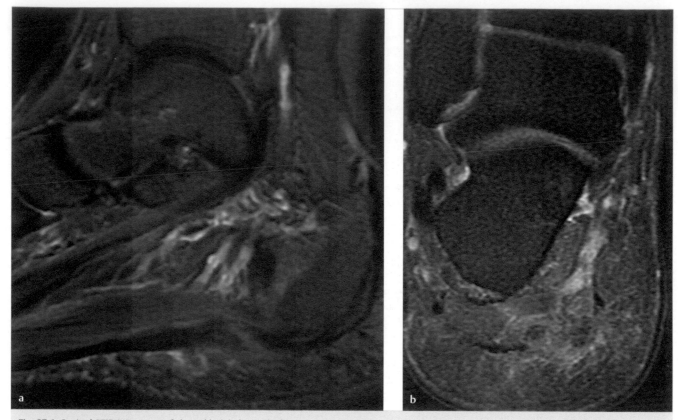

Fig. 67.1 Sagittal STIR MR image of the ankle **(a)** shows thickening and focal disruption in the central cord of plantar fascia. Coronal fat-suppressed, proton density-weighted MR image of the ankle **(b)** reveals focal area of increased signal along the medial aspect of central cord of plantar fascia.

■ **Clinical History**

A 45-year-old female with acute on chronic heel pain (▶ Fig. 67.1).

■ Key Finding

Plantar fascial abnormality.

■ Top 3 Differential Diagnoses

- **Plantar fasciitis:** Plantar fasciitis is the most common cause of plantar heel pain. This condition can arise either from stress of repetitive trauma or as an enthesopathy in association with seronegative spondyloarthropathies. Radiographs may reveal a plantar calcaneal spur. MR imaging characteristics include fusiform fascial thickening that involves the proximal portion, extending to the calcaneal insertion. The normal plantar fascia appears as a thin (2–4 mm), low-signal intensity band. In plantar fasciitis, there is increased signal intensity of the proximal plantar fascia, with intermediate signal on T1-weighted and proton density images, and high-signal on T2 weighted and short tau inversion recovery (STIR) sequences. Associated MR imaging findings include edema of the adjacent fat pad and underlying soft tissues, and focal bone marrow edema within the medial calcaneal tuberosity. Plantar fasciitis related to seronegative arthropathies is usually bilateral.
- **Plantar fascia tear/rupture:** This relatively uncommon condition is most commonly seen in competitive athletes who are engaged in sports like running and jumping, but may also occur as a result of repetitive minor trauma to the aponeurosis in recreational running and jumping. Spontaneous rupture of plantar aponeurosis can be seen in patients with prior plantar fasciitis, especially in patients treated with local steroid injections. Traumatic tears manifest as sudden plantar heel pain, and a palpable tender mass is detected at the site of injury. On MRI, there is partial or complete interruption of the normally low-signal intensity fascia, with areas of increased signal intensity on T2-weighted and STIR images, likely representing edema and hemorrhage. Perifascial fluid accumulations are commonly seen on T2-weighted images. Tears of the plantar fascia commonly involve the underlying flexor digitorum brevis muscle.
- **Plantar fibromatosis (Ledderhose disease):** Plantar fibromatosis is a relatively uncommon, benign, but locally invasive lesion, characterized by fibrous proliferation arising from the plantar fascia. It can be associated with other superficial fibromatosis, mainly palmar fibromatosis. Central and medial portions of the plantar fascia are usually involved. On MRI, lesions appear as single or multiple nodular areas of thickening of the inferior margin of the plantar fascia, usually measuring less than 3 cm. Nodules have low-to-intermediate signal intensity on T1- and T2-weighted images. Larger lesions tend to have a heterogeneous signal intensity. A spectrum of enhancement patterns corresponding to the cellular portions of the lesion may be seen. Infiltration of the plantar musculature can be seen in aggressive or deep fibromatosis.

■ Diagnosis

Plantar fascial tear.

✓ Pearls

- Plantar fasciitis is seen as thickening and increased signal of proximal part of plantar fascia.
- Plantar fascial rupture presents as focal interruption of aponeurosis with surrounding edema.
- Plantar fibromas are low-to-intermediate signal intensity lesions and can show variable enhancement.

■ Suggested Readings

Narváez JA, Narváez J, Ortega R, Aguilera C, Sánchez A, Andía E. Painful heel: MR imaging findings. Radiographics. 2000; 20(2):333–352

Theodorou DJ, Theodorou SJ, Farooki S, Kakitsubata Y, Resnick D. Disorders of the plantar aponeurosis: a spectrum of MR imaging findings. AJR Am J Roentgenol. 2001; 176(1):97–104

Case 68

Paulomi Kanzaria and Jasjeet Bindra

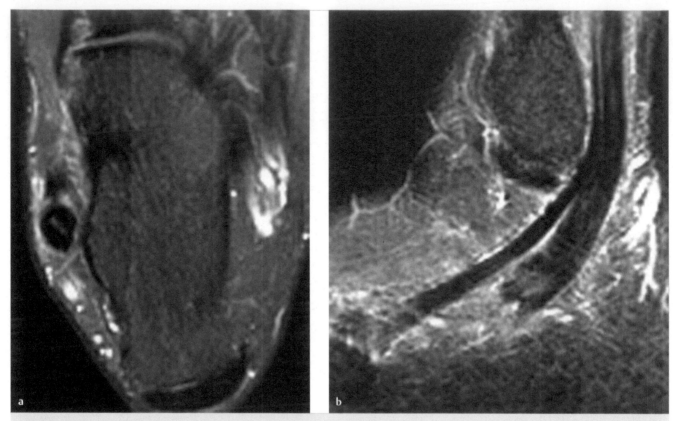

Fig. 68.1 Axial fat-suppressed, proton density-weighted, MR image of the ankle **(a)** shows a high-signal cleft in the peroneus longus tendon. Sagittal STIR MR image **(b)** of the same ankle shows the cleft along its length.

■ Clinical History

A 55-year-old male with chronic lateral ankle pain (▶ Fig. 68.1).

■ Key Finding

Peroneal tendon disease at the ankle.

■ Top 3 Differential Diagnoses

- **Peroneal tenosynovitis:** Acute peroneal tenosynovitis is commonly seen in ballet dancers and in athletes who resume activity after a layoff. It is thought to be secondary to increased stress around fixed pulleys such as the retromalleolar groove, peroneal tubercle, or undersurface of the cuboid bone. In chronic peroneal tenosynovitis, MR imaging shows fluid accumulation in the common peroneal tendon sheath. A sliver of fluid within the tendon sheath can be seen normally. However, distension of the tendon sheath with circumferential synovial fluid indicates tenosynovitis. Acute calcaneofibular ligamentous tear can mimic tenosynovitis with fluid in the sheath.

  Stenosing tenosynovitis occurs with synovial proliferation, and fibrosis around the tendons prevents their free excursion. MR imaging shows thickened synovium with linear areas of intermediate- or low-signal intensity within the synovial fluid.

- **Peroneus brevis (PB) tendon tear (peroneal split syndrome):** Peroneus brevis is susceptible to degenerative tears due to its position between the bony retromalleolar groove and the peroneus longus tendon, where it gets compressed with dorsiflexion of the foot. Axial MR images reveal a typical C-shaped configuration or boomerang shape of the torn tendon, with medial and lateral limbs partially enveloping the peroneus longus tendon and thinning of the tendon anterior to the peroneal longus tendon. The presence of accessory peroneus quartus muscle can cause crowding in the retromalleolar groove, predisposing to PB tendon disease.

- **Peroneus longus (PL) tendon tear:** PL tears are often associated with PB tendon tears at the retromalleolar groove. Isolated tears of PL tendon are more frequently seen at the midfoot. Tendon rupture may be associated with avulsion fracture of the os peroneum. On MR imaging, high- or intermediate-signal intensity is seen at the tear site, while tendon ruptures show complete discontinuity of fibers. Split tears are frequently seen with a hypertrophied peroneal tubercle, and MR imaging may also show a hypertrophic peroneal tubercle and bone marrow edema of the tubercle. Calcaneal fractures predispose to partial tears, dislocation, and entrapment of both PL and PB tendons. Dislocation of the peroneal tendons can also occur secondary to injury of the superficial peroneal retinaculum.

■ Diagnosis

Peroneus longus tear.

✓ Pearls

- Fluid accumulation in the peroneal tendon sheath, secondary to calcaneofibular ligament tear, may mimic chronic peroneal tenosynovitis.

- The peroneal tendons may be dislocated, secondary to injury to the superior peroneal retinaculum.
- Peroneus longus tendon abnormalities may be associated with painful os peroneum syndrome (POPS).

■ Suggested Readings

Donovan A, Rosenberg ZS, Bencardino JT, et al. Plantar tendons of the foot: MR imaging and US. Radiographics. 2013; 33(7):2065–2085

Rosenberg ZS, Beltran J, Bencardino JT. MD. MR Imaging of the ankle and foot. Radiographics. 2000; 20:S153–S179

Wang X-T, Rosenberg ZS, Mechlin MB, Schweitzer ME. Normal variants and diseases of the peroneal tendons and superior peroneal retinaculum: MR imaging features. Radiographics. 2005; 25(3):587–602. PubMed PMID: 15888611

Case 69

Jasjeet Bindra

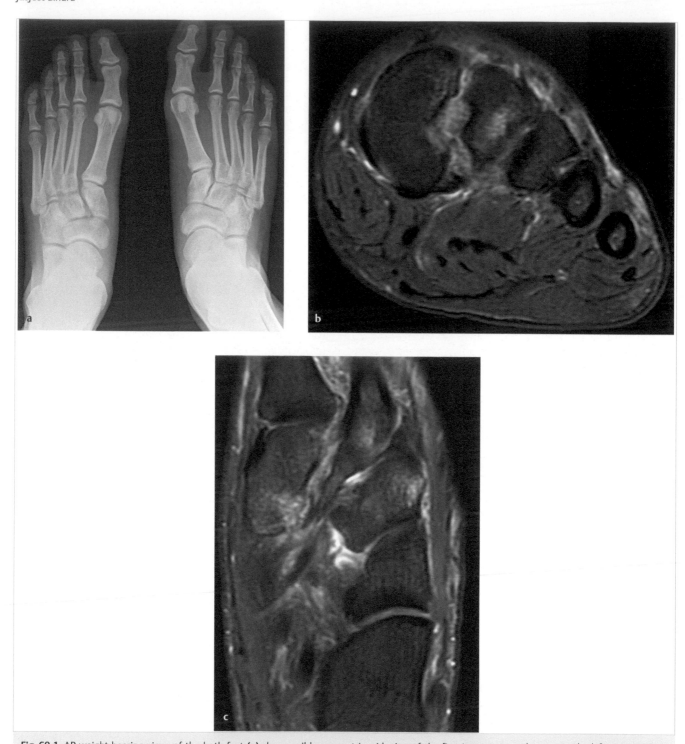

Fig. 69.1 AP weight-bearing view of the both feet **(a)** shows mild asymmetric widening of the first intermetatarsal space on the left. Coronal fat-suppressed, T2-weighted and axial fat-suppressed, proton density-weighted, MR images **(b, c)** of the midfoot view show edema and disruption of ligament complex between medial cuneiform and second metatarsal base.

■ Clinical History

A 68-year-old female with twisting injury of the foot, followed by pain and inability to bear weight (▶ Fig. 69.1).

■ Key Finding

Midfoot ligamentous or osseous injury.

■ Top 3 Differential Diagnoses

- **Lisfranc joint complex injury:** The Lisfranc joint consists of the tarsometatarsal (TMT) joint complex. The stability of the Lisfranc joint complex is derived from osseous relationships and ligamentous support. Ligamentous structures can be divided into tarsometatarsal, intertarsal, and intermetatarsal ligaments. The Lisfranc ligament joins the second metatarsal base to the medial cuneiform, securing the medial column to the intermediate and lateral columns. The Lisfranc ligament has three components—the relatively weak dorsal ligament, interosseous ligament, and the strong plantar ligament. Traumatic injuries to the joint complex can occur in both high-energy and low-energy trauma. High-energy trauma is usually secondary to motor vehicle collisions or falls from a height. Low-energy injuries or midfoot sprains are more difficult to diagnose. Findings on radiography could include dorsal soft tissue swelling, small avulsion fractures at the base of the second metatarsal or first cuneiform, and signs of subtle malalignment at second TMT. MR imaging permits direct evaluation of ligamentous and osseous injuries. Primary signs of ligamentous injury include ligament irregularity or frank disruption and abnormal signal intensity within the ligament.
- **Chopart joint injury:** The Chopart joint complex is formed by calcaneocuboid and talocalcaneonavicular joints. It is stabilized by multiple ligaments, including the spring ligament, bifurcate ligament, and long and short plantar ligaments. Traumatic injuries of the Chopart joint range from pure ligamentous injuries and small avulsion fractures to rare fracture dislocations. The bifurcate ligament is a dorsolateral ligament with two components: the medial calcaneonavicular ligament and lateral calcaneocuboid ligament. These can be visualized on the sagittal MR images. Tiny avulsion fractures at the anterior process of calcaneus or cuboid may indicate injury of the bifurcate ligament. The spring ligament, also called the plantar calcaneonavicular ligament, supports the head of the talus and stabilizes the medial longitudinal arch. Pathology of spring ligament is usually degenerative but can occasionally be traumatic. Marrow contusions and ligamentous disruptions at the Chopart joint can be optimally visualized with MR imaging.
- **Navicular fracture:** Acute fractures of navicular are relatively infrequent. Dorsal avulsion fractures are the most common navicular fractures, typically related to plantar flexion injury. Navicular is the most common midfoot bone involved with stress fractures, which typically involves the middle third because of its sparse blood supply. Radiographs have low-sensitivity. CT and MR have much higher sensitivity.

■ Additional Diagnostic Consideration

- **Cuboid fracture:** Isolated cuboid fractures are rare. A nutcracker mechanism has been described in the setting of eversion injury, in which the cuboid is crushed between the fourth and fifth metatarsal bases and the anterior process of calcaneus.

■ Diagnosis

Lisfranc joint complex injury.

✓ Pearls

- The Lisfranc ligament extends between the medial cuneiform and second metatarsal base.
- Bifurcate ligament can be visualized on sagittal MR images of ankle or midfoot.
- Stress fractures of navicular most commonly involve the middle third because of its sparse blood supply.

■ Suggested Readings

Benirschke SK, Meinberg E, Anderson SA, Jones CB, Cole PA. Fractures and dislocations of the midfoot: Lisfranc and Chopart injuries. J Bone Joint Surg Am. 2012; 94(14):1325–1337

Tafur M, Rosenberg ZS, Bencardino JT. MR imaging of the midfoot including Chopart and Lisfranc joint complexes. Magn Reson Imaging Clin N Am. 2017; 25(1): 95–125

Case 70

Jasjeet Bindra

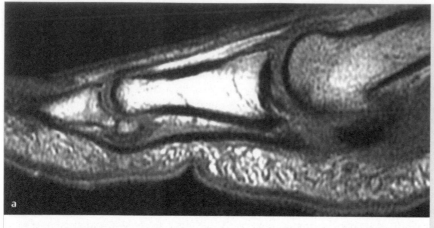
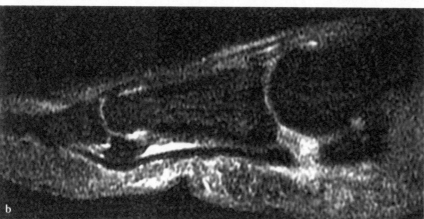

Fig. 70.1 Sagittal T1-weighted and STIR MR images of the great toe (**a, b**) show a tear of the medial sesamoid phalangeal ligament with slight proximal retraction of the medial hallux sesamoid.

■ Clinical History

A 22-year-old athlete with acute pain and inability to bear weight following a hyperextension injury to great toe (▶ Fig. 70.1).

■ **Key Finding**

Hallux sesamoid abnormality.

■ **Top 3 Differential Diagnoses**

• **Plantar plate injury (Turf toe):** Turf toe, a hyperextension injury of the first metatarsophalangeal (MTP) joint, is most commonly seen in football players who play on artificial turf and wear lightweight, flexible shoes. It may result in partial or complete disruption of the plantar plate, a fibrocartilaginous thickening of the plantar aspect of capsule of the first MTP. This plantar plate in conjunction with the hallucal sesamoid complex and adjacent tendinous structures play a vital role in providing stability to the first MTP joint. The injury is usually located just distal to the sesamoids and may allow sesamoid retraction or proximal migration. Radiographs may demonstrate soft-tissue swelling, avulsion fractures, sesamoid fractures, diastasis of bipartite sesamoids, or proximal migration of sesamoids. The plantar plate and hallucal sesamoids are best analyzed on sagittal and coronal short-axis planes on MRI. On MR, there may be soft-tissue edema, partial or complete disruption of plantar plate, and associated sesamoid pathology like edema, fracture, diastasis or proximal migration of sesamoids. Concomitant tendinous and cartilaginous injuries may also be seen.

• **Sesamoiditis:** Sesamoiditis is a nonspecific term referring to any painful inflammatory condition of the sesamoid bones.

Sesamoiditis occurs in the setting of repetitive trauma to the plantar aspect of the forefoot, or it may occur in the context of osteoarthritis, inflammatory arthropathy or avascular necrosis (AVN). Radiographs may be normal or may demonstrate fragmentation and sclerosis of the involved sesamoid. MR imaging will demonstrate diffuse marrow edema. MR imaging permits more specific diagnosis of fracture, AVN or underlying pathology, and thus imaging modality of choice.

• **Sesamoid fracture:** Most acute sesamoid fractures involve the tibial sesamoid. Radiographic signs include irregular margins, with unequal separation of sesamoid fragments, absence of similar findings on the contralateral side, or evidence of attempted healing. It can be difficult to differentiate a bipartite or multipartite sesamoid from a fracture on radiography, and in those cases, CT or MR can help. A bipartite sesamoid will demonstrate rounded fragments with smooth sclerotic margins. On MR imaging, the fracture will be seen as low-signal intensity line on T1-weighted imaging, and as high- or low-signal intensity line on T2-weighted imaging. MR will also show diffuse marrow edema.

■ **Additional Diagnostic Consideration**

• **Sesamoid AVN:** Avascular necrosis of hallucal sesamoids is relatively uncommon. Repetitive trauma is the probable cause in most cases. Radiographs may show fragmentation, stippled appearance, and increased density. Early MR imaging usually shows marrow edema, but late MR imaging will show fragmentation and mixed signal on T1- and T2-weighted images from sclerosis intermixed with edema.

■ **Diagnosis**

Turf toe.

✓ **Pearls**

• Plantar plate is best analyzed on sagittal and coronal (short axis) MR images.
• A fractured sesamoid will demonstrate irregular, nonsclerotic margins of the fragments.

• Early MR findings of AVN are similar to the findings of sesamoiditis and stress related changes.

■ **Suggested Readings**

Ashman CJ, Klecker RJ, Yu JS. Forefoot pain involving the metatarsal region: differential diagnosis with MR imaging. Radiographics. 2001; 21(6):1425–1440

Sanders TG, Rathur SK. Imaging of painful conditions of the hallucal sesamoid complex and plantar capsular structures of the first metatarsophalangeal joint. Radiol Clin North Am. 2008; 46(6):1079–1092, vii

Case 71

Robert D. Boutin

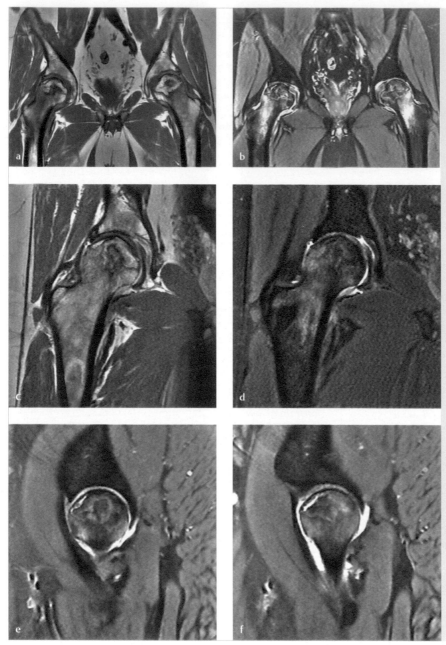

Fig. 71.1 Coronal T1-weighted (**a**) and coronal fat-suppressed T2 (**b**) images of the pelvis show bilateral geographic signal with a sclerotic-appearing rim in the femoral heads on T1 imaging, and extensive adjacent bone edema extending into the intertrochanteric regions. Small field-of-view coronal proton density-weighted (**c**), coronal fat-suppressed T2-weighted (**d**), sagittal fat-suppressed T2-weighted (**e**) images of the right hip show subtle (<2 mm) flattening of the subchondral bone plate anterolaterally. Sagittal fat-suppressed T2 images of the right (**e**) and left (**f**) hips show that the femoral head collapse is accompanied by a subchondral crescent of hyperintense signal that is bilaterally symmetric.

■ Clinical History

A 34-year-old man with a history of "unremarkable radiographs 3 months ago" and continued bilateral hip pain (▶ Fig. 71.1).

■ Key Finding

Subchondral crescent sign–Roentgen classic.

■ Diagnosis

Osteonecrosis (AVN): Osteonecrosis is defined as ischemic death of the cellular constituents of bone and marrow. Other related terms include "bone infarct" (usually reserved for metaphyseal and diaphyseal involvement) and avascular necrosis (AVN, commonly used for subarticular involvement).

AVN has a propensity to occur in the femoral head, presumably because of a potentially precarious blood supply. Pathogenic mechanisms responsible for AVN generally involve 1. traumatic disruption of blood vessels (e.g., femoral neck fracture, hip dislocation, or hip subluxation) or 2. "systemic" causes (e.g., intraosseous hypertension with vascular stasis or thromboembolic abnormalities). Risk factors associated with nontraumatic AVN include corticosteroids, alcoholism, pancreatitis, hemoglobinopathies, radiation therapy, and barotrauma. Importantly, the nontraumatic conditions that are associated with AVN generally place *multiple* bones at risk for osteonecrosis.

With femoral head AVN, radiographs may be falsely negative, especially prior to collapse of the subchondral bone plate (pre-collapse radiographic sensitivity and specificity are generally substantially <70% and <90%, respectively). Therefore, a high-index of suspicion for AVN is appropriate when a younger patient (age <50 years) presents with hip pain and negative radiographs. MRI is generally the next diagnostic imaging test of choice, with a sensitivity and specificity for diagnosing femoral head AVN substantially >90%.

On MRI, femoral head AVN is commonly seen as a demarcated zone of altered signal that extends typically to the superior subchondral bone plate and has a serpentine border of low-signal.

Bone marrow edema (BME) adjacent to areas of AVN is strongly associated with pain (compared to "clinically silent" AVN). BME often indicates femoral head collapse (often subtle) is present. With femoral head collapse, joint-preserving procedures (e.g., core decompression with or without adjuvants) are not effective; total hip arthroplasty then becomes the most reliable long-term treatment.

There is no universal consensus on a staging system for femoral head AVN. Therefore, reports should document the most important findings of AVN, regardless of the staging system: (1) femoral head collapse (e.g., presence and extent); (2) size of AVN (e.g., estimate of percentage of femoral head affected); (3) acetabular changes (e.g., subchondral cysts and sclerosis). The crescent sign is also a key finding, since it may indicate femoral head collapse has occurred.

✓ Pearls

- Osteonecrosis is highly associated with hip trauma, chronic corticosteroid use, and alcoholism, as well as many other less common conditions (e.g., metabolic and coagulation disorders).
- Femoral head AVN can be present in young adults with hip pain and normal radiographs; therefore, a high index of clinical suspicion may be appropriate.

- MRI may be appropriate to diagnose femoral head AVN prior to collapse. Early treatment improves the chances of hip survival (up to 80% at 5 years).

■ Suggested Readings

Boutin RD. MR imaging of the hip. In: McCarthy SM, ed. RSNA Categorical Course in Diagnostic Radiology. Chicago, Illinois: Radiological Society of North America. 1999;201–217

Chee CG, Cho J, Kang Y, et al. Diagnostic accuracy of digital radiography for the diagnosis of osteonecrosis of the femoral head, revisited. Acta Radiol. 2019; 60(8): 969–976

Grecula MJ. CORR Insights: which classification system is most useful for classifying osteonecrosis of the femoral head? Clin Orthop Relat Res. 2018; 476(6): 1250–1252

Lamb JN, Holton C, O'Connor P, Giannoudis PV. Avascular necrosis of the hip. BMJ. 2019; 365:l2178

Larson E, Jones LC, Goodman SB, Koo KH, Cui Q. Early-stage osteonecrosis of the femoral head: where are we and where are we going in year 2018? Int Orthop. 2018; 42(7):1723–1728

Steinberg ME, Oh SC, Khoury V, Udupa JK, Steinberg DR. Lesion size measurement in femoral head necrosis. Int Orthop. 2018; 42(7):1585–1591

Case 72

Robert D. Boutin and Jasjeet Bindra

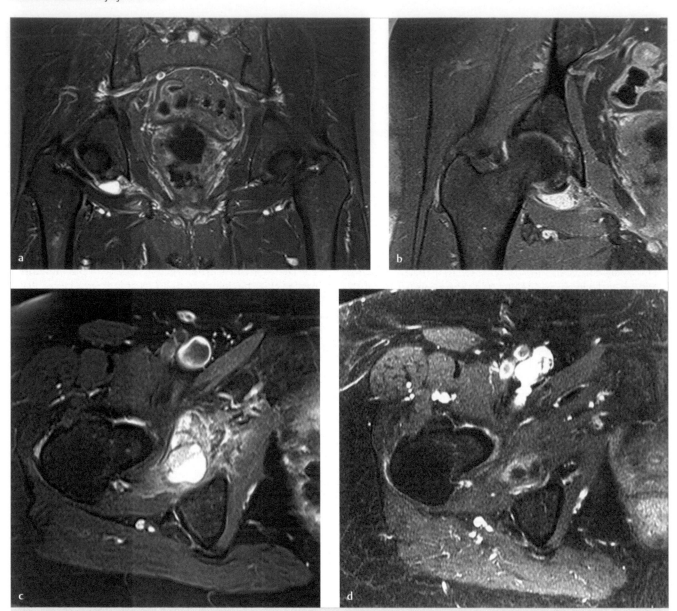

Fig. 72.1 Coronal fat-suppressed T2-weighted **(a, b)** images show a rounded collection of fluid signal inferomedial to the right hip joint, with a thin pedicle extending back to the hip joint. Axial fat-suppressed T2-weighted **(c)** image shows the rounded collection of fluid-like signal inferomedial to the right hip joint at the baseline. At follow-up imaging 6 months later, the axial postcontrast fat-suppressed T1-weighted **(d)** image shows the lesion is smaller and displays only a mild peripheral rim of enhancement.

■ Clinical History

A 78-year-old woman with a history of a lung cancer and right hip pain (▸ Fig. 72.1).

■ Key Finding

Fluid collection at the inferomedial aspect of the hip–Roentgen classic.

■ Diagnosis

Obturator externus bursa fluid collection: The obturator externus bursa is located inferomedial to the hip joint, at the superior aspect of the obturator externus muscle.

The externus bursa is a synovial-lined potential space or recess that communicates with the hip joint through a narrow opening between the ischiofemoral capsular ligament (superiorly) and the zona orbicularis (inferiorly).

Like the well-known iliopsoas bursa, the obturator externus bursa normally communicates with the hip joint in a minority of individuals. With a chronic hip joint effusion, however, the frequency of fluid decompressing into these adjacent bursae increases. Chronic hip joint effusions can be seen with many conditions, including osteoarthritis, osteonecrosis, and synovial osteochondromatosis. Direct irritation of the obturator externus bursa might also occur with an obturator externus impingement syndrome between the obturator externus muscle and the acetabular cup after total hip arthroplasty.

Periarticular bursal fluid collections in the obturator externus bursa are less common than in the iliopsoas bursa, but they are not rare. With MR arthrography, communication between the hip joint and the obturator externus bursa is observed in 6% of patients.

✓ Pearls

- Fluid may collect in the obturator externus bursa, which is located at the inferomedial aspect of the hip joint.
- Distension of the obturator externus bursa may be an incidental finding or may be secondary to a chronic increase in the intra-articular hip joint pressure that causes fluid decompression into the adjacent obturator externus bursa.
- The characteristic location and appearance of communication between the hip joint and the obturator externus bursa helps in making a confident diagnosis, and avoids misdiagnosis of a ganglion, paralabral cyst, or neoplasm.

■ Suggested Readings

Gudena R, Alzahrani A, Railton P, Powell J, Ganz R. The anatomy and function of the obturator externus. Hip Int. 2015; 25(5):424–427

Kassarjian A, Llopis E, Schwartz RB, Bencardino JT. Obturator externus bursa: prevalence of communication with the hip joint and associated intra-articular findings in 200 consecutive hip MR arthrograms. Eur Radiol. 2009; 19(11):2779–2782

Müller M, Dewey M, Springer I, Perka C, Tohtz S. Relationship between cup position and obturator externus muscle in total hip arthroplasty. J Orthop Surg Res. 2010; 5:44

Robinson P, White LM, Agur A, Wunder J, Bell RS. Obturator externus bursa: anatomic origin and MR imaging features of pathologic involvement. Radiology. 2003; 228(1):230–234

Robinson P, White LM, Kandel R, Bell RS, Wunder JS. Primary synovial osteochondromatosis of the hip: extracapsular patterns of spread. Skeletal Radiol. 2004; 33(4):210–215

Case 73

Robert D. Boutin

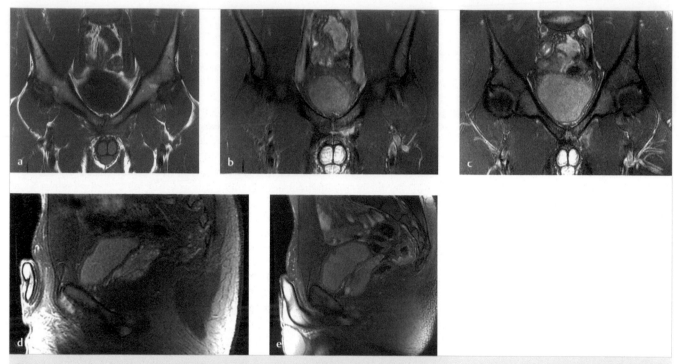

Fig. 73.1 Coronal T1-weighted **(a)** and coronal fat-suppressed T2-weighted **(b, c)** images show a T2-hyperintense signal completely disrupting the adductor longus tendon and the adjacent aponeurotic plate attachment at the pubic body on the left. A cleft of T2-hyperintense signal also undermines the midline pubic plate. On the left of midline, sagittal fat-suppressed T2-weighted **(d)** image confirms the presence of focal hyperintense signal undermining the insertion of the rectus abdominis–adductor aponeurosis onto the pubic body. On the right of midline, sagittal fat-suppressed T2-weighted **(e)** image shows the normal low-signal intensity insertion of the rectus abdominis–adductor aponeurosis at the anterior aspect of the pubic bone.

▪ Clinical History

A 21-year-old elite college football player with pubic symphysis pain, particularly on the left (▶ Fig. 73.1).

■ Key Finding

Cleft of T2-hyperintense signal at the attachment of the rectus abdominis–adductor aponeurosis–Roentgen classic.

■ Diagnosis

Tear at the rectus abdominis–adductor aponeurosis: The center of the "musculoskeletal core" is the pubic symphysis, with adjacent osseous, musculotendinous, aponeurotic, and ligamentous structures that help maintain normal biomechanical stability.

The interconnectedness of the musculoskeletal core is an important concept, because a "central core injury" at or anterior to the pubic symphysis can destabilize the pubic symphysis region, resulting in a vicious cycle of progressively abnormal biomechanics associated with athletic pubalgia. Such groin pain associated with sports is typically seen with shearing forces imposed by kicking, stretching, or cutting maneuvers (e.g., soccer, hockey, or football).

There are multiple causes of athletic pubalgia, including core injuries due to detachment at the pubic insertion of a strong anterior prepubic aponeurosis. Core injuries may originate in the *midline* at the "midline pubic plate" (a thin fibrous aponeurosis anterior to the pubic symphysis) or *unilaterally* at the adjacent "rectus abdominis–adductor aponeurosis" (formed by the distal rectus abdominis and proximal adductor longus fibers, converging to attach to the anterior periosteum of the pubic bones).

The location and extent of injuries in this region vary, and therefore high-resolution images and knowledge of anatomy are important. Focused sonographic and radiographic techniques may be used in diagnostic evaluations among many athletes, but MRI is often utilized to simultaneously display all relevant bone and soft-tissue structures.

On MRI, a cleft of T2-hyperintense signal undermining the normal midline or paramedian aponeurotic attachment is a common finding, diagnostic of a detachment or tear. With athletic pubalgia, additional imaging findings affecting treatment and prognosis include adjacent tendinosis, myotendinous strain, tendon tear, stress reaction (bone marrow edema), stress fracture, and osteoarthritis. Concomitant apophysitis and calcific tendinitis are also possible.

✓ Pearls

- Pain in the pubic region can result from a wide array of disorders involving osteoarticular, musculotendinous, aponeurotic and ligamentous structures, as well as gastrointestinal, neurologic, urologic, and gynecologic sources.
- Musculoskeletal core injuries in athletes are commonly centered at the aponeurotic plate inserting onto the anterior symphyseal region, particularly involving the rectus abdominis and adductor longus.
- For athletes with pubalgia, treatment choice and prognosis (e.g., return to play) are strongly influenced by the location, extent, and chronicity of imaging findings.

■ Suggested Readings

Agten CA, Sutter R, Buck FM, Pfirrmann CW. Hip imaging in athletes: sports imaging series. Radiology. 2016; 280(2):351–369

Delic JA, Ross AB, Blankenbaker DG, Woo K. Incidence and implications of fracture in core muscle injury. Skeletal Radiol. 2019; 48(12):1991–1997

Emblom BA, Mathis T, Aune K. Athletic pubalgia secondary to rectus abdominis adductor longus aponeurotic plate injury: diagnosis, management, and operative treatment of 100 competitive athletes. Orthop J Sports Med. 2018; 6 (9):2325967118798333

Hegazi TM, Belair JA, McCarthy EJ, Roedl JB, Morrison WB. Sports injuries about the hip: what the radiologist should know. Radiographics. 2016; 36(6):1717–1745

Lee SC, Endo Y, Potter HG. Imaging of groin pain: magnetic resonance and ultrasound imaging features. Sports Health. 2017; 9(5):428–435

Mizrahi DJ, Poor AE, Meyers WC, Roedl JB, Zoga AC. Imaging of the pelvis and lower extremity: demystifying uncommon sources of pelvic pain. Radiol Clin North Am. 2018; 56(6):983–995

Case 74

Robert D. Boutin and Jasjeet Bindra

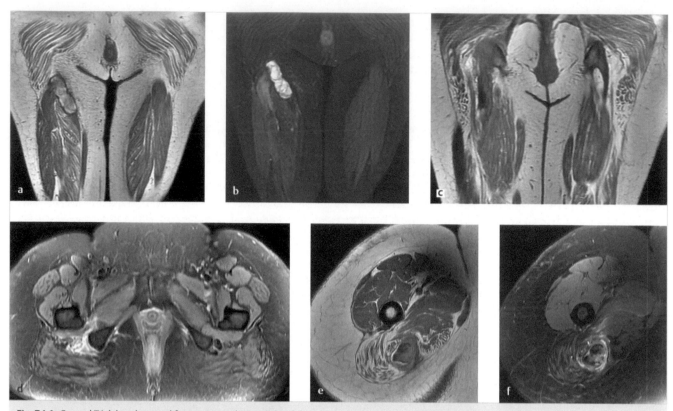

Fig. 74.1 Coronal T1 **(a)** and coronal fat-suppressed T2-weighted **(b)** images at the posterior thigh region show a mildly heterogeneous ovoid lesion of predominantly hyperintense signal, with a thin rim of low T2 signal intensity. Coronal T1 **(c)** and axial fat-suppressed T2-weighted **(d)** images of the pelvis region show abnormally increased signal intensity at the proximal attachment site of the hamstring tendons on the right ischial tuberosity. Small field-of-view axial T1-weighted **(e)** and axial fat-suppressed T2-weighted **(f)** images of the proximal thigh show the retracted tendon stump surrounded by edema and subtle fibrotic tissue (immediately medial to the sciatic nerve).

■ Clinical History

A 66-year-old woman with a history of an injury 1 month earlier and continued pain (▶ Fig. 74.1).

■ Key Finding

Hamstring tendon discontinuity, with subacute hematoma–Roentgen classic.

■ Diagnosis

Complete hamstring tendon tear: The hamstrings consist of the semitendinosus, semimembranosus, and biceps femoris. Proximal hamstring injuries are a common cause of buttock/thigh pain, and they may also be associated with knee flexion weakness and sciatic neuralgia.

The mechanism for these injuries is typically eccentric hamstring contraction during forced flexion of the hip while the knee is extended (e.g., affecting the "leading leg" when inadvertently forced into performing "the splits"). Most commonly, this occurs during sporting activities (e.g., waterskiing or soccer) or injuries during activities of daily living (especially in older patients).

For purposes of diagnosis and management, injuries involving the proximal hamstrings can be classified according to the location and extent (type 1: osseous avulsions; type 2: tear at the musculotendinous junction; type 3: incomplete avulsion from bone; type 4: complete avulsion with only minimal retraction; and type 5: complete avulsion with retraction >2 cm). The pattern of injury is often associated with patient age: osseous avulsion of the ischial apophysis characteristically occurs in adolescent athletes, myotendinous strains often occur in young adult athletes, and tendon disruption at the ischial attachment is most common after age 30.

The initial diagnostic imaging test of choice is often radiography to evaluate an ischial tuberosity avulsion fracture and enthesopathy. To confirm or rule out an injury amenable to surgical repair, additional imaging with MRI (or sonography) should be performed in a timely manner.

On MRI, complete proximal hamstring ruptures are characterized by discontinuity of the tendon(s) with hematoma.

Scarring (often subtle on MRI) can develop relatively rapidly, resulting in loss of myotendinous elasticity and tethering to the sciatic nerve. In contradistinction, partial-thickness tendon tears in older adults are typically displayed as a thin curvilinear band of T2 hyperintensity ("sickle sign") over the surface of the ischial tuberosity footprint, without any tendon retraction.

The most common indication for acute surgical repair (<1 month after injury) is either a two-tendon tear/avulsion with >2 cm retraction or a complete tear/avulsion involving all three tendons. In the chronic setting, surgery is often more technically demanding and results in more complications because of hamstring retraction and fibrosis. Furthermore, because a simple repair procedure may not be effective in the chronic setting, it may be deemed necessary to perform a complex reconstruction procedure (e.g., with Achilles tendon allograft).

Treatment of partial-thickness tears at the proximal hamstring tendon origin varies in accordance with the patient and physician. If patients fail nonoperative management, some surgeons advocate repair of partial hamstring insertion tears using an endoscopic transtendinous repair technique (this is similar to repairs of other partial-thickness, nonretracted tendon tears, such as with the supraspinatus and gluteus medius tendons). However, it is important to recognize that partial-thickness tears at the proximal hamstring tendon origin are very common with aging both in symptomatic and asymptomatic individuals. Symptomatic patients are more likely to have adjacent peritendinous soft-tissue edema and ischial tuberosity bone edema.

✓ Pearls

- After an acute injury, a high-index of clinical suspicion for complete proximal hamstring ruptures is appropriate, because expedited surgery generally results in better outcomes than delayed surgery.
- With recent rupture of hamstring tendons, hematoma formation is common and should not be confused with neoplasm.

- Partial-thickness tears at the proximal hamstring attachment to the ischial tuberosity are very common with aging, with variable management primarily based on patient symptoms.

■ Suggested Readings

Belk JW, Kraeutler MJ, Mei-Dan O, Houck DA, McCarty EC, Mulcahey MK. Return to sport after proximal hamstring tendon repair: a systematic review. Orthop J Sports Med. 2019; 7(6):2325967119853218

Bowman KF, Jr, Cohen SB, Bradley JP. Operative management of partial-thickness tears of the proximal hamstring muscles in athletes. Am J Sports Med. 2013; 41 (6):1363–1371

De Smet AA, Blankenbaker DG, Alsheik NH, Lindstrom MJ. MRI appearance of the proximal hamstring tendons in patients with and without symptomatic proximal hamstring tendinopathy. AJR Am J Roentgenol. 2012; 198(2):418–422

Irger M, Willinger L, Lacheta L, Pogorzelski J, Imhoff AB, Feucht MJ. Proximal hamstring tendon avulsion injuries occur predominately in middle-aged patients with distinct gender differences: epidemiologic analysis of 263 surgically treated cases. Knee Surg Sports Traumatol Arthrosc. 2020; 28(4):1221–1229

Thompson SM, Fung S, Wood DG. The prevalence of proximal hamstring pathology on MRI in the asymptomatic population. Knee Surg Sports Traumatol Arthrosc. 2017; 25(1):108–111

Wood DG, Packham I, Trikha SP, Linklater J. Avulsion of the proximal hamstring origin. J Bone Joint Surg Am. 2008; 90(11):2365–2374

Part 5

Arthropathies

Case 75

Robert D. Boutin and Geoffrey M. Riley

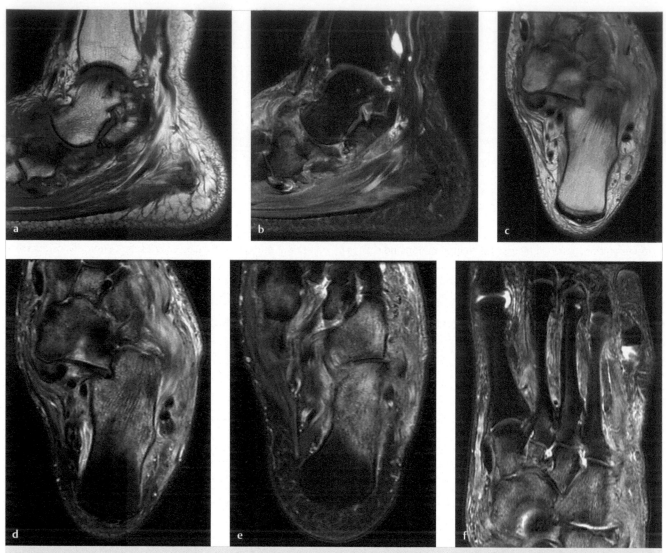

Fig. 75.1 Sagittal T1-weighted (**a**) and sagittal fat-suppressed T2-weighted (**b**) images of the ankle and adjacent foot show the navicular is displaced plantarly relative to the talus and cuneiform bone. Corresponding axial proton density-weighted (**c**), and axial fat-suppressed T2-weighted (**d–f**) images show intense, diffuse edema in the bones and soft tissues that are centered at the midfoot. Notably, there is no soft-tissue ulceration, sinus tract, or fluid collection.

■ Clinical History

A 45-year-old man with bilateral foot swelling, redness, and warmth, but no history of trauma or pain (▶ Fig. 75.1).

■ Key Finding

Intense, diffuse, nontraumatic bone and soft-tissue edema centered at the midfoot.

■ Top 3 Differential Diagnoses

- **Charcot arthropathy:** Charcot arthropathy, also referred to as *neuropathic osteoarthropathy*, is secondary to neuropathy. Reduced proprioception and pain sensation are associated with repetitive microtrauma and alterations in the sympathetic nervous system. Charcot foot is most commonly seen in patients with a history of diabetes mellitus (type I or II) for at least 10 years, but can be due to other causes (e.g., neurosyphilis). Charcot foot can be missed by over 90% of providers prior to foot specialist referral, and it is often debilitating when it is not managed effectively in its early stages.

  Charcot arthropathy classically involves the midfoot, with involvement of the tarsometatarsal and tarsal joints in at least 80% of cases. The "active phase" is characterized initially by inflammation, followed by osseous fragmentation and collapse of the longitudinal arch of the foot. These imaging findings precede more extensive osteoarticular destruction (often with bone proliferation) and deformity (e.g., rocker-bottom foot).

  Radiographs may be normal or nondiagnostic during the early stage of Charcot foot. MRI can be useful for early diagnosis, monitoring disease activity, and assessing complications, such as infection.
- **Infection:** Cellulitis and osteomyelitis commonly cause intense edema in the soft tissues and bone marrow of the foot. Since bone edema on MRI is entirely nonspecific, soft-tissue defects should always be sought. In the absence of deep ulceration or penetrating trauma, foot osteomyelitis is rare. Notably, soft-tissue ulcers may be seen in some patients with Charcot foot, and therefore osteomyelitis and Charcot foot may coexist. In addition to deep ulceration and cellulitis, other MRI findings associated with osteomyelitis may include a sinus tract, abscess, and cortical erosion.

  Clinically, high-laboratory inflammatory marker levels (e.g., erythrocyte sedimentation rate [ESR], C-reactive protein [CRP]) are more consistent with acute infection rather than Charcot foot.
- **Arthritis:** Arthritis, especially osteoarthritis and gout, may target the midfoot and cause bone edema. Clinically, osteoarthritis and gout are not associated with warmth and peripheral neuropathy (unlike Charcot foot).

  With imaging of osteoarthritis, typical findings of degenerative joint disease are seen, including osteophytes and subchondral cysts. With gout, tophi and osseous erosions with overhanging edges are characteristic. With both osteoarthritis and gout, bone fragmentation with severe malalignment (which are typical of advanced Charcot foot) are generally absent.

■ Diagnosis

Charcot arthropathy (neuropathic osteoarthropathy).

✓ Pearls

- Bone marrow edema is a nonspecific finding that may be due to inflammation, infection, and/or altered biomechanics.
- In the foot, unless there is a deep ulcer or penetrating trauma, osteomyelitis is almost never present.
- Osteoarthritis and gout are known to affect the midfoot, but imaging findings are generally different from Charcot foot and osteomyelitis.

■ Suggested Readings

Dodd A, Daniels TR. Charcot neuroarthropathy of the foot and ankle. J Bone Joint Surg Am. 2018; 100(8):696–711

Holmes C, Schmidt B, Munson M, Wrobel JS. Charcot stage 0: A review and considerations for making the correct diagnosis early. Clin Diabetes Endocrinol. 2015; 1(1):18

Rosskopf AB, Loupatatzis C, Pfirrmann CWA, Böni T, Berli MC. The Charcot foot: a pictorial review. Insights Imaging. 2019; 10(1):77

Schmidt BM, Holmes CM. Updates on diabetic foot and Charcot osteopathic arthropathy. Curr Diab Rep. 2018; 18(10):74

Case 76

Robert D. Boutin

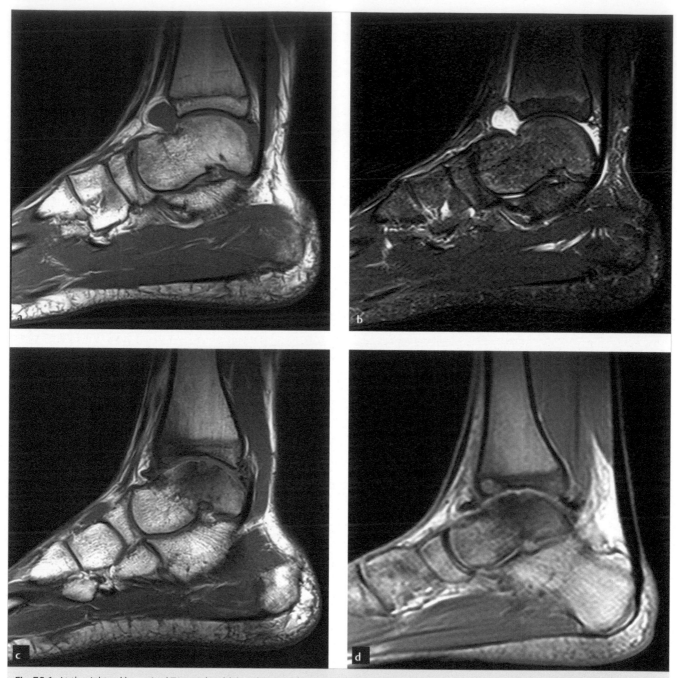

Fig. 76.1 At the right ankle, sagittal T1-weighted **(a)** and sagittal fat-suppressed T2-weighted **(b)** images show a moderate joint effusion (nonspecific). At the left ankle, sagittal T1-weighted **(c)** and sagittal T2* gradient-echo **(d)** images show arthropathy, with chondrosis and subchondral reactive changes at both the talar dome and the tibial plafond. Although there is no joint effusion on the left, there is low-signal intensity in the anterior and posterior recesses of the ankle (best seen on the gradient-echo image).

■ Clinical History

A 14-year-old boy with bilateral ankle pain, but no history of trauma (▶ Fig. 76.1).

■ Key Finding

Polyarticular arthritis in an adolescent, with "blooming" intra-articular hemosiderin.

■ Top 3 Differential Diagnoses

- **Juvenile idiopathic arthritis (JIA):** JIA refers to heterogeneous forms of arthritis of unknown etiology that begin prior to the age of 16 years and persist for more than 6 weeks. JIA is considered the most common rheumatic disease in children (with population prevalence similar to type 1 diabetes mellitus).

  Although JIA nomenclature continues to evolve as more is understood about these idiopathic conditions, the major subtypes of JIA currently include systemic arthritis, polyarthritis, oligoarthritis, enthesitis-related arthritis, and psoriatic arthritis.

  JIA can affect essentially any joint, including the knee, ankle/foot, and wrist/hand. Imaging is important in early diagnosis (e.g., ruling out other disorders that may mimic JIA) and assessing risk of erosive damage. If initial treatments fail, patients often benefit from more aggressive pharmacologic treatment (e.g., disease-modifying antirheumatic drugs [DMARDS]) during a therapeutic "window of opportunity," before advanced arthritis occurs. If untreated, growth disturbances may occur (e.g., hyperemia can be associated with epiphyseal overgrowth and premature fusion of physes).

  Both MRI and sonography may be complementary to clinical examination and radiography by showing subclinical synovitis, erosions, and enthesitis. MRI is the only imaging method that detects bone marrow edema, which is an important independent predictor of erosive damage and functional impairment.

- **Hemophilic arthropathy:** Hemophilia can cause spontaneous, recurrent intra-articular hemorrhages that cause arthropathy. This X-linked inherited disorder only occurs in males.

  The most commonly targeted joints include the knees, ankles, and elbows. The later stages of hemophilic arthropathy are well-evaluated by radiography, including epiphyseal overgrowth/deformity and diffuse joint space loss. In the early stages, however, radiography underestimates the extent of joint involvement compared to MRI.

  MRI shows findings that resemble an inflammatory arthritis (e.g., JIA), including effusion and synovitis, followed by erosion and cartilage destruction. With hemophilic arthropathy (like JIA), multiple joints are often involved. However, with hemophilic arthropathy (unlike JIA), MRI can show low-T2 signal in joints that "bloom" with gradient-echo MRI. The differential diagnosis of hemosiderin confined to a *single* joint includes tenosynovial giant cell tumor (formerly termed pigmented villonodular synovitis), which is a *monoarticular* process.

- **Infectious arthritis:** The differential diagnosis of arthritis can be extensive. Any inflammatory arthritis can show imaging findings associated with periarticular soft-tissue swelling, effusion, periarticular demineralization, erosions, and uniform joint space narrowing.

  Infectious arthritis is particularly important to consider when there is an unexplained inflammatory arthritis confined to a *single* joint. However, in as many as 20% of cases, *multiple* joints may be involved. Infectious arthritis typically is caused by hematogenous spread of bacteria (e.g., *Staph aureus*).

  The joints most frequently affected by septic arthritis in children include the hip and knee; other joints like the ankle and elbow are less common. Imaging shows nonspecific findings, including joint effusion and synovitis, periarticular edema, periarticular osteopenia, erosion, and eventually joint space narrowing. Therefore, if a joint effusion is demonstrated in a patient clinically suspected of an infectious arthritis, then joint aspiration should be performed to assess for an infectious etiology.

■ Diagnosis

Hemophilic arthropathy.

✓ Pearls

- If arthritis involves multiple joints, a systemic arthritis must be considered.
- If arthritis involves multiple joints and intra-articular hemosiderin is present, consider hemophilia causing hemophilic arthropathy.

- If arthritis affects multiple joints for more than 6 weeks in a patient younger than 16 years, consider JIA (a diagnosis of exclusion).

■ Suggested Readings

Jacobson JA, Girish G, Jiang Y, Sabb BJ. Radiographic evaluation of arthritis: degenerative joint disease and variations. Radiology. 2008; 248(3):737–747

Malattia C, Tzaribachev N, van den Berg JM, Magni-Manzoni S. Juvenile idiopathic arthritis–the role of imaging from a rheumatologist's perspective. Pediatr Radiol. 2018; 48(6):785–791

Sudoł-Szopińska I, Jans L, Jurik AG, Hemke R, Eshed I, Boutry N. Imaging features of the juvenile inflammatory arthropathies. Semin Musculoskelet Radiol. 2018; 22(2):147–165

von Drygalski A, Moore RE, Nguyen S, et al. Advanced hemophilic arthropathy: sensitivity of soft tissue discrimination with musculoskeletal ultrasound. J Ultrasound Med. 2018; 37(8):1945–1956

Wyseure T, Mosnier LO, von Drygalski A. Advances and challenges in hemophilic arthropathy. Semin Hematol. 2016; 53(1):10–19

Case 77

Robert D. Boutin

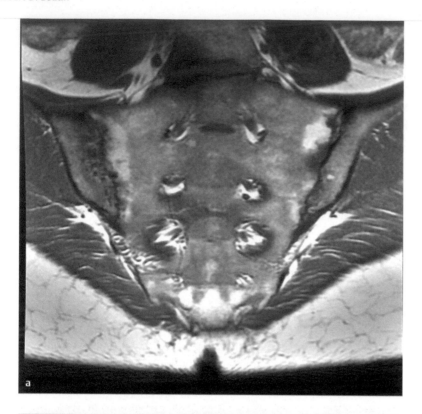

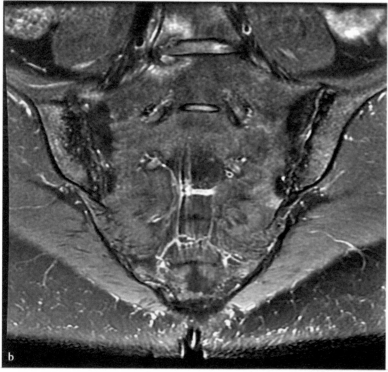

Fig. 77.1 Coronal-oblique T1-weighted (**a**) and coronal fat-suppressed T2-weighted (**b**) images of sacroiliac (SI) joints demonstrate erosion (loss of cortical integrity), extensive subchondral sclerosis, adjacent bone marrow edema, and fat metaplasia involving the SI joints bilaterally. Vertebral body corner inflammatory lesions are observed on both sides of the L5–S1 endplate on the right.

■ Clinical History

A 43-year-old woman was diagnosed with "chronic pain syndrome" for 15 years (▶ Fig. 77.1).

■ Key Finding

Bilateral sacroiliitis.

■ Top 3 Differential Diagnoses

- **Spondyloarthritis:** Spondyloarthritis is a group of a chronic inflammatory rheumatic diseases that include ankylosing spondylitis (most common), psoriatic arthritis, reactive arthritis, and inflammatory bowel disease-associated arthritis. The differentiation into these types has become less important in light of the 2019 Assessment in SpondyloArthritis International Society classification criteria. For the past decade, spondyloarthritis has been generally classified into two forms, based on its main clinical manifestation– axial and peripheral.

  Axial spondyloarthritis primarily targets the sacroiliac (SI) joints and spine, commonly presenting in patients aged <40–45 years with inflammatory back pain (IBP). IBP is defined as presence of back pain with four out of five of the following parameters: age of onset <40 years, insidious onset, improvement with exercise, no improvement with rest, and pain at night (improved by getting up).

  Population prevalence in the USA is approximately 1%. Delay in diagnosis is a major problem (averaging up to 14 years), and therefore familiarity with diagnostic criteria is important. It is currently recommended that patients should be referred to a rheumatologist if ≥ one of three features of spondyloarthritis are present (IBP, HLA-B27 positivity, imaging evidence of sacroiliitis). Although serum biomarkers are commonly used (HLA-B27 and C-reactive protein), MRI of the SI joints is considered the most sensitive imaging biomarker. MRI facilitates earlier diagnosis and earlier treatment, which may include exercise, nonsteroidal anti-inflammatory drugs (NSAIDs), and biologic drugs (disease-modifying antirheumatic drugs [DMARDs]). Axial spondyloarthritis usually starts in the SI joints and only later involves the spine.

  Ankylosing spondylitis is the most common cause of bilateral sacroiliitis. In the classic description of spondyloarthritis, sacroiliitis is characteristically symmetrical with ankylosing spondylitis and inflammatory bowel disease-associated arthritis, whereas with psoriatic and reactive arthritis, sacroiliitis may be unilateral, asymmetrical, or symmetrical.

- **Sacroiliitis-like changes:** The SI joints can be affected bilaterally by a wide variety of mechanical and systemic disorders affecting other synovial or fibrous joints.

  Mechanical (e.g., degenerative or posttraumatic) changes involving the SI joints are frequent. Most commonly, these include osteoarthritis, osteitis condensans ilii, and stress reaction. In addition to imaging features, clinical context and laboratory markers are helpful in differentiating true inflammatory sacroiliitis from mechanical changes.

  Bilateral sacroiliitis caused by spondyloarthritis must be differentiated from systemic or metabolic conditions. *Hyperparathyroidism* causes subperiosteal resorption in a distribution that is bilateral and greater on the iliac side of the joint (like ankylosing spondylitis), but it does not cause joint space narrowing or ankylosis. *Calcium pyrophosphate disease* (CPPD) is seen in older patients with chondrocalcinosis who may develop bilateral SI joint subchondral cysts/erosions, sclerosis, and joint space narrowing.

- **Anatomical variations:** Anatomical and physiological variations in the SI joints may be considered in the differential diagnosis of sacroiliitis and mechanical changes involving the SI joints.

  Anatomical variations occur most commonly in women, and they can be seen in almost one-third of SI joint MRI examinations. These variations can be unilateral (28%) or bilateral (72%), and they can involve the cartilaginous or ligamentous part of the SI joint. Of five different types of anatomical variations, the "dysmorphic SI joint" (prevalence, 17%) and the "accessory SI joint" (prevalence, 11%) are most frequently associated with edematous and/or structural changes that could be mistaken for inflammatory sacroiliitis.

■ Diagnosis

Axial spondyloarthritis (ankylosing spondylitis).

✓ Pearls

- Bilateral sacroiliitis is associated with axial spondyloarthritis, most commonly ankylosing spondylitis.
- The SI joints may be affected bilaterally by conditions that may mimic sacroiliitis, particularly mechanical (e.g., degenerative or posttraumatic) changes and systemic disorders (e.g., hyperparathyroidism or CPPD).

- Anatomical variations can be seen in almost one-third of SI joint MRI examinations, and they may be associated with edematous and/or structural changes that could be confused with sacroiliitis.

■ Suggested Readings

Bray TJP, Jones A, Bennett AN, et al. Recommendations for acquisition and interpretation of MRI of the spine and sacroiliac joints in the diagnosis of axial spondyloarthritis in the UK. Rheumatology (Oxford). 2019; 58(10):1831–1838

Danve A, Deodhar A. Axial spondyloarthritis in the USA: diagnostic challenges and missed opportunities. Clin Rheumatol. 2019; 38(3):625–634

El Rafei M, Badr S, Lefebvre G, et al. Sacroiliac joints: anatomical variations on MR images. Eur Radiol. 2018; 28(12):5328–5337

Eshed I, Hermann KA, Zejden A, Sudoł-Szopińska I. Imaging to differentiate the various forms of seronegative arthritis. Semin Musculoskelet Radiol. 2018; 22(2):189–196

Maksymowych WP, Lambert RG, Østergaard M, et al. MRI lesions in the sacroiliac joints of patients with spondyloarthritis: an update of definitions and validation by the ASAS MRI working group. Ann Rheum Dis. 2019; 78(11):1550–1558

Tsoi C, Griffith JF, Lee RKL, Wong PCH, Tam LS. Imaging of sacroiliitis: current status, limitations and pitfalls. Quant Imaging Med Surg. 2019; 9(2):318–335

Case 78

Robert D. Boutin

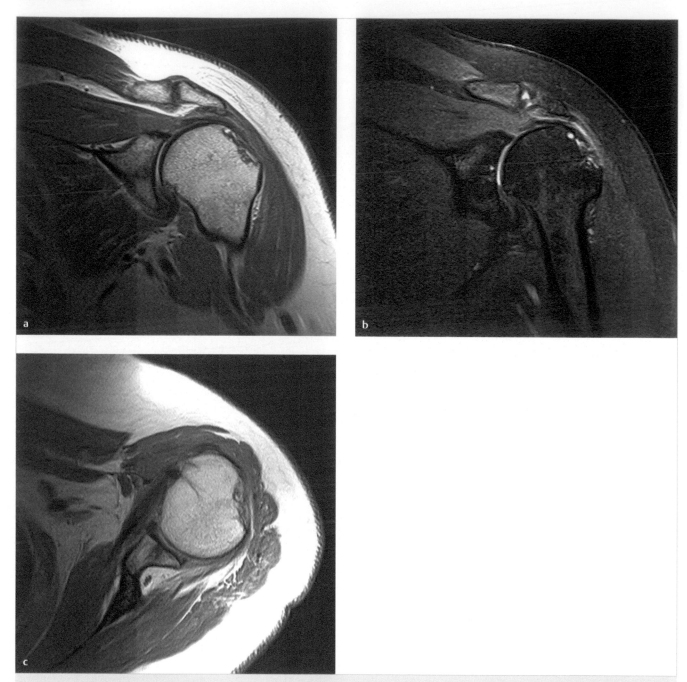

Fig. 78.1 Coronal proton density-weighted **(a)**, coronal fat-suppressed T2-weighted **(b)**, and axial proton density-weighted **(c)** images of the shoulder show an apparent flattening deformity at the posterolateral aspect of the humeral head.

■ Clinical History

A 37-year-old patient with nontraumatic shoulder pain
(▶ Fig. 78.1).

■ Key Finding

Contour defect at the posterolateral humeral head.

■ Top 3 Differential Diagnoses

- **Erosive arthritis:** In patients with inflammatory arthritis, the shoulder is often involved (up to approximately two-thirds of the patients with rheumatoid arthritis and one-third of patients with chronic ankylosing spondylitis). Shoulder involvement can include rotator cuff pathology, synovitis, and erosion.

  With ankylosing spondylitis, the shoulder joint is the second most frequently targeted peripheral joint (after the hip joint). In some patients with ankylosing spondylitis, the entire superolateral/posterolateral aspect of the humeral head becomes eroded. This erosive process results in a characteristic defect of the humeral head which can mimic a Hill–Sachs lesion, which has been termed the "hatchet sign".

- **Hill–Sachs lesion:** A Hill–Sachs lesion is an impaction fracture deformity that occurs in at least two-thirds of anterior shoulder dislocations. The posttraumatic deformity is located at the posterosuperolateral aspect of the humeral head.

  The Hill–Sachs lesion is often defined as significant ("engaging") if it is in a position that allows it to engage with the anterior glenoid when the arm is abducted 90° and externally rotated 90°. Engagement of a Hill–Sachs lesion is a better predictor of recurrent instability than defect size alone. Although this topic continues to be an active area of investigation, engaging Hill–Sachs lesions are generally observed to be off the glenoid track (the glenoid track = 0.83 D − d, where D is the diameter of the inferior glenoid and d is the bone loss).

  In addition to treating any glenoid injury (e.g., Bankart lesion), an engaging Hill–Sachs lesion may be treated with a remplissage procedure, which involves filling of the Hill–Sachs defect with the joint capsule and infraspinatus tendon (i.e., arthroscopic posterior capsulodesis and infraspinatus tenodesis, respectively).

- **Cystic lesion in the posterosuperior humeral head:** Numerous types of cystic-appearing foci may occur in the bone at the margin of the humeral head. Humeral head cysts have been associated with many articular disorders and rotator cuff disorders. In addition, incidental cystic changes close to the bare area of the humerus, associated with degenerative changes and vascular channels at the posterolateral humeral head, also are commonly observed. Finally, in the posterosuperior portions of the humeral head (i.e., at the bare area or just posterior to the greater tuberosity), tiny (≤4 mm) pseudocysts lined with collagen connective tissue may occur and are thought likely to be a normal variant.

■ Diagnosis

Erosive arthritis (hatchet sign due to ankylosing spondylitis).

✓ Pearls

- With ankylosing spondylitis, a characteristic pattern of erosion at the superolateral/posterolateral aspect of the humeral head termed the "hatchet sign" can mimic a Hill–Sachs lesion.
- A Hill–Sachs lesion is an impaction fracture deformity that occurs frequently after a shoulder dislocation. In some cases, it may be implicated in recurrent dislocations and treated surgically.
- In the posterosuperior portions of the humeral head, tiny pseudocysts are likely an incidental normal variant.

■ Suggested Readings

Fox JA, Sanchez A, Zajac TJ, Provencher MT. Understanding the Hill–Sachs lesion in its role in patients with recurrent anterior shoulder instability. Curr Rev Musculoskelet Med. 2017; 10(4):469–479

Gyftopoulos S, Beltran LS, Bookman J, Rokito A. MRI evaluation of bipolar bone loss using the on-track off-track method: a feasibility study. AJR Am J Roentgenol. 2015; 205(4):848–852

Jin W, Ryu KN, Park YK, Lee WK, Ko SH, Yang DM. Cystic lesions in the posterosuperior portion of the humeral head on MR arthrography: correlations with gross and histologic findings in cadavers. AJR Am J Roentgenol. 2005; 184(4):1211–1215

Maio M, Sarmento M, Moura N, Cartucho A. How to measure a Hill–Sachs lesion: a systematic review. EFORT Open Rev. 2019; 4(4):151–157

Sankaye P, Ostlere S. Arthritis at the shoulder joint. Semin Musculoskelet Radiol. 2015; 19(3):307–318

Soker G, Bozkirli ED, Soker E, et al. Magnetic resonance imaging evaluation of shoulder joint in patients with early stage of ankylosing spondylitis: A case-control study. Diagn Interv Imaging. 2016; 97(4):419–424

Case 79

Michael A. Tall

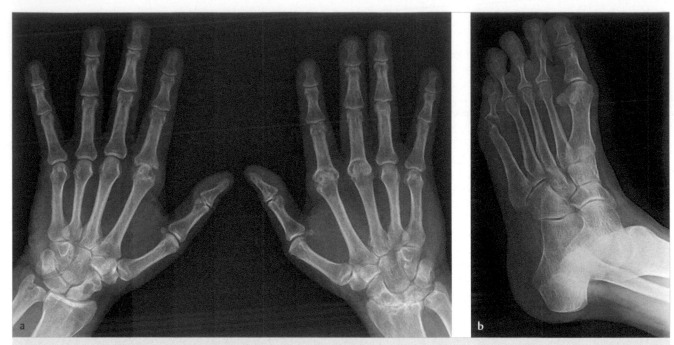

Fig. 79.1 Dorsovolar radiograph of bilateral hands **(a)** shows erosive changes and joint space narrowing at some of the metacarpophalangeal joints with severe joint space loss at the right radiocarpal joint and cystic lucencies scattered over both wrists. Oblique radiograph of the left foot **(b)** reveals marked erosive changes at the 5th metatarsophalangeal joint.

■ Clinical History

A 54-year-old female with stiffness and pain in her hands and feet (▶ Fig. 79.1).

■ Key Finding

Proximal arthropathy affecting primarily the metacarpophalangeal joints.

■ Top 3 Differential Diagnoses

- **Rheumatoid arthritis (RA):** The common radiographic manifestations of RA consist of periarticular osteopenia, uniform joint space loss with marginal erosions, subchondral cyst formation, and subluxations. Unlike psoriatic and reactive arthritis, there is a lack of bone formation. In the hand, the distribution primarily involves the metacarpophalangeal joints(MCPs), proximal interphalangeal (PIP) joints, and carpal bones in a fairly bilateral symmetric fashion. In the feet, often the earliest erosive changes are seen along the lateral aspect of the fifth metatarsal heads. In the feet, target sites of RA include metatarsophalangeal, PIP, and intertarsal joints. As the disease progresses, joint subluxations occur predominantly at the MCPs. Hand involvement precedes involvement of the feet in the vast majority of patients.
- **Crystalline arthropathy: Calcium pyrophosphate deposition (CPPD) arthropathy** is the most common crystalline arthropathy. The radiographic appearance resembles osteoarthropathy.

Symmetric joint space narrowing, subchondral cysts, and osteophytes may be present, but unlike rheumatoid arthritis, erosions are absent. In the hand, the arthropathy is usually confined to the MCP joints. Chondrocalcinosis is often present, most frequently in the triangular fibrocartilage of the wrist. **Gout** is a crystalline arthropathy that primarily involves the hands and feet. The distribution is sporadic and bilateral involvement, when present, is asymmetric. Unlike rheumatoid arthritis, the erosions in gout demonstrate sclerotic borders with characteristic overhanging edges. Soft-tissue tophi occur in chronic disease. Bony mineralization is usually normal.

- **Collagen vascular disease: Systemic lupus erythematosus (SLE)** is the most common of the collagen vascular diseases. Radiographic findings of SLE include juxta-articular osteopenia, joint subluxations and dislocations. Unlike RA, erosions are not typically present.

■ Additional Diagnostic Consideration

- **Hemochromatosis:** In hemochromatosis, there is a predilection for the second and third MCP joints in the hands with subchondral cysts and hooked osteophytes. Bony mineralization is

preserved, and there are no erosions. As in CPPD arthropathy, chondrocalcinosis may be present.

■ Diagnosis

Rheumatoid arthritis.

✓ Pearls

- Rheumatoid arthritis demonstrates uniform joint space loss, marginal erosions, and subchondral cysts.
- Erosions in gout demonstrate sclerotic borders, often with overhanging edges; tophi may also be present.

- SLE demonstrates periarticular osteopenia, and subluxations without erosions.
- Hemochromatosis results in joint space narrowing, hooked osteophytes, and chondrocalcinosis.

■ Suggested Readings

Brower AC, FlemmingDJ. Arthritis: in Black and White. 3rd ed. Philadelphia, PA: Saunders Elsevier; 2012

Gupta KB, Duryea J, Weissman BN. Radiographic evaluation of osteoarthritis. Radiol Clin North Am. 2004; 42(1):11–41, v

Jacobson JA, Girish G, Jiang Y, Resnick D. Radiographic evaluation of arthritis: inflammatory conditions. Radiology. 2008; 248(2):378–389

Case 80

Michael A. Tall

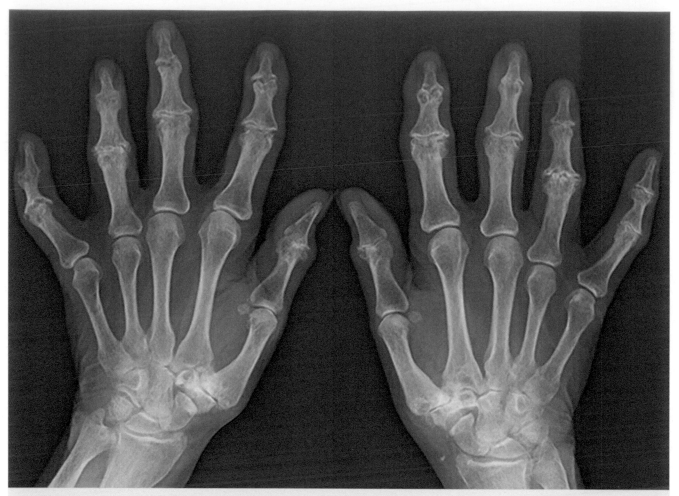

Fig. 80.1 Dorsovolar radiograph of the hands demonstrates joint space narrowing, irregularity, subchondral sclerosis, osteophytosis, and central erosions involving several proximal interphalangeal (PIP) and distal interphalangeal (DIP) joints of both hands. A few DIP joints show fusion. Bony mineralization is preserved.

■ Clinical History

A 71-year-old female with a history of longstanding bilateral hand and finger pain (▶ Fig. 80.1).

■ Key Finding

Distal arthropathy primarily affecting the interphalangeal joints.

■ Top 3 Differential Diagnoses

- **Osteoarthritis:** Primary osteoarthritis in the hand involves the distal interphalangeal (DIP) and proximal interphalangeal (PIP) joints with relative sparing of the metacarpophalangeal (MCP) joints. There is nonuniform joint space loss with subchondral sclerosis and osteophyte development in the areas of greatest cartilage loss. The soft-tissue swelling around the DIP joint, associated with osteophyte formation, is called the Heberdon's node, while that around the PIP joint is called the Bouchard node. Erosions and ankylosis are not present.
- **Erosive osteoarthritis:** Erosive osteoarthritis is primarily seen in postmenopausal females. It has the same distribution in the hand that primary osteoarthritis has, with involvement of the DIP and PIP joints in the fingers and the first carpometacarpal (CMC) joint. In addition to osteophytes, central erosions characteristically produce two convexities of the joint surface, likened to the wings of a seagull. Ankylosis of the joints may also occur.
- **Psoriatic arthritis:** The hands are most commonly involved in psoriatic arthritis. There are three different patterns of distribution. The first pattern is primarily DIP and PIP involvement. The second pattern is ray involvement, wherein one to three fingers will be involved in all joints, while the other fingers are spared. The third pattern is similar to rheumatoid arthritis (RA) but there is usually DIP involvement and/or evidence of bone proliferation, which is in contradistinction to RA. Erosions occur initially at the margins of the joint but eventually progress to involve the entire joint. The ends of the bones may become pointed and saucerized and give the classic "pencil in cup" appearance. Bony mineralization is usually preserved, even with severe erosive disease. Bone proliferation is one of the most important features of psoriatic arthritis and is almost always present in some form.

■ Additional Diagnostic Considerations

- **Reactive arthritis:** Lower extremity involvement is more common. Upper extremity involvement, when present, typically occurs in the hands. The specific radiographic changes are essentially identical to psoriatic arthritis, with erosive changes and new bone formation. This is often limited to just one digit. The PIP joints are more frequently involved than the DIPs or the MCPs.
- **Rheumatoid arthritis:** The common radiographic manifestations consist of periarticular osteopenia, progressing to generalized osteoporosis, uniform joint space loss with marginal erosions, subchondral cyst formation, and subluxations. Unlike psoriatic and reactive arthritis, there is a lack of bone formation. The distribution primarily involves the PIPs, MCPs, and carpal bones in a primarily symmetric fashion.

■ Diagnosis

Erosive osteoarthritis.

✓ Pearls

- The hallmarks of osteoarthritis include joint space narrowing, sclerosis, and osteophyte formation.
- Central erosions in the interphalangeal joints are characteristic of erosive osteoarthropathy.
- Marginal erosions and new bone formation are characteristic of reactive and psoriatic arthropathy.
- Advanced psoriatic arthritis may result in the classic "pencil-in-cup" deformity in the phalanges.

■ Suggested Readings

Brower AC, Flemming DJ. Arthritis: in Black and White. 3rd ed. Philadelphia, PA: Saunders Elsevier; 2012

Gupta KB, Duryea J, Weissman BN. Radiographic evaluation of osteoarthritis. Radiol Clin North Am. 2004; 42(1):11–41, v

Jacobson JA, Girish G, Jiang Y, Sabb BJ. Radiographic evaluation of arthritis: degenerative joint disease and variations. Radiology. 2008; 248(3):737–747

Case 81

Michael A. Tall and Jasjeet Bindra

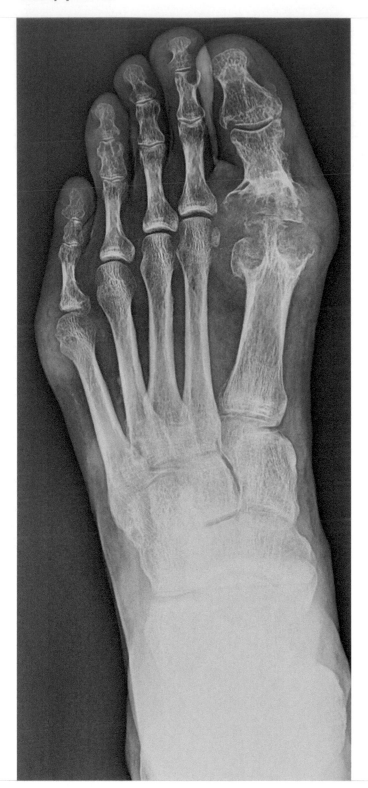

Fig. 81.1 Frontal radiograph of the foot demonstrates erosions at multiple joints in the forefoot. Prominent erosions at the 1st metatarsophalangeal (MTP) joint have sclerotic borders and overhanging edges. There are soft-tissue, mass-like lesions with faintly increased density along the joints, especially the 1st and 5th MTP joints.

■ Clinical History

A 74-year-old male with long-standing history of foot pain which is most pronounced at the great toe (▶ Fig. 81.1).

■ Key Finding

Erosive arthropathy involving the foot.

■ Top 3 Differential Diagnoses

- **Rheumatoid arthritis (RA):** RA is characterized by a fairly bilateral symmetric distribution, uniform joint space narrowing, periarticular osteopenia, marginal erosions, and joint subluxations. The feet are involved in 80 to 90% of cases and usually lag behind the findings in the hands. The lateral aspect of the 5th metatarsal head is often the earliest site of involvement. Metatarsophalangeal (MTP), proximal interphalangeal (PIP), and intertarsal joint involvement can be seen with sparing of distal interphalangeal (DIP) joints. Retrocalcaneal bursitis with erosions and Achilles tendonitis are also common findings.
- **Gout:** Gouty arthritis is caused by the accumulation of monosodium urate crystals. It most commonly affects older males. Characteristic radiographic findings include well-defined, punched-out erosions, often with a sclerotic border and overhanging edges, along with soft-tissue tophi. Bone mineralization is usually normal and joint spaces are preserved until late in the disease. The distribution is typically polyarticular and asymmetric. The 1st MTP joint is the most common joint involved and is referred to as podagra.
- **Reactive arthritis:** Early in the disease process, juxta-articular osteoporosis predominates. This may affect only a single joint. Normal bony mineralization may return. Later, uniform joint space narrowing, marginal erosions, and adjacent bone proliferation occur. Eventually, ankylosis may occur; however, it does not occur as frequently as in psoriatic arthritis. Small joints of the foot and the calcaneus are the most frequently involved joints, with preferential involvement of the MTP joints and 1st IP joint.

■ Additional Diagnostic Consideration

- **Psoriatic arthritis:** The hands are most commonly involved in psoriatic arthritis, but the feet may be involved as well. Marginal erosions coupled with bony proliferation are the hallmarks of the disease. Erosive changes may become so severe that they result in "pencil-in-cup" deformity. Diffuse, soft-tissue swelling of an entire digit may also occur, which is referred to as a "sausage digit" deformity. Ankylosis is common in the hands and feet. Characteristic distribution in feet involves IP joints, MTP joints, and posterior calcaneus. DIP involvement tends to be seen early and more severe than PIP or MTP joints.

■ Diagnosis

Tophaceous gout.

✓ Pearls

- The first MTP joint is the most commonly affected joint in gout and is referred to as podagra.
- Bony mineralization is normal, and the joint spaces are generally preserved until late in the course of gout.
- RA has symmetric joint space narrowing, marginal erosions, and periarticular osteopenia.
- Reactive arthritis involves the feet with joint space narrowing, marginal erosions, and bony proliferation.

■ Suggested Readings

Brower AC, Flemming DJ. Arthritis: in Black and White. 3rd ed. Philadelphia, PA: Saunders Elsevier;2012

Girish G, Glazebrook KN, Jacobson JA. Advanced imaging in gout. AJR Am J Roentgenol. 2013; 201(3):515–525

Monu JU, Pope TL, Jr. Gout: a clinical and radiologic review. Radiol Clin North Am. 2004; 42(1):169–184

Case 82

William T. O'Brien, Sr.

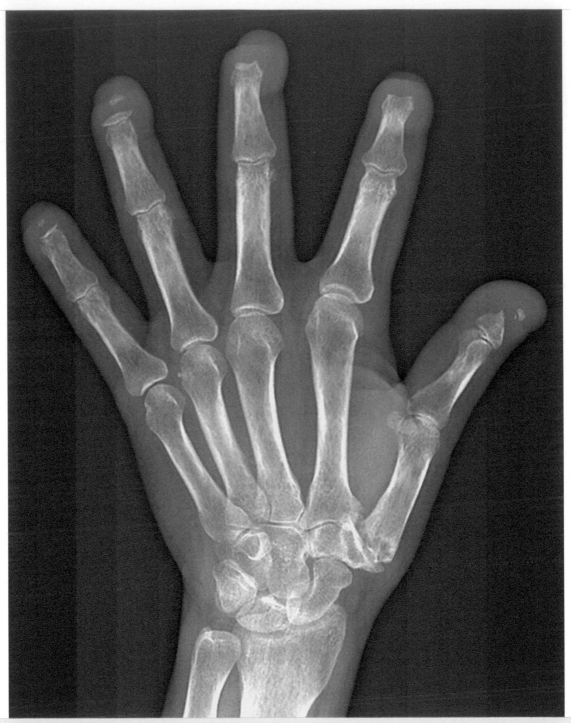

Fig. 82.1 Frontal plain radiograph of the left hand demonstrates resorption of all terminal phalangeal tufts (acro-osteolysis). There is complete resorption of terminal phalanges of the second and third digits.

■ Clinical History

A 49-year-old female with chronic bilateral hand pain and ulcerations (▶ Fig. 82.1).

■ Key Finding

Acro-osteolysis.

■ Top 3 Differential Diagnoses

- **Hyperparathyroidism:** Hyperparathyroidism is a systemic abnormality of calcium homeostasis which can be primary (overproduction by the parathyroid glands), secondary (caused by renal failure or malabsorption), or tertiary (autonomous production by the parathyroid glands due to chronic renal failure or malabsorption). Subperiosteal resorption of bone, especially along the radial aspect of the second and third middle phalanges of the hands, is virtually diagnostic of hyperparathyroidism. Additional osseous abnormalities include resorption of the distal clavicles, band-likeosteosclerosis of the vertebral bodies referred to as "rugger jersey" spine, brown tumors, and resorption of the terminal phalanges.
- **Scleroderma:** Scleroderma is a systemic connective tissue disorder that results in characteristic musculoskeletal abnormalities that are most prominent in the hands. The most common manifestations include bony erosions and soft-tissue resorption along the distal phalanges. Severe cases result in tapering or complete destruction of the distal phalanges (acro-osteolysis). Soft-tissue calcifications are evident in approximately 10 to 30% of patients. CREST syndrome is a variant of scleroderma consisting of calcinosis, Raynaud's phenomenon, esophageal dysmotility, sclerodactyly, and telangiectasias.
- **Trauma:** Thermal injury refers to either cold injury (frostbite) or burn injury. Both processes cause vascular occlusion and ischemia, resulting in soft-tissue and osseous abnormalities. Osseous manifestations include osteoporosis, periostitis, and resorption of the distal phalanges. In the setting of frostbite, the findings are typically bilateral, with sparing of the thumbs secondary to clenched fists, and the digits protecting the thumbs. Premature growth plate fusion is a complication in children.

■ Additional Diagnostic Considerations

- **Psoriasis:** Psoriatic arthritis is a polyarticular arthritis with multiple variants. Although the distribution is variable, psoriasis has a predilection for the distal interphalangeal (DIP) joints of the hands. Musculoskeletal involvement of the hand includes soft-tissue swelling, periarticular erosions, "fluffy" periostitis, and resorption of the distal phalanges. Bone mineralization is usually normal. Classic radiographic findings include the "sausage digit" (diffuse soft tissue swelling) and the "pencil-in-cup" deformity from resorption and tapering of the distal aspect of the phalanges. Psoriasis may also involve the feet and sacroiliac joints.
- **Hajdu-Cheney syndrome:** Hajdu–Cheney is a rare syndrome that may occur sporadically or with an autosomal dominant familial inheritance. Patients have dysmorphic facies and cranial abnormalities, including an enlarged sellaturcica, wormian bones, and basilar invagination. Hearing deficits and speech impediments are common. Osteolysis occurs within the distal phalanges of the hands and feet with classic band-likelucencies that isolate proximal and distal osseous fragments in the terminal tufts.

■ Diagnosis

Scleroderma.

✓ Pearls

- Hyperparathyroidism results in radial-sided subperiosteal resorption of the 2nd and 3rd middle phalanges.
- Scleroderma may result in soft-tissue resorption and calcifications with distal phalangeal acro-osteolysis.
- Thermal (burn and frostbite) injuries may manifest as osteoporosis, periostitis, and acro-osteolysis.
- Hajdu–Cheney is a rare syndrome with dysmorphic facies and band-like acro-osteolysis.

■ Suggested Readings

Avouac J, Guerini H, Wipff J, et al. Radiological hand involvement in systemic sclerosis. Ann Rheum Dis. 2006; 65(8):1088–1092

Resnick D, Kransdorf MJ. Bone and Joint Imaging. 3rd ed. Philadelphia, PA: Elsevier Saunders;2005

Case 83

M. Jason Akers

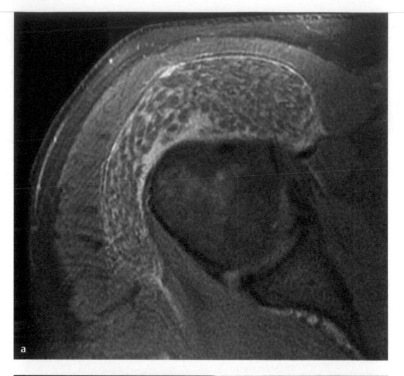

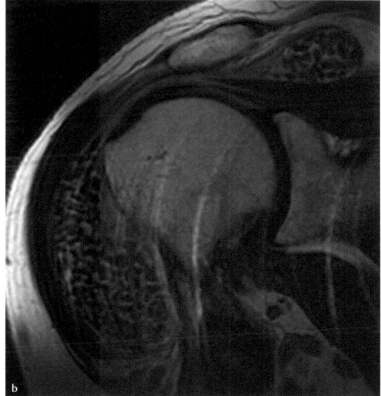

Fig. 83.1 Axial fat-suppressed T2-weighted MR image of the shoulder (**a**) and coronal T2-weighted image (**b**) of the same shoulder show marked distension of subacromia–subdeltoid bursa with fluid containing multiple small iso- to hypointense nodules or bodies.

■ **Clinical History**

71-year-old male with shoulder pain and swelling (▶ Fig. 83.1).

■ Key Finding

Loose bodies.

■ Top 3 Differential Diagnoses

- **Synovial (osteo)chondromatosis:** Synovial (osteo)chondromatosis is a disease of the synovium, resulting from synovial metaplasia, the cause of which is unknown. It is seen in men between the ages of 20 and 50 years and is most commonly intra-articular but may also occur in tendon sheaths and bursae. Occasionally, conglomerate masses may extend into the extracapsular soft tissues. The disease is typically monoarticular with the knee, elbow, shoulder, and hip joints most commonly involved. Synovial metaplasia results in the formation of synovial villonodular projections that grow to form nodules. If the nodules remain attached to the synovium, they develop a blood supply and may become ossified. If the nodules break off, they are nourished by synovial fluid and become cartilaginous. As much as 85% have sufficient calcification to be detected on radiographs, appearing as multiple, round, similar-sized calcified bodies. The bodies are of variable MR signal, depending on the proportion of calcium, chondroid, and mature ossific tissue, ranging from low-signal on all sequences to marrow signal on all sequences. Mechanical articular cartilage destruction results in well-marginated erosions. Malignant degeneration is rare. Treatment involves resection of the bodies along with synovectomy. Recurrences after surgical debridement can occur.
- **Pigmented villonodular synovitis (PVNS):** PVNS is a benign neoplastic process of the synovium. It can occur intra-articularly and involve the joint diffusely or focally. It may also occur extra-articularly in a bursa or tendon sheath (giant cell tumor of the tendon sheath). The intra-articular form is characterized by villonodular proliferation of the synovium with associated hemorrhage. It is monoarticular with common locations including the knee and hip joints. On radiographs, PVNS manifests as a large joint effusion with or without associated erosions and subchondral cysts. Joint spaces are usually preserved. MRI shows a joint effusion and focal or diffuse synovial thickening that is low-signal on T1 and T2 due to hemosiderin deposition. The hemosiderin causes susceptibility artifact and subsequent blooming on gradient echo sequences. Treatment involves synovectomy; incomplete resection is associated with high-recurrence rates.
- **Rice bodies:** Multiple small, loose bodies can occur within joints affected by rheumatoid arthritis, which are are termed "rice bodies" due to their resemblance to polished grains of rice. "Rice bodies" are small fragments of fibrous tissue that occur as a nonspecific response to synovial inflammation. The exact cause is unknown, but one theory postulates that "rice bodies" represent detached fragments of infarcted synovium. First described in association with tuberculous arthritis, "rice bodies" are now more frequently associated with rheumatoid arthritis. They can, however, also be seen in the absence of any underlying systemic disorder. On MR, "rice bodies" are hypointense on T2 due to their fibrous nature and are associated with a joint effusion, synovial hypertrophy, and synovial enhancement after gadolinium administration.

■ Diagnosis

Rice bodies.

✓ Pearls

- Synovial (osteo)chondromatosis is a synovial metaplasia that results in loose bodies; 85% are calcified.
- PVNS shows low-signal synovial thickening on T1 and T2 with blooming on gradient due to hemosiderin.
- "Rice bodies" are small, loose bodies that are most frequently associated with rheumatoid arthritis.

■ Suggested Readings

Chung C, Coley BD, Martin LC. Rice bodies in juvenile rheumatoid arthritis. AJR Am J Roentgenol. 1998; 170(3):698–700

Cheung HS, Ryan LM, Kozin F, McCarty DJ. Synovial origins of rice bodies in joint fluid. Arthritis Rheum. 1980; 23(1):72–76

Dürr HR, Stäbler A, Maier M, Refior HJ. Pigmented villonodular synovitis. Review of 20 cases. J Rheumatol. 2001; 28(7):1620–1630

Murphey MD, Vidal JA, Fanburg-Smith JC, Gajewski DA. Imaging of synovial chondromatosis with radiologic-pathologic correlation. Radiographics. 2007; 27(5): 1465–1488

Stoller DW, Bredella MA, Phillip FJ. Diagnostic Imaging: Orthopaedics, Salt Lake City, UT: Amirsys; 2004

Case 84

Robert D. Boutin

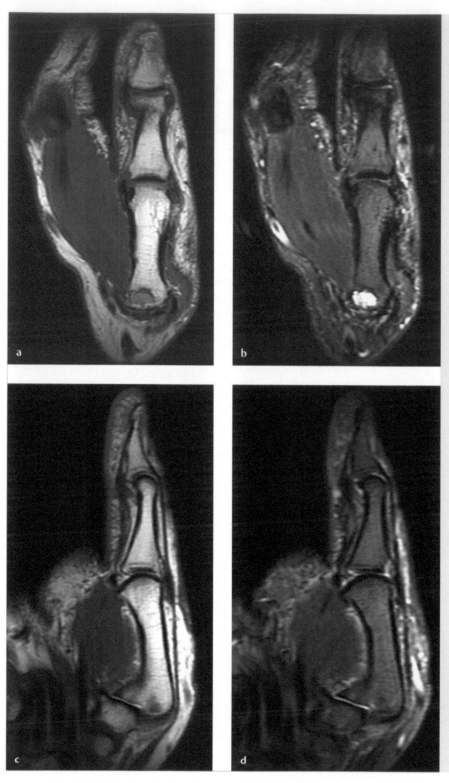

Fig. 84.1 Coronal proton density-weighted (**a**) and coronal fat-suppressed T2-weighted (**b**) images of the thumb show a subchondral cyst in the 1st metacarpal base. The intermetacarpal ligament was clearly disrupted on sequential coronal images. Sagittal proton density-weighted (**c**) and sagittal fat-suppressed T2-weighted (**d**) images of the thumb demonstrate diffuse high-grade articular cartilage loss at the carpometa-carpal (CMC) joint, with disruption of the anterior oblique ligament and dorsal subluxation of the metacarpal base relative to the trapezium.

■ Clinical History

A 64-year-old man with basilar thumb joint pain (► Fig. 84.1).

■ Key Finding

Articular cartilage thinning, subchondral cyst formation, and dorsal subluxation of the first metacarpal base–Roentgen classic.

■ Diagnosis

Osteoarthritis (OA) of the thumb carpometacarpal (CMC) joint: OA of the thumb CMC joint is a common cause of pain and significant functional disability in older adults (e.g., after age 75 years, affecting up to 25% of men and 40% of women).

With radiography, hallmarks of OA include joint space narrowing, subchondral cysts, subchondral sclerosis, and osteophytes. At the thumb CMC joint, OA is also manifested by the significant dorsal (or dorsoradial) subluxation compared to control subjects. This subluxation is not related to a history of trauma, but it is likely rather the result of ligamentous laxity/dysfunction. Indeed, in symptomatic patients with thumb CMC OA, several ligaments may be disrupted. MRI most often shows combined disruption of the anterior oblique ligament (also termed the palmar beak ligament) and the intermetacarpal ligament.

Currently, most symptomatic CMC OA is treated conservatively, unless it becomes severe. There are numerous invasive surgical techniques to treat end-stage thumb CMC OA, such as a trapeziectomy with ligament reconstruction and tendon interposition. Although radiography is the initial imaging test of choice, there is a great deal of work assessing other imaging techniques for optimizing OA diagnosis and management. Sonography has been used to show inflammatory soft-tissue features of OA, such as synovitis and effusion. MRI also shows inflammatory features associated with symptomatic OA, including bone marrow edema, and is more sensitive for evaluating CMC OA than radiography.

A thumb base OA MRI scoring system ("TOMS") for the assessment of inflammatory and structural abnormalities has been developed to assess patient outcomes. In addition to subluxation, the specific imaging features used for MRI scoring are synovitis, subchondral bone defects (including erosions, cysts, and bone attrition), osteophytes, cartilage, and bone marrow lesions on a 0 to 3 scale (normal to severe).

✓ Pearls

- The thumb CMC joint is an extremely common target site for OA. Arthritis at this articulation is generally due to OA, not other etiologies (e.g., rheumatoid arthritis).
- In the past decade, the use of sonography and MRI for assessing arthritis in the hand has increased. Compared to radiography, these modalities are more sensitive for detecting pathological features, including active inflammatory changes (e.g., synovitis, effusion, or bone marrow edema).
- With thumb CMC OA, subluxation is a nontraumatic finding that is commonly associated with disruption of more than one ligament.

■ Suggested Readings

Dumont C, Lerzer S, Vafa MA, et al. Osteoarthritis of the carpometacarpal joint of the thumb: a new MR imaging technique for the standardized detection of relevant ligamental lesions. Skeletal Radiol. 2014; 43(10):1411–1420

Hirschmann A, Sutter R, Schweizer A, Pfirrmann CW. The carpometacarpal joint of the thumb: MR appearance in asymptomatic volunteers. Skeletal Radiol. 2013; 42(8):1105–1112

Kroon FPB, Conaghan PG, Foltz V, et al. Development and reliability of the OMERACT thumb base osteoarthritis magnetic resonance imaging scoring system. J Rheumatol. 2017; 44(11):1694–1698

Marshall M, Watt FE, Vincent TL, Dziedzic K. Hand osteoarthritis: clinical phenotypes, molecular mechanisms and disease management. Nat Rev Rheumatol. 2018; 14(11):641–656

Melville DM, Taljanovic MS, Scalcione LR, et al. Imaging and management of thumb carpometacarpal joint osteoarthritis. Skeletal Radiol. 2015; 44(2):165–177

van Beest S, Kroon FPB, Kroon HM, et al. Assessment of osteoarthritic features in the thumb base with the newly developed OMERACT magnetic resonance imaging scoring system is a valid addition to standard radiography. Osteoarthritis Cartilage. 2019; 27(3):468–475

Part 6

Infection

Case 85

Robert D. Boutin

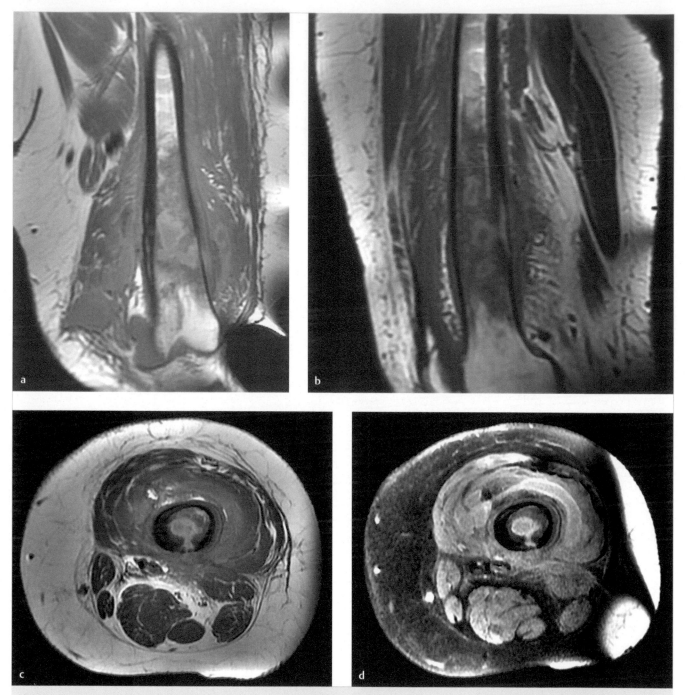

Fig. 85.1 Coronal T1-weighted **(a)**, sagittal T1-weighted **(b)**, and axial T1-weighted **(c)** images show a rounded thin rim or "penumbra" of mildly hyperintense signal intensity within the femoral shaft and in the adjacent soft tissues. Axial fat-suppressed T1-weighted **(d)** image also shows subtle intrinsically increased signal intensity in the same distribution.

■ Clinical History

A 30-year-old obese man with ongoing left thigh pain (▶ Fig. 85.1).

■ Key Finding

Penumbra sign.

■ Top 3 Differential Diagnoses

- **Subacute osteomyelitis:** Unlike acute infection that commonly presents with overt clinical and laboratory findings, subacute and chronic infections may only present with pain, nonspecific inflammatory markers (e.g., elevated C-reactive protein), and nonspecific radiographic findings.

  MRI can be helpful in differentiating infection from neoplasm when a penumbra sign is present. The penumbra sign is a thin layer of granulation tissue that rims an abscess and is characteristically seen with subacute osteomyelitis. For subacute osteomyelitis, the reported diagnostic sensitivity and specificity of the penumbra sign are approximately 75% and >90%, respectively. The penumbra sign may also be associated with chronic osteomyelitis, soft-tissue abscess, and "acute on chronic" musculoskeletal infections.

  The penumbra sign is reported most frequently in the metaphysis and metadiaphysis of long bones. The "penumbra" (halo) of increased signal on unenhanced T1 images (hyperintense to the abscess and isointense to normal muscle) may be caused by high-protein content within granulation tissue, which can be easily overlooked. If contrast is administered intravenously, this rim of vascularized, inflamed granulation tissue around the abscess enhances avidly.

- **Subchondral ganglion/cyst:** Benign cystic-appearing lesions of bone, such as an intraosseous ganglion, can show findings reminiscent of a penumbra. Unlike most cases of osteomyelitis, subchondral cysts are commonly associated with overlying chondrosis and located in epiphyseal regions.

- **Tumors:** Benign or malignant tumors may show findings interpreted as a penumbra sign. Specifically, reports have included cases of eosinophilic granuloma, chondroblastoma, leiomyosarcoma, and even Ewing sarcoma (in the presence of a bulky soft tissue mass). In some cases, this phenomenon of T1 hyperintensity may be due to a pathologic fracture with subacute hematoma.

■ Diagnosis

Subacute osteomyelitis.

✓ Pearls

- Musculoskeletal infection in the subacute and chronic setting can be difficult to differentiate from neoplasm, both with clinical evaluation and with imaging.
- The penumbra sign is considered highly characteristic of musculoskeletal infection, most commonly subacute osteomyelitis.

- The penumbra sign is a thin halo of relatively hyperintense signal on unenhanced T1 images caused by granulation tissue that rims an abscess.

■ Suggested Readings

Crundwell N, O'Donnell P, Saifuddin A. Non-neoplastic conditions presenting as soft-tissue tumours. Clin Radiol. 2007; 62(1):18–27

Davies AM, Grimer R. The penumbra sign in subacute osteomyelitis. Eur Radiol. 2005; 15(6):1268–1270

Kasalak Ö, Overbosch J, Adams HJ, et al. Diagnostic value of MRI signs in differentiating Ewing sarcoma from osteomyelitis. Acta Radiol. 2019; 60(2):204–212

McCarville MB, Chen JY, Coleman JL, et al. Distinguishing osteomyelitis from Ewing sarcoma on radiography and MRI. AJR Am J Roentgenol. 2015; 205(3):640–650, quiz 651

McGuinness B, Wilson N, Doyle AJ. The "penumbra sign" on T1-weighted MRI for differentiating musculoskeletal infection from tumour. Skeletal Radiol. 2007; 36 (5):417–421

Shimose S, Sugita T, Kubo T, Matsuo T, Nobuto H, Ochi M. Differential diagnosis between osteomyelitis and bone tumors. Acta Radiol. 2008; 49(8):928–933

Case 86

Michael A. Tall

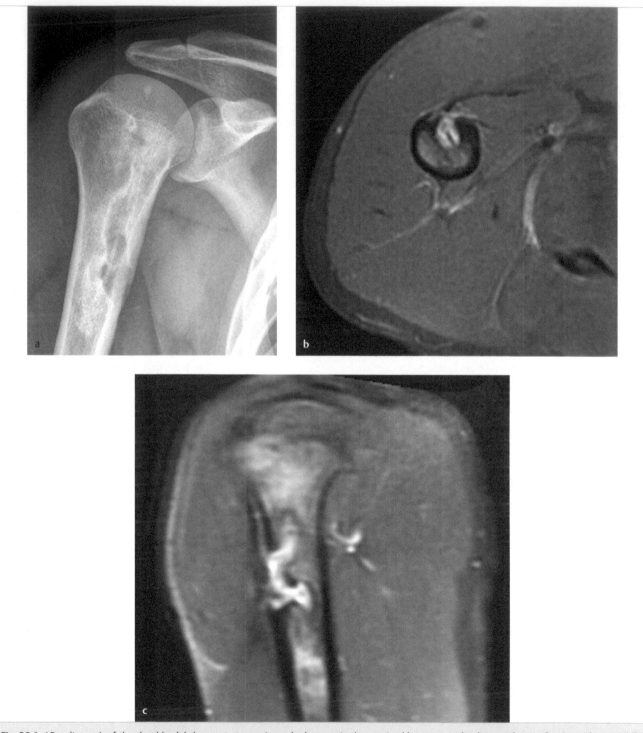

Fig. 86.1 AP radiograph of the shoulder (**a**) demonstrates an irregular lucency in the proximal humerus with a linear sclerotic density within. Axial (**b**) and sagittal (**c**) contrast-enhanced, fat-suppressed, T1-weighted images through the proximal humerus show a centrally located, nonenhancing bony sequestrum surrounded by enhancing granulation tissue (involucrum). A cloaca is present, extending from the involucrum to the overlying cortex.

■ Clinical History

A 23-year-old male with arm pain, swelling, and fevers (▶ Fig. 86.1).

■ Key Finding

Sequestrum.

■ Top 3 Differential Diagnoses

- **Osteomyelitis:** A sequestrum in the setting of osteomyelitis refers to a segment of dead, sclerotic bone that is separated from living bone by granulation tissue. The sequestrum may reside within the marrow and become a source of focal infection that can cause repeated flare-ups of acute osteomyelitis. A rim of living bone that surrounds the sequestrum is referred to as an involucrum. The involucrum may be permeated by a cloaca through which pus and the sequestrum itself may be expelled to the skin surface through a draining sinus tract.
- **Langerhans cell histiocytosis (LCH):** Eosinophilic granuloma is a subset of LCH which is characterized by multiple, predominantly lytic lesions throughout the axial and appendicular skeleton of children and young adults (<30 years of age). It accounts for approximately 70 percent of cases of LCH.

Lesions within the long bones are characterized as lytic lesions with endosteal scalloping and occasionally periosteal reaction. Cranial involvement classically consists of a lytic lesion with beveled edges due to asymmetric involvement of the inner and outer tables. Lytic lesions of cranial vault sometimes contain a central and radiodense fragment of bone, referred to as "button sequestrum."
- **Osteoid osteoma:** The classic radiographic findings in an osteoid osteoma are a centrally located oval or round radiolucent nidus surrounded by a uniform region of sclerotic bone. The central lucency is highly vascularized and is the target of surgical debridement or radiofrequency ablation. In 80% of cases, the nidus contains variable amounts of calcification. Common sites include the long bones of the lower extremities and spine.

■ Additional Diagnostic Considerations

- **Lymphoma:** Both Hodgkin and nonHodgkin lymphoma can affect the bones in both primary and widespread diseases. Primary nonHodgkin lymphoma most commonly presents in the appendicular skeleton as an aggressive osteolytic lesion with poorly defined margins. Osteosclerosis, when evident, is more commonly found in Hodgkin disease, which can present with osteolytic lesions, osteosclerotic lesions, or a mixture of

both. Sequestrum is more commonly seen in the Hodgkin variant.
- **Fibrosarcoma:** Fibrosarcomas are characterized by osteolytic foci with a geographic, moth-eaten, or permeative pattern of bone destruction. There is little osteosclerosis and a striking absence of a significant osseous reaction despite the bone destruction. Occasionally, a sequestrum may be evident.

■ Diagnosis

Osteomyelitis.

✓ Pearls

- Osteomyelitis may demonstrate a sequestrum surrounded by an involucrum and permeated by a cloaca.
- LCH results in lytic calvarial lesions with beveled edges and button sequestrum.

- Osteoid osteomas typically demonstrate a round or oval radiolucent nidus surrounded by sclerotic bone.
- The central nidus in osteoid osteoma is highly vascularized and is the target of radiofrequency ablation.

■ Suggested Readings

Helms CA. Fundamentals of Skeletal Radiology. 4th ed. Philadelphia, PA: Elsevier Saunders; 2014

Jennin F, Bousson V, Parlier C, Jomaah N, Khanine V, Laredo JD. Bony sequestrum: a radiologic review. Skeletal Radiol. 2011; 40(8):963–975

Krasnokutsky MV. The button sequestrum sign. Radiology. 2005; 236(3):1026–1027

Resnick D, Kransdorf MJ. Bone and Joint Imaging. 3rd ed. Philadelphia, PA: Elsevier Saunders; 2005

Case 87

Robert D. Boutin

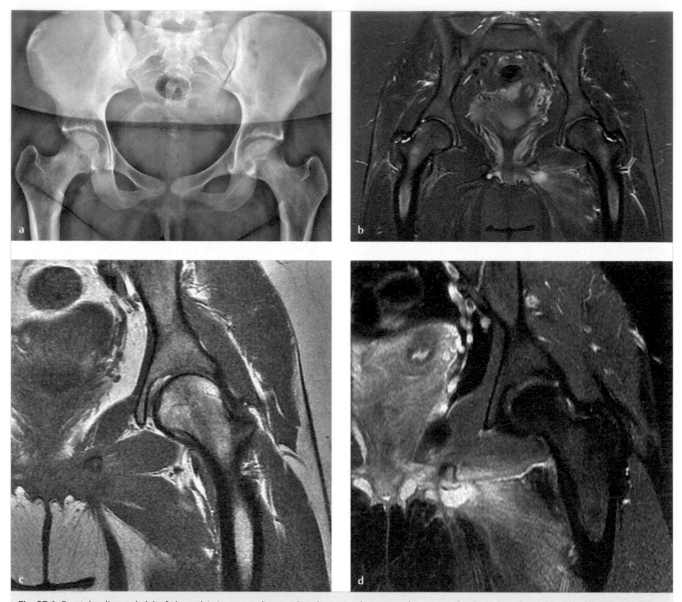

Fig. 87.1 Frontal radiograph **(a)** of the pelvis is unrevealing, with only minimal contour alteration inferolateral to the pubic symphysis on the left. Coronal fat-suppressed T2-weighted **(b)**, coronal T1 **(c)**, and coronal STIR **(d)** images demonstrate bone and muscle edema at the left inferior pubic ramus region, in addition to a small rounded collection of fluid signal.

■ **Clinical History**

A 15-year-old obese, sedentary female with a history of left groin pain and limp (▶ Fig. 87.1).

■ Key Finding

Fluid collection with edema at metaphyseal-equivalent location (prior to skeletal maturity).

■ Top 3 Differential Diagnoses

- **Apophysitis:** An apophysis is defined as a secondary ossification center connected to a parent bone by an associated cartilaginous physis. Apophyses (also called traction epiphyses) occur at tendon attachment sites and are considered "epiphyseal equivalent" structures.

  Repetitive muscle contraction (e.g., overuse with sports) can result in microavulsive injury with inflammatory changes, often referred to as "apophysitis." This type of chronic overuse injury is most common in the pelvis, with imaging findings that may include physeal widening, osseous irregularity, and associated edema.

  The progression of ossification and age of complete fusion varies at the different ossification centers. Familiarity with the imaging appearance of ossification centers throughout childhood is fundamental for differentiating normal versus pathologic findings. In the pelvis, the secondary ossification centers of the symphysis pubis appear later than all other apophyses. Closure of the symphysis pubis secondary ossification centers occur late in the process of skeletal maturation, usually in early adulthood.

- **Avulsion:** The pelvis has numerous apophyses. Prior to ossification, an apophysis is purely cartilaginous and therefore derangements generally go undetected on radiography. With acute biomechanical overload, the typical point of failure ("weakest leak" in the musculoskeletal unit) is the apophyseal physis.

  Traction-related avulsion fractures can affect any apophysis in the pelvis. These avulsions most commonly occur in adolescent athletes at the ischial apophysis, anterior inferior iliac spine, and anterior superior iliac spine.

- **Infection:** Osteomyelitis in adolescent patients is typically spread hematogenously and targets highly vascularized metaphyses of long bones. In the pelvis of skeletally immature patients, osteomyelitis occurs preferentially in metaphyseal-equivalent locations at the junction of bone and cartilage. Typical imaging findings of osteomyelitis are often accompanied by abscess and myositis.

■ Diagnosis

Infection(osteomyelitis, abscess, and myositis).

✓ Pearls

- Radiography is generally the initial imaging test of choice for suspected musculoskeletal derangements.
- After radiography, imaging with sonography and MRI may be preferred over CT for many musculoskeletal conditions, even though improvements have been made with radiation dose reduction with CT.
- The pelvis has numerous apophyses that dynamically change with normal skeletal maturation. Apophyseal regions may be affected by various pain generators, including apophysitis, avulsion fracture, and infection.

■ Suggested Readings

Arnaiz J, Piedra T, de Lucas EM, et al. Imaging findings of lower limb apophysitis. AJR Am J Roentgenol. 2011; 196(3):W316:25

Bayer J, Neubauer J, Saueressig U, Südkamp NP, Reising K. Age- and gender-related characteristics of the pubic symphysis and triradiate cartilage in pediatric computed tomography. Pediatr Radiol. 2016; 46(12):1705–1712

Grissom LE, Harty MP, Guo GW, Kecskemethy HH. Maturation of pelvic ossification centers on computed tomography in normal children. Pediatr Radiol. 2018; 48 (13):1902–1914

Jaramillo D, Dormans JP, Delgado J, Laor T, St Geme JW, III. Hematogenous osteomyelitis in infants and children: imaging of a changing disease. Radiology. 2017; 283 (3):629–643

Nguyen JC, Sheehan SE, Davis KW, Gill KG. Sports and the growing musculoskeletal system: sports imaging series. Radiology. 2017; 284(1):25–42

Parvaresh KC, Pennock AT, Bomar JD, Wenger DR, Upasani VV. Analysis of acetabular ossification from the triradiate cartilage and secondary centers. J Pediatr Orthop. 2018; 38(3):e145–e150

Case 88

Robert D. Boutin

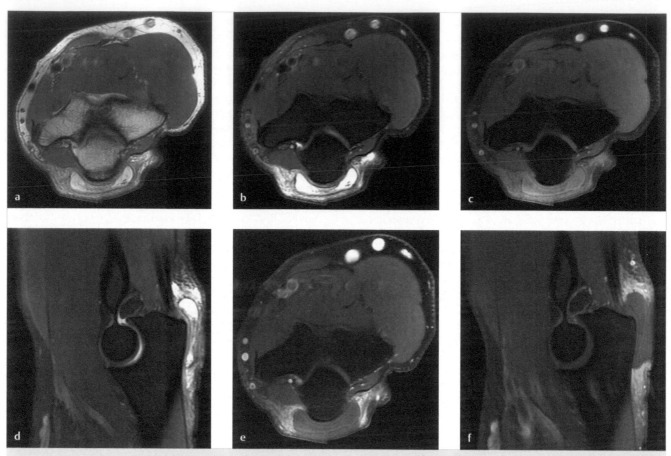

Fig. 88.1 Axial proton density-weighted **(a)**, axial fat-suppressed T2-weighted **(b)**, axial fat-suppressed T1-weighted **(c)**, and sagittal fat-suppressed T2-weighted **(d)** images of the elbow show a crescentic lesion with perilesional edema signal in the superficial soft tissue. The lesion signal intensity is similar to fluid, but it is mildly hyperintense to muscle on T1 imaging and contains tissue of intermediate signal on the other images. After IV contrast administration, axial **(e)**, sagittal **(f)** fat-suppressed T1-weighted images show only peripheral enhancement.

▪ Clinical History

A 49-year-old man with a history of chemotherapy for chronic lymphocytic leukemia and a posterior elbow mass (▶ Fig. 88.1).

■ Key Finding

Space-occupying lesion posterior to the olecranon.

■ Top 3 Differential Diagnoses

- **Olecranon bursitis, noninfectious (nonseptic):** Bursae are sac-like structures that normally have a thin synovial lining, but can become inflamed and distended with many different types of acute and chronic derangements (e.g., blunt trauma, repetitive microtrauma, inflammatory arthritis such as rheumatoid arthritis, and crystal-induced arthropathy such as gout).

  Clinically, swelling and inflammation at the dorsal aspect of the elbow are nonspecific findings. Bursal fluid aspiration may be useful for laboratory analysis (e.g., assess for monosodium urate crystals and rule out infection). More than two-thirds of olecranon bursitis cases are noninfectious. However, of patients with infectious bursitis, about one-third have a history of a previous episode of noninfectious olecranon bursitis.

- **Olecranon bursitis, infectious (septic):** Two superficial bursae are located in the subcutaneous fat layer and are prone to infection in the setting of penetrating trauma: the olecranon bursa and the prepatellar bursa. Direct inoculation of pathogens into these bursae classically occurs with a puncture wound or abrasion. Septic olecranon bursitis is much more common than septic elbow arthritis in adults. Impaired immunity is an important risk factor in up to half of all cases of septic olecranon bursitis (e.g., alcohol abuse, diabetes, malignancy such as chronic lymphocytic leukemia, and medications such as chemotherapy, corticosteroids and anti-TNF drugs).

  Imaging may be used to assess the underlying bone and joint (e.g., rule out osteomyelitis and joint effusion). There is considerable overlap in the imaging findings of infectious and noninfectious olecranon bursitis (e.g., volume of bursal fluid, bursal septation, or olecranon bone marrow signal changes). However, septic olecranon bursitis can be excluded in the absence of bursal and soft-tissue enhancement.

- **Neoplasm:** Neoplasms may occur superficial to the fascia in the subcutaneous layer, and they may be evaluated by diagnostic imaging. When MRI is performed, IV contrast material can be very helpful to differentiate cystic versus solid lesions.

  Proper imaging before sarcoma surgery is of paramount importance, because initial optimal wide resection is one of the most important factors for avoiding local recurrence (usually ranging from 11–23%). Because sarcomas start out as small tumors and may be superficial, radiologists can help surgeons avoid problematic "unplanned excisions" (also referred to as "whoops surgeries") by maintaining a high level of suspicion if an indeterminant solid lesion is present.

■ Diagnosis

Olecranon bursitis, infectious.

✓ Pearls

- If a patient has a history of skin disruption over the olecranon or impaired immunity, a higher index of suspicion for an infectious form of olecranon bursitis is appropriate.
- The cause of bursitis may not necessarily be determined based on clinical findings or imaging findings in isolation.
- Aspiration of bursal contents for laboratory analysis may be appropriate.
- Although superficial soft-tissue masses are often benign, it is important to recall that subcutaneous soft-tissue sarcomas are sometimes small and mismanaged.

■ Suggested Readings

Blackwell JR, Hay BA, Bolt AM, Hay SM. Olecranon bursitis: a systematic overview. Shoulder Elbow. 2014; 6(3):182–190

Boutin FJ, Boutin RD, Boutin FJ Jr. Bursitis. In: Chapman MW, Madison M, eds. Operative Orthopaedics. 2nd ed.Philadelphia: Lippincott;1993:3419–3432

Dyrop HB, Safwat A, Vedsted P, et al. Characteristics of 64 sarcoma patients referred to a sarcoma center after unplanned excision. J Surg Oncol. 2016; 113(2):235–239

Endo M, Setsu N, Fujiwara T, et al. Diagnosis and management of subcutaneous soft tissue sarcoma. Curr Treat Options Oncol. 2019; 20(7):54

Floemer F, Morrison WB, Bongartz G, Ledermann HP. MRI characteristics of olecranon bursitis. AJR Am J Roentgenol. 2004; 183(1):29–34

Morel M, Taïeb S, Penel N, et al. Imaging of the most frequent superficial soft-tissue sarcomas. Skeletal Radiol. 2011; 40(3):271–284

Reilly D, Kamineni S. Olecranon bursitis. J Shoulder Elbow Surg. 2016; 25(1):158–167

Case 89

Robert D. Boutin

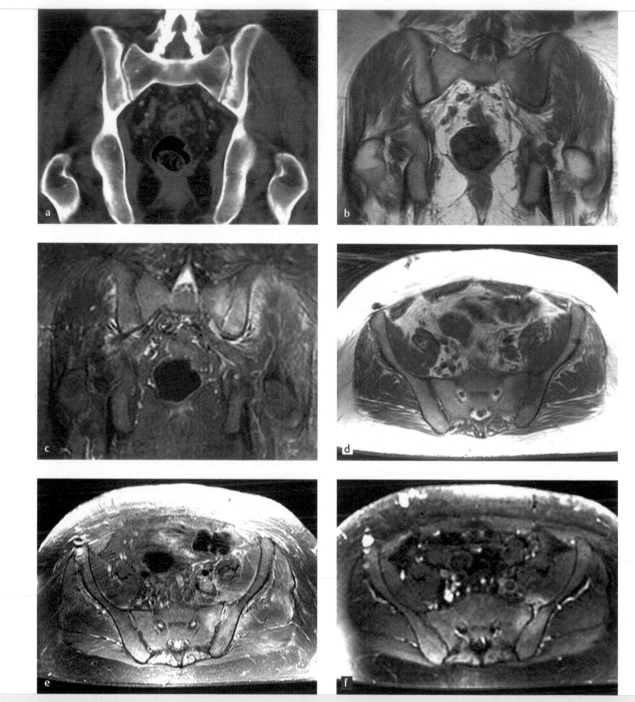

Fig. 89.1 Coronal pelvis CT (**a**) shows subtle subchondral sclerosis and irregularity at the lateral aspect of the left sacroiliac (SI) joint. Follow-up pelvis MRI utilizing coronal T1-weighted (**b**), coronal fat-suppressed T2-weighted (**c**), axial T1-weighted (**d**), and axial fat-suppressed T2-weighted (**e**) images demonstrate bone edema on both sides of the left SI joint as well as periarticular muscle edema. After contrast administration, the axial fat-suppressed T1-weighted (**f**) image shows enhancing bone edema and capsular thickening/capsulitis anteriorly.

■ **Clinical History**

A 34-year-old woman with low back and buttock pain (▶ Fig. 89.1).

■ Key Finding

Unilateral sacroiliitis.

■ Top 3 Differential Diagnoses

- **Spondyloarthritis:** Unilateral sacroiliitis is most commonly caused by spondyloarthritis, particularly psoriatic arthritis, reactive arthritis, and the early stages of ankylosing spondylitis.

  Radiographs are not sensitive or specific in the diagnosis of early sacroiliitis. When positive, the characteristic findings of sacroiliitis on radiography and CT are subchondral erosion and sclerosis, often particularly affecting the iliac side of the joint.

  MRI is often the diagnostic imaging test of choice to assess for active sacroiliitis in patients with suspected spondyloarthritis. The ASAS (Assessment of SpondyloArthritis international Society) criteria for a positive MRI examination include active inflammatory features such as bone marrow edema, synovitis (joint space enhancement), capsulitis, and enthesitis. With time, the MRI findings can evolve to include signs of structural change such as erosion, subchondral sclerosis, fat metaplasia in the subchondral bone (best seen on nonfat-suppressed T1 images), and ankylosis.

- **Infectious sacroiliitis:** Infectious sacroiliitis is not common, and it constitutes only <2% of all causes of sacroiliitis. However, it is important to recognize this cause of sacroiliitis because diagnosis is often missed initially, and the treatment is so much different than with other causes of sacroiliitis. The clinical picture is often not determinative, with only about half of all patients having a fever and inflammatory blood markers that are often nonspecific (e.g., WBC count, ESR, CRP). Potential risk factors may include concurrent infection (e.g., urinary tract infection), postpartum state, IV drug use, or immunocompromised state.

  MRI is highly sensitive in the detection of infectious sacroiliitis, but there are some overlapping features such as bone edema and erosions. In general, MRI findings of bone edema and periarticular edema are particularly intense with infection, but are more mild with spondyloarthritis. In addition, infectious sacroiliitis is specifically suggested by MRI findings of extensive extracapsular, soft-tissue abnormalities, including periarticular muscle edema, thick capsulitis (>5 mm), extracapsular fluid collections, and bone erosions measuring >1 cm. Of these findings, periarticular muscle edema is the single most important predictor of infectious sacroiliitis. Furthermore, periarticular fluid collections are almost exclusively seen with infectious sacroiliitis (highly specific, but not sensitive).

- **Degenerative and posttraumatic:** Osteoarthritis (OA) commonly affects the sacroiliac (SI) joints, most often in older adults. Although it is often seen bilaterally, it can be asymmetric or even unilateral occasionally. Altered stresses that predispose to a unilateral phenomenon can include a history of trauma or altered biomechanics (e.g., scoliosis, transitional lumbosacral segment, or athletic pelvic stress injury). SI joints may also be affected by other insults, including radiation therapy to the pelvis, sometimes with superimposed osteonecrosis or the insufficiency type of stress fracture.

  The primary findings of SI OA include joint space narrowing (especially inferiorly), subchondral sclerosis (especially at the ilium), osteophytes (especially anteriorly), and vacuum phenomenon (gas within the joint). Intra-articular osseous ankylosis is not a feature of OA. Bone marrow edema involving the SI joints and mimicking sacroiliitis has been found in almost one-third of athletes or patients who have a nonspondyloarthritis type of inflammatory, low-back pain.

■ Diagnosis

Infectious sacroiliitis.

✓ Pearls

- Sacroiliitis is often the first manifestation of spondyloarthritis.
- Unilateral sacroiliitis is most commonly caused by spondyloarthritis (e.g., psoriatic arthritis, reactive arthritis, early ankylosing spondylitis).
- Infectious sacroiliitis is specifically suggested by MRI findings of extensive extracapsular soft-tissue abnormalities (e.g., periarticular muscle edema, thick capsulitis, or extracapsular fluid collections) and bone erosions measuring >1 cm.

■ Suggested Readings

Kang Y, Hong SH, Kim JY, et al. Unilateral sacroiliitis: differential diagnosis between infectious sacroiliitis and spondyloarthritis based on MRI findings. AJR Am J Roentgenol. 2015; 205(5):1048–1055

Kanna RM, Bosco A, Shetty AP, Rajasekaran S. Unilateral sacroiliitis: differentiating infective and inflammatory etiology by magnetic resonance imaging and tissue studies. Eur Spine J. 2019; 28(4):762–767

Maksymowych WP, Lambert RG, Østergaard M, et al. MRI lesions in the sacroiliac joints of patients with spondyloarthritis: an update of definitions and validation by the ASAS MRI working group. Ann Rheum Dis. 2019; 78(11):1550–1558

Sieper J, Rudwaleit M, Baraliakos X, et al. The Assessment of SpondyloArthritis international Society (ASAS) handbook: a guide to assess spondyloarthritis. Ann Rheum Dis. 2009; 68 Suppl 2:ii1–ii44

Sondag M, Gete K, Verhoeven F, Aubry S, Prati C, Wendling D. Analysis of the early signs of septic sacroiliitis on computed tomography. Eur J Rheumatol. 2019; 6(3):122–125

Case 90

Robert D. Boutin

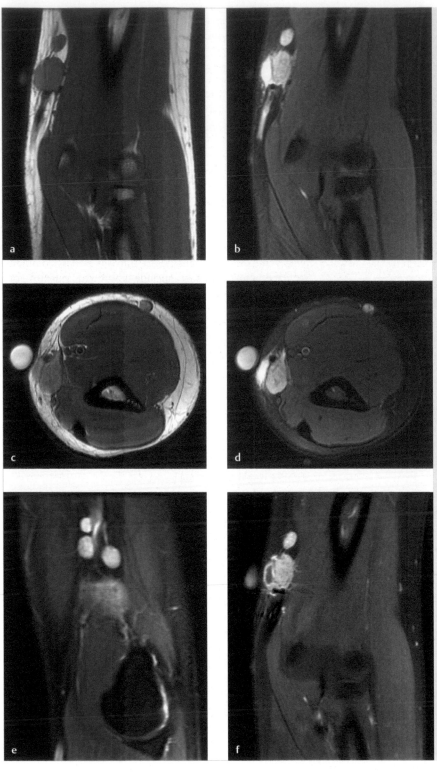

Fig. 90.1 Coronal T1-weighted (**a**) and fat-suppressed T2-weighted (**b**) images of the elbow demonstrate small, nodular, soft-tissue masses (approximately 3 cm proximal to the medial humeral epicondyle). Corresponding axial proton density-weighted (**c**), axial fat-suppressed T2-weighted (**d**), and sagittal fat-suppressed T2-weighted (**e**) images show the main epitrochlear mass and its satellites are superficial to the brachial fascia and posterior to the basilic vein. After contrast administration, a coronal fat-suppressed T1-weighted (**f**) image shows there is generally enhancement, except at the site of a small nonenhancing fluid collection (immediately deep to the skin marker).

■ Clinical History

A 19-year-old woman with a moderately painful mass near the elbow for 3 months (▶ Fig. 90.1).

■ Key Finding

Epitrochlear lymphadenopathy.

■ Top 3 Differential Diagnoses

- **Infection:** Infectious etiologies include viral, bacterial, myco bacterial, fungal, or parasitic diseases. In the past, epitrochlear adenopathy was commonly associated with tuberculosis or other mycobacteria. Now, in children and young adults who have exposure to cats (but no other medical history), the most common cause of a painful epitrochlear mass is the Gram negative bacteria *Bartonella henselae*. This is commonly referred to as "cat scratch disease" because inoculation occurs via the scratch or bite of a cat.

  With *cat scratch disease*, key imaging features help differentiate lymph nodes in the medial epitrochlear location from other causes of soft-tissue masses. Specifically, the anatomic location of epitrochlear lymph nodes is posterior to the basilic vein and superficial to the brachialis muscle fascia. This fascia separates epitrochlear lymph nodes from deeper neurovascular structures (i.e., neurovascular bundles containing the ulnar nerve, median nerve and brachial artery), and therefore allows exclusion of common intermuscular lesions like peripheral nerve sheath tumors and primary intramuscular masses. Other characteristic imaging features of epitrochlear lymphadenopathy include oval shape (>90% of cases), one or more satellite nodes (>50%), and small fluid collection (abscess, >33%).

- **Inflammation:** Inflammatory (noninfectious) causes of epitrochlear lymphadenopathy include foreign material (e.g., related to IV drug use), sarcoidosis, and Kimura disease.

  Sarcoidosis is a systemic inflammatory disease characterized by the immune granulomas that form most commonly in the lungs and the lymphatic system.

  Kimura disease is an idiopathic chronic inflammatory disorder characterized by subcutaneous lymphoid masses involving the head, neck, or upper extremities, typically affecting young men of Asian descent.

- **Neoplasm:** Neoplastic conditions can cause epitrochlear lymph node enlargement (>5–10 mm). The most commonly reported neoplastic causes include lymphoma, leukemia, and melanoma, in addition to various metastases.

■ Diagnosis

Cat scratch disease.

✓ Pearls

- Lymphadenopathy can be caused most commonly by infectious etiologies, noninfectious inflammatory conditions (e.g., autoimmune diseases), and neoplastic disorders. Appropriate workup may include blood tests, imaging, and biopsy.
- The epitrochlear lymph nodes drain the superficial lymphatic systems at the ulnar aspect of the hand and forearm.

- Although soft-tissue masses at the medial aspect of the elbow are often referred to specialists with a concern for neoplasm, the imaging appearance of epitrochlear lymphadenopathy is distinct from lesions arising from nerves and vessels.

■ Suggested Readings

Bernard SA, Walker EA, Carroll JF, Klassen-Fischer M, Murphey MD. Epitrochlear cat scratch disease: unique imaging features allowing differentiation from other soft tissue masses of the medial arm. Skeletal Radiol. 2016; 45(9):1227–1234

Gaddey HL, Riegel AM. Unexplained lymphadenopathy: evaluation and differential diagnosis. Am Fam Physician. 2016; 94(11):896–903

Grunewald J, Grutters JC, Arkema EV, Saketkoo LA, Moller DR, Müller-Quernheim J. Sarcoidosis. Nat Rev Dis Primers. 2019; 5(1):45

Lam AC, Au Yeung RK, Lau VW. A rare disease in an atypical location–Kimura's disease of the upper extremity. Skeletal Radiol. 2015; 44(12):1833–1837

Muthu V, Sehgal IS, Dhooria S, Agarwal R. Clinical significance and epidemiological evolution of epitrochlear lymphadenopathy in pre- and post-highly active antiretroviral therapy era: A systematic review of the literature. Lung India. 2018; 35 (2):150–153

Case 91

Robert D. Boutin

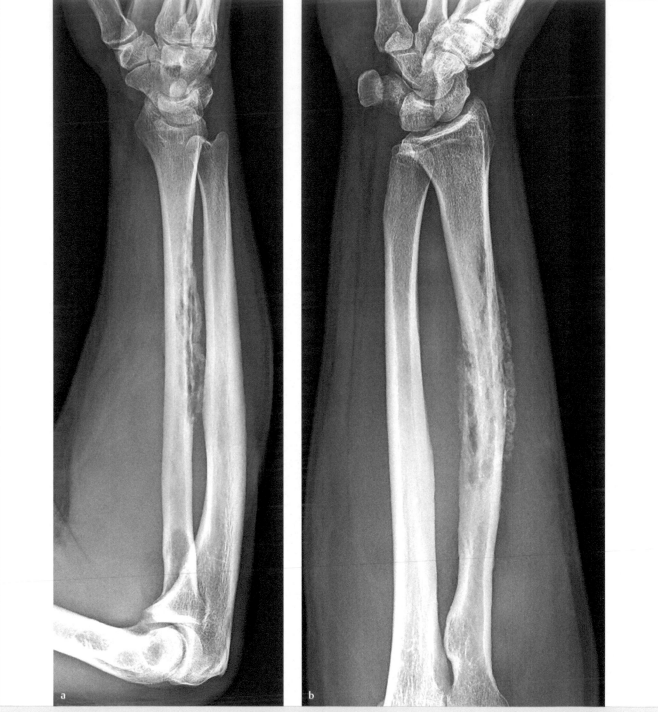

Fig. 91.1 Lateral **(a)** and frontal **(b)** radiographs of the forearm show aggressive, cortically-based osteolysis and periosteal reaction at the radial shaft.

■ Clinical History

A 57-year-old man with persistent forearm pain after a puncture wound at work (▶ Fig. 91.1).

■ Key Finding

Aggressive, cortically-based osteolysis and periosteal reaction at the diaphysis of an adult long bone.

■ Top 3 Differential Diagnoses

- **Osteomyelitis:** Osteomyelitis (infection of bone) may be classified by route of infection (hematogenous vs. nonhematogenous), duration of infection (acute vs. chronic), and organism (e.g., pyogenic vs. atypical).

  Osteomyelitis in the extremities of adults is encountered most commonly in diabetic feet with overlying, soft-tissue ulcerations. In the absence of clinical and laboratory findings to suggest osteomyelitis, the radiographic appearance may be confused with neoplasm.

  Although radiography is the initial imaging test of choice, cross-sectional imaging may be helpful to evaluate relevant findings in a patient with infection (e.g., abscess, sequestrum, sinus tract, gas, foreign material, halo sign). Cross-sectional imaging also can help determine the extent of an inflammatory/infectious process in the medullary bone and regional soft tissues.

- **Malignant neoplasm:** Aggressive, cortically-based osteolysis and periosteal reaction at the diaphysis of a long bone can be caused by various "small, round blue cell neoplasms." A differential diagnostic list of "small, round blue cell lesions" is long. In musculoskeletal radiology, some of the most common conditions can be recalled with the following mnemonic "LEMON": Lymphoma/Leukemia/LCH, Ewing sarcoma, Multiple myeloma/plasmacytoma/metastasis, Osteomyelitis, and Neuroblastoma.

  When accounting for the anatomic location and patient age, the differential diagnosis can be honed further.

- **Miscellaneous:** In the differential diagnosis for an unknown process, you can quickly consider all the major categories of disease to ensure you are not forgetting something important. Many physicians like using a "universal differential diagnosis" mnemonic such as "VINDICATE": Vascular, Inflammation/Infection, Neoplastic/Neurologic, Degenerative/Drugs, Iatrogenic/Idiopathic, Congenital, Autoimmune, Trauma, and Endocrine/metabolic.

  For example, in a case of cortically-based osteolysis, considerations sometimes might include "drugs" (e.g., sequelae of IV drug use), "iatrogenic" conditions (e.g., atypical appearance after hardware removal or bone curettage), "idiopathic" conditions (e.g., Gorham–Stout disease, also referred to as "vanishing bone disease"), and "endocrine/metabolic" conditions (e.g., hyperparathyroidism).

■ Diagnosis

Osteomyelitis.

✓ Pearls

- After radiography, cross-sectional imaging in a patient with infection is commonly helpful to assess for abscess, sequestrum, sinus tract, gas, foreign material, and halo sign.
- The differential diagnosis of an aggressive, cortically-based osteolysis and periosteal reaction at the diaphysis of a long bone in an adult primarily focuses on osteomyelitis versus malignant neoplasm.
- Biopsy is often necessary to establish a definitive diagnosis. Accurate identification of a specific infectious pathogen or specific tumor histology is crucial in guiding optimal treatment and establishing a prognosis.

■ Suggested Readings

Chadayammuri V, Herbert B, Hao J, et al. Diagnostic accuracy of various modalities relative to open bone biopsy for detection of long bone posttraumatic osteomyelitis. Eur J Orthop Surg Traumatol. 2017; 27(7):871–875

Dellinger MT, Garg N, Olsen BR. Viewpoints on vessels and vanishing bones in Gorham-Stout disease. Bone. 2014; 63:47–52

Glaudemans AWJM, Jutte PC, Cataldo MA, et al. Consensus document for the diagnosis of peripheral bone infection in adults: a joint paper by the EANM, EBJIS, and ESR (with ESCMID endorsement). Eur J Nucl Med Mol Imaging. 2019; 46(4):957–970

Govaert GA, IJpma FF, McNally M, McNally E, Reininga IH, Glaudemans AW. Accuracy of diagnostic imaging modalities for peripheral post-traumatic osteomyelitis - a systematic review of the recent literature. Eur J Nucl Med Mol Imaging. 2017; 44 (8):1393–1407

Rosen RA, Morehouse HT, Karp HJ, Yu GS. Intracortical fissuring in osteomyelitis. Radiology. 1981; 141(1):17–20

Case 92

Robert D. Boutin

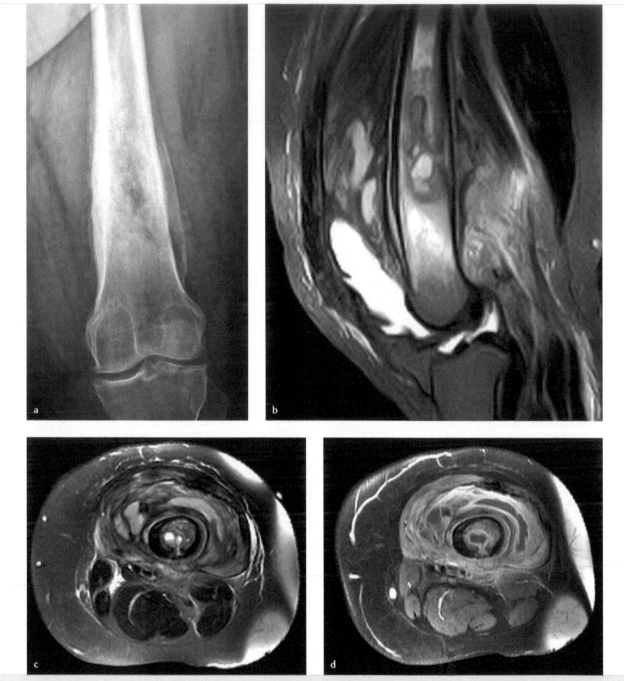

Fig. 92.1 Frontal radiograph (**a**) of the femur shows a "moth-eaten" pattern of patchy osteolysis with ill-defined margins, a broad zone of transition, as well as lamellated periosteal reaction. Sagittal fat-suppressed T2-weighted (**b**) and axial fat-suppressed T2-weighted (**c**) images show rounded fluid-like signal in both the medullary bone and the overlying soft tissues. Axial postcontrast fat-suppressed T1-weighted (**d**) image shows peripheral enhancement of these findings, as well as tiny, very thin linear channels that perforate the posterior cortex.

■ Clinical History

A young adult man presented to the emergency department with thigh pain (▸ Fig. 92.1).

■ Key Finding

Abscesses in bone and adjacent to bone, with thin perforations in cortex–Roentgen classic.

■ Diagnosis

Infection: Musculoskeletal infections can have protean imaging manifestations. The imaging findings may vary according to infection acuity (acute, subacute, or chronic), patient age, route of bone contamination (i.e., hematogenous, contiguous spread, or direct contamination), and infectious organism.

Given that the presentation of musculoskeletal infection can vary significantly, depending on the duration, location, and cause, it is prudent to synthesize all pertinent data for an accurate diagnosis, including clinical history, laboratory results, and radiographic/imaging findings.

MRI is generally considered sensitive for the detection of early osteomyelitis. Diagnostic specificity of MRI, however, may be limited; diminished T1 and increased T2 signal intensity in bone marrow can be caused by a wide variety of etiologies.

Although MRI signal intensity changes are often not specific for osteomyelitis, some imaging findings should be recognized as highly characteristic. In particular, with hematogenous seeding of osteomyelitis in a long bone, a peripherally enhancing abscess in the medullary bone can be accompanied by cortical perforation and abscess formation overlying the cortex (under the periosteum in children or in the adjacent soft tissue in adults). With contiguous spread of infection (classically seen in the diabetic foot), a soft-tissue defect may abut the bone and be associated with cortical disruption and underlying marrow changes.

■ Diagnosis

Osteomyelitis with cloaca and abscesses (intraosseous and soft tissue).

✓ Pearls

- For the diagnosis of osteomyelitis, MRI is highly sensitive and sometimes specific. The specificity of MRI for active infection may be particularly limited with certain conditions, including neuropathic (Charcot) osteoarthropathy, prior surgery, and some neoplasms.

- MRI findings with high specificity for osteomyelitis include the presence of a cortical perforation (cloaca) connecting abscesses in bone and adjacent to bone.
- IV contrast material can help to delineate cloacae and sinus tracts, differentiate abscesses from phlegmon, and show areas of devitalized (necrotic) tissue.

■ Suggested Readings

Boutin RD, Brossmann J, Sartoris DJ, Reilly D, Resnick D. Update on imaging of orthopedic infections. Orthop Clin North Am. 1998; 29(1):41–66

Desimpel J, Posadzy M, Vanhoenacker F. The many faces of osteomyelitis: a pictorial review. J Belg Soc Radiol. 2017; 101(1):24

Jaramillo D, Dormans JP, Delgado J, Laor T, St Geme JW III. Hematogenous osteomyelitis in infants and children: imaging of a changing disease. Radiology. 2017; 283 (3):629–643

Kompel A, Murakami A, Guermazi A. Magnetic resonance imaging of nontraumatic musculoskeletal emergencies. Magn Reson Imaging Clin N Am. 2016; 24(2):369–389

Lee YJ, Sadigh S, Mankad K, Kapse N, Rajeswaran G. The imaging of osteomyelitis. Quant Imaging Med Surg. 2016; 6(2):184–198

Sconfienza LM, Signore A, Cassar-Pullicino V, et al. Diagnosis of peripheral bone and prosthetic joint infections: overview on the consensus documents by the EANM, EBJIS, and ESR (with ESCMID endorsement). Eur Radiol. 2019; 29(12):6425–6438

Part 7

Soft Tissue Tumors

Case 93

Robert D. Boutin

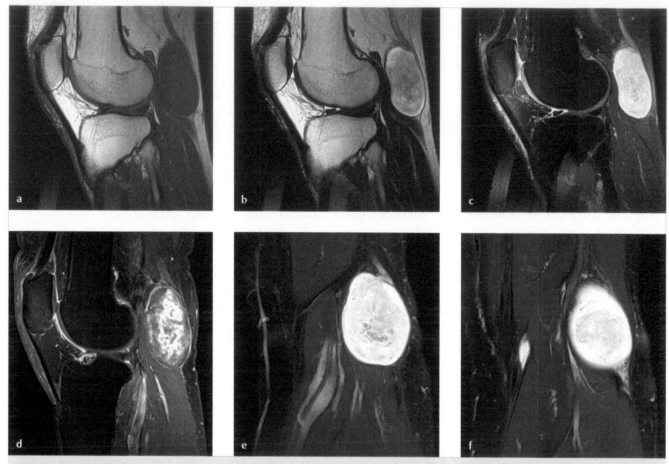

Fig. 93.1 Sagittal T1-weighted (**a**), sagittal T2-weighted (**b**), sagittal fat-suppressed T2-weighted (**c**), and sagittal postcontrast fat-suppressed T1-weighted (**d**) images of the knee show a lesion in the popliteal fossa. Although the fat-suppressed T2-weighted image displays the lesion as hyperintense (similar to fluid), there is more heterogeneous, diminished signal within the lesion on the T2 image without fat suppression and enhancement on the postcontrast image. Sagittal images also show longitudinal linear signal (isointense with the lesion) entering the posterior-superior margin of the mass. Coronal fat-suppressed T2-weighted images confirm the appearance of a stalk-like structure that eccentrically enters (**e**) and exits (**f**) the mass.

▪ Clinical History

A 51-year-old man referred for a history of a "firm, slowly growing popliteal cyst" (▶ Fig. 93.1).

■ Key Finding

Fusiform mass, with longitudinal "tail" entering and exiting eccentrically.

■ Top 3 Differential Diagnoses

- **Benign peripheral nerve sheath tumor:** Benign peripheral nerve sheath tumors (BPNSTs) are classified into two general types among patients without neurofibromatosis: schwannomas (also termed neurilemmomas) and neurofibromas.

  Both types of BPNSTs can show contrast enhancement and *features distinctive to neurogenic neoplasms*, including a fusiform shape with a "tail sign" (i.e., nerve entering and exiting the mass), a "target sign" (i.e., central hypointense signal surrounded by hyperintense signal on T2 images), a "fascicular sign" (i.e., fascicular nerve bundles seen as small, round intermediate signal structures surrounded by higher signal intensity on T2 images), or a "split-fat sign" (i.e., rind of fat, often best seen over the proximal and distal poles of the mass on long-axis images).

  With schwannomas (unlike neurofibromas) arising from larger nerves, the mass is characteristically seen *eccentric* to the nerve, which facilitates surgical resection and sparing of the nerve.

- **Malignant peripheral nerve sheath tumor:** Malignant peripheral nerve sheath tumors (MPNSTs) typically affect large nerves and have a strong association with neurofibromatosis type 1 (lifetime prevalence, ~10%).

  Although MPNSTs can be difficult to differentiate from BPNSTs (particularly plexiform neurofibromas in patients with neurofibromatosis), the *three MRI findings most associated with MPNSTs* include large size (>5 cm), infiltrative margins (associated with perilesional edema and perilesional enhancement) and heterogeneous signal on T1, T2, and postcontrast images (due to intratumoral necrosis and bleeding).

- **Vascular derangement:** Vascular derangements can include aneurysm, pseudoaneurysm, thrombosis, and venous varicosity.

  True aneurysms involve all layers of the vessel wall (intima, media, and adventitia), and occur most commonly in older men with atherosclerosis or hypertension. Popliteal aneurysms are the most common type of peripheral artery aneurysm (70%), bilateral in at least 50% of patients, and typically undergo repair when >1.5 to 2 cm.

  Pseudoaneurysms (also referred to as false aneurysms) occur when a blood vessel wall is injured (e.g., with surgery or an adjacent osteochondroma), and the leaking blood collects in the perivascular soft tissue (often contained by the media or adventitia). These lesions arise from the popliteal artery and may contain lamellated thrombus with areas of high-T1 signal (due to methemoglobin) and low-T2 signal (due to hemosiderin or flow void).

■ Diagnosis

Schwannoma (BPNST) of the common peroneal nerve.

✓ Pearls

- A *neurogenic neoplasm* should be considered when a fusiform mass is observed in the distribution of a nerve, especially when long-axis images show a "tail" of the mass entering proximally and exiting distally.

- Compared to most solitary BPNSTs, *MPNSTs* are highly associated with neurofibromatosis type 1 and are characterized by large size, perilesional edema, and intratumoral necrosis.

- Like neurogenic tumors, popliteal vessel derangements occur in the intermuscular fat plane and have longitudinally-oriented, tail-like structures emanating from the proximal and distal poles of the lesion.

■ Suggested Readings

Ahlawat S, Fayad LM. Imaging cellularity in benign and malignant peripheral nerve sheath tumors: utility of the "target sign" by diffusion weighted imaging. Eur J Radiol. 2018; 102:195–201

Baptista E, Kubo R, Santos DC, Taneja AK. A teenager presenting with pain and popliteal mass. Pseudoaneurysm of the popliteal artery secondary to a distal femoral osteochondroma. Skeletal Radiol. 2017; 46(6):805–806, 841–842

Leake AE, Segal MA, Chaer RA, et al. Meta-analysis of open and endovascular repair of popliteal artery aneurysms. J Vasc Surg. 2017; 65(1):246–256.e2

Matsumine A, Kusuzaki K, Nakamura T, et al. Differentiation between neurofibromas and malignant peripheral nerve sheath tumors in neurofibromatosis 1 evaluated by MRI. J Cancer Res Clin Oncol. 2009; 135(7):891–900

Miettinen MM, Antonescu CR, Fletcher CDM, et al. Histopathologic evaluation of atypical neurofibromatous tumors and their transformation into malignant peripheral nerve sheath tumor in patients with neurofibromatosis 1-a consensus overview. Hum Pathol. 2017; 67:1–10

Yu YH, Wu JT, Ye J, Chen MX. Radiological findings of malignant peripheral nerve sheath tumor: reports of six cases and review of literature. World J Surg Oncol. 2016; 14:142

Case 94

Robert D. Boutin

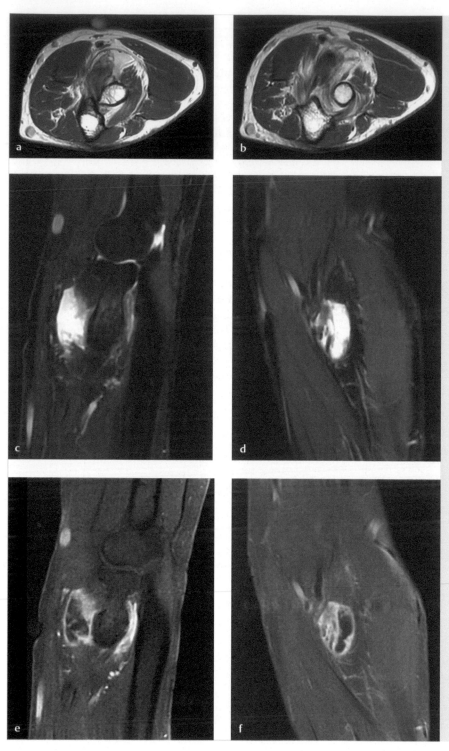

Fig. 94.1 Axial proton density-weighted images **(a, b)** of the elbow show biceps tendinopathy, with osseous hypertrophy narrowing of the radioulnar interspace and bicipitoradial bursal fluid extending between the biceps tendon and its insertion onto the radial tuberosity. Sagittal **(c)** and coronal **(d)** fat-suppressed T2-weighted images show a rounded collection of fluid signal containing synovial thickening and thin septation. After IV contrast administration, sagittal **(e)** and coronal **(f)** fat-suppressed T1-weighted images show peripheral and septal enhancement, with extension between the radius and ulna in **(e)**.

■ Clinical History

A 59-year-old woman with a lump anterior to the elbow for 1 year. The patient reports the lump is "soft in morning, but it increases in size and firmness by the end of the day" (▶ Fig. 94.1).

■ Key Finding

Complex fluid collection in the bicipitoradial bursa.

■ Top 3 Differential Diagnoses

- **Bicipitoradial bursitis:** The bicipitoradial bursa is located between the biceps tendon and the radial tuberosity. The role of this synovial-lined bursa is to reduce friction between the tendon and bone during pronation and supination.

  Bursal inflammation and enlargement may occur secondary to numerous etiologies. The most common cause is chronic mechanical friction in association with biceps tendinopathy or partial tearing. Less common etiologies include synovial-based inflammatory processes (e.g., rheumatoid arthritis), indolent infection (e.g., tuberculosis), neoplastic conditions (e.g., synovial chondromatosis), and metabolic disorders (e.g. tumoral calcinosis). Patients sometimes notice that non-neoplastic fluid collections (e.g., bursitis, cysts) wax and wane in size.
- **Periarticular cyst:** A periarticular cyst (or ganglion) may arise from the elbow, most commonly at the anterior aspect of the radiocapitellar joint. Such cysts are often identified at the elbow joint line proximal to the arcade of Frohse (proximal edge of the supinator muscle), with a thin pedicle that allows a confident diagnosis.

Cysts can exert mass effect on the radial nerve or its branches, most often the superficial (sensory) branch of the radial nerve, compressing it against the extensor carpi radialis brevis muscle, with clinical symptoms that may mimic lateral epicondylitis. When the deep (motor) branch of the radial nerve (posterior interosseous nerve) is affected, symptoms are related to weakness in the extensor muscles, and MRI can show denervation changes in the affected muscles.

- **Hematoma:** Blood may collect in the antecubital region after tissue trauma. In the acute setting, such blood may be related to common injuries (e.g., biceps tendon rupture) or uncommon injuries (e.g., brachialis muscle rupture with full-thickness anterior capsule tear associated with a transient elbow dislocation). Percutaneous tissue trauma (e.g., iatrogenic or IV drug use) may occasionally be complicated by hematoma and/or infection.

  After an elbow dislocation event, characteristic concomitant injuries should be sought, including collateral ligament rupture, osseous injury (e.g., coronoid process fracture), and neurovascular injury (e.g., brachial artery occlusion).

■ Diagnosis

Bicipitoradial bursitis.

✓ Pearls

- Non-neoplastic conditions can mimic soft-tissue neoplasms. Knowledge of the characteristic anatomic sites for bursae can be helpful in avoiding misdiagnosis.
- Although the bicipitoradial bursa is not normally identified on MRI, it can become inflamed and distended. Bicipitoradial bursitis often presents clinically as a soft-tissue mass, and it

may cause compression of the adjacent radial nerve branches.
- Unlike a ganglion cyst (which often arises at the anterior aspect of the radiocapitellar joint), bicipitoradial bursitis invariably extends between the biceps tendon and radial tuberosity.

■ Suggested Readings

Luokkala T, Temperley D, Basu S, Karjalainen TV, Watts AC. Analysis of magnetic resonance imaging-confirmed soft tissue injury pattern in simple elbow dislocations. J Shoulder Elbow Surg. 2019; 28(2):341–348

Rodriguez Miralles J, Natera Cisneros L, Escolà A, Fallone JC, Cots M, Espiga X. Type A ganglion cysts of the radiocapitellar joint may involve compression of the superficial radial nerve. Orthop Traumatol Surg Res. 2016; 102(6):791–794

Schreiber JJ, Potter HG, Warren RF, Hotchkiss RN, Daluiski A. Magnetic resonance imaging findings in acute elbow dislocation: insight into mechanism. J Hand Surg Am. 2014; 39(2):199–205

Skaf AY, Boutin RD, Dantas RW, et al. Bicipitoradial bursitis: MR imaging findings in eight patients and anatomic data from contrast material opacification of bursae followed by routine radiography and MR imaging in cadavers. Radiology. 1999; 212(1):111–116

Yamazaki H, Kato H, Hata Y, Murakami N, Saitoh S. The two locations of ganglions causing radial nerve palsy. J Hand Surg Eur Vol. 2007; 32(3):341–345

Yap SH, Griffith JF, Lee RKL. Imaging bicipitoradial bursitis: a pictorial essay. Skeletal Radiol. 2019; 48(1):5–10

Case 95

Robert D. Boutin

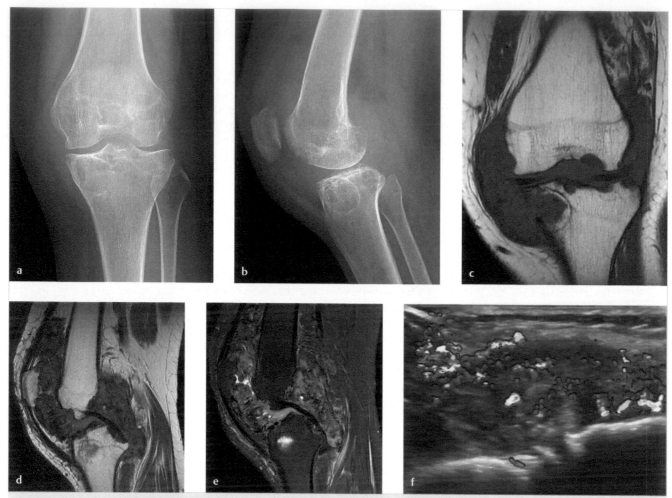

Fig. 95.1 Knee AP (**a**) and lateral (**b**) radiographs show soft-tissue fullness in the joint, erosions, osseous demineralization, and relatively preserved joint spaces. Coronal T1-weighted (**c**), sagittal proton density-weighted (**d**), and fat-suppressed T2-weighted (**e**) images of the knee show a bulky soft-tissue mass of intermediate-to-low signal intensity on all pulse sequences. The mass distends the joint and causes osseous erosions. Doppler sonography (**f**) shows vascularity within the mass.

■ Clinical History

A 42-year-old woman with recurrent knee pain and fullness 10 years after arthroscopic synovectomy (▶ Fig. 95.1).

■ Key Finding

Infiltrative intra-articular mass of low-T2 signal intensity, with erosions.

■ Top 3 Differential Diagnoses

- **Tenosynovial giant cell tumor (TSGCT), diffuse type:** Tenosynovial giant cell tumor is a synovial-based proliferative disorder that can target the synovial lining of a joint, tendon sheath, or bursa.

  Since revision of nomenclature by the World Health Organization in 2013, the umbrella term TSGCT is used to apply to giant cell-containing neoplasms that were formerly known as "pigmented villonodular synovitis (PVNS)" and "giant cell tumor of the tendon sheath." Currently, the favored lexicon for the family of TSGCT lesions describes the tumors by extent as either localized (nodular) or diffuse (infiltrative).

  With the diffuse-type of TSGCT, the most common presentation is a monoarticular process in the knee. Any synovial joint can be affected, including the hip, ankle, and elbow. With radiography, the intra-articular soft-tissue mass is characteristically nonmineralized. With MRI, the hallmark is a low-T2 mass infiltrating the joint recesses, with hemosiderin-containing tissue that shows susceptibility ("blooming") artifact on gradient-echo images and enhancement after contrast administration. With sonography, vascularity can be seen in the mass. These nonmalignant neoplasms can be locally aggressive, with adjacent osseous erosions and recurrence after surgery.

  Treatment with surgery alone is associated with recurrence rates of 30 to 40%. Promising results are now reported for surgery combined with a new generation of immune-oncology drugs.

- **Synovial chondromatosis, primary:** Like TSGCT, primary synovial chondromatosis is generally considered a monoarticular process that most commonly presents in young to middle-aged patients and often targets the knee (70%). Secondary synovial chondromatosis is a term that is sometimes used to refer to loose bodies that occur secondary to a chronic arthritis, typically osteoarthritis.

  With primary synovial chondromatosis, intra-articular cartilaginous loose bodies are shed into the joint. These nodular fragments are typically small (<1 cm) and relatively similar in size. At the time of presentation, no radiographically visible mineralization (calcification or ossification) is present in one-third of cases. The imaging findings are considered pathognomonic when innumerable mineralized bodies of similar size and shape are observed in a joint with preserved articular cartilage.

- **Hemophilic arthropathy:** Hemophilic arthropathy can result in low-T2 signal with thickening of the synovium and can often affect the knee. Like TSGCT, hemosiderin in the joint "blooms" on gradient-echo MRI, and there is no mineralization on radiographic examinations. Unlike TSGCT and synovial chondromatosis, hemophilic arthropathy is often polyarticular and only affects males.

■ Diagnosis

Tenosynovial giant cell tumor, diffuse type (pigmented villonodular synovitis).

✓ Pearls

- With MRI, hypointense signal on T2 images is generally caused by a lesion containing calcification, hemosiderin, or fibrous tissue. Radiography is helpful in differentiating mineralized versus nonmineralized tissue.
- The classic presentation of a diffuse type of TSGCT is an infiltrative soft-tissue mass with T2-hypointense signal, most commonly as a monoarticular process involving the knee joint.

- Primary synovial chondromatosis is nonmineralized in one-third of cases. In the remaining cases, the diagnosis can generally be made when innumerable mineralized bodies of similar size and shape are observed in a joint with preserved articular cartilage.

■ Suggested Readings

Boutin RD, Bindra J, Canter RJ. Imaging soft tissue tumors. In: Chapman MW, James MA, eds. Chapman's Comprehensive Orthopaedic Surgery. 4th ed. New Delhi: Jaypee; 2019

Evenski AJ, Stensby JD, Rosas S, Emory CL. Diagnostic imaging and management of common intra-articular and peri-articular soft tissue tumors and tumor like conditions of the knee. J Knee Surg. 2019; 32(4):322–330

Gounder MM, Thomas DM, Tap WD. Locally aggressive connective tissue tumors. J Clin Oncol. 2018; 36(2):202–209

Papakonstantinou O, Isaac A, Dalili D, Noebauer-Huhmann IM. T2-weighted hypointense tumors and tumor-like lesions. Semin Musculoskelet Radiol. 2019; 23(1): 58–75

Wadhwa V, Cho G, Moore D, Pezeshk P, Coyner K, Chhabra A. T2 black lesions on routine knee MRI: differential considerations. Eur Radiol. 2016; 26(7):2387–2399

Case 96

Robert D. Boutin and Jasjeet Bindra

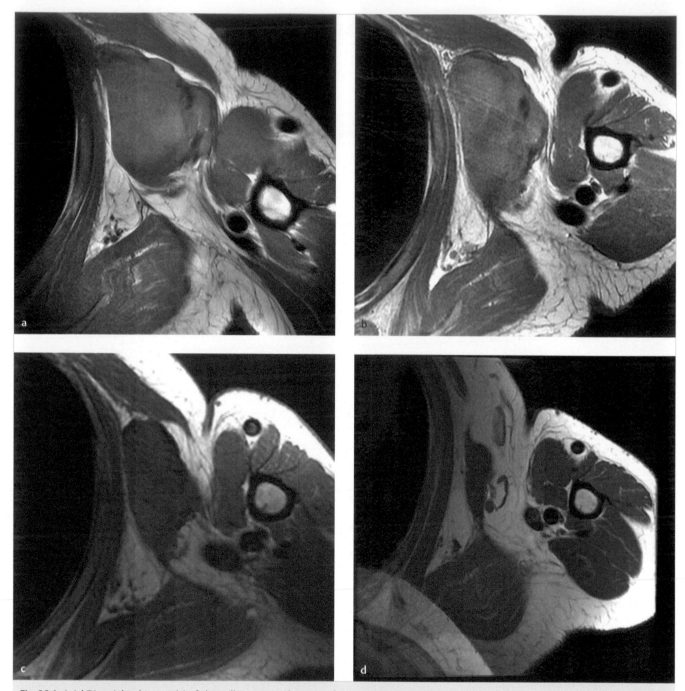

Fig. 96.1 Axial T1-weighted image (**a**) of the axillary region shows a soft-tissue mass at presentation that contains collagenous bands of low-signal intensity and has a radiating linear hypointense strand ("tail sign" or "band sign") posteriorly. During medical treatment only, the mass becomes progressively smaller and diffusely hypointense on corresponding follow-up T1 images at 6 months (**b**), and 12 months (**c**), and 18 months (**d**).

■ Clinical History

A 31-year-old patient with negative radiographs and an a traumatic, firm axillary mass. The patient presents with serial MRI examinations for tumor surveillance while on systemic treatment that includes nonsteroidal anti-inflammatory drugs (NSAIDs) and tyrosine kinase inhibitors (sorafenib) (▶ Fig. 96.1).

■ Key Finding

Nonmineralized, soft-tissue mass with an infiltrative border ("tail sign") that responds favorably to nonoperative treatment.

■ Top 3 Differential Diagnoses

- **Desmoid tumor:** Desmoid-type fibromatosis is a locally aggressive mesenchymal neoplasm that produces fibrotic tissue and grows with infiltrative margins. Although these are considered intermediate-grade neoplasms and do not metastasize, they can cause significant morbidity because of their infiltrative growth and tendency to recur locally after surgery.

  On MRI, desmoid tumors typically contain areas of intermediate and low-T1 signal. As these lesions evolve and respond to treatment, signal intensity tends to progressively decrease on T2 and postcontrast images (reflecting changes from cellular neoplasm to collagenous scar). Favorable treatment response is also shown by progressive decrease in tumor volume over time. Characteristic band-like linear extension along a fascial plane ("tail sign") at the tumor margin is seen in approximately 80% of cases. Intralesional necrosis is generally absent (unlike many sarcomas).

  The three most common extra-abdominal locations for desmoid-type fibromatosis are the extremities (60%), paraspinal/chest wall region (25%), and head/neck (15%). The compartment of origin and local extent (e.g., involvement of crucial structures, neurovascular bundles, bones) are the prime determinants of treatment and prognosis. Multicentric lesions occur in a small minority of patients (~10%); this is classically associated with familial adenomatous polyposis and the diagnosis commonly referred to as Gardner syndrome.

  Treatment is tailored to the individual patient. First-line therapy generally favors close observation and systemic treatment (e.g., NSAIDs, hormonal blockade, cytotoxic chemotherapy, tyrosine-kinase inhibitors), rather than surgery or radiation therapy.
- **Tenosynovial giant cell tumor:** When radiographs do not show any mineralization, the MRI differential diagnosis of a hypointense mass with an infiltrative margin most commonly includes tenosynovial giant cell tumor. Tenosynovial giant cell tumors are classically observed along a tendon sheath ("giant cell tumor of the tendon sheath") or in a synovial joint ("pigmented villonodular synovitis").
- **Miscellaneous fibrous soft-tissue tumors:** With negative radiographs, uncommon miscellaneous fibrous tumors can be in the differential diagnosis of a hypointense mass with an infiltrative margin. These fibrous (fibroblastic or myofibroblastic) tumors include fascia-based lesions, particularly nodular fasciitis, desmoplastic fibroma, and fibrosarcoma.

■ Diagnosis

Desmoid tumor (aggressive fibromatosis).

✓ Pearls

- Imaging has a crucial role in the diagnosis, local staging, and management of desmoid-type fibromatosis.
- Management of desmoid-type fibromatosis often begins with systemic treatment, rather than surgery or radiation.
- Favorable response to systemic treatment is shown by decreased volume and decreased signal intensity on serial MRI examinations.

■ Suggested Readings

Benech N, Walter T, Saurin JC. Desmoid tumors and celecoxib with sorafenib. N Engl J Med. 2017; 376(26):2595–2597

Braschi-Amirfarzan M, Keraliya AR, Krajewski KM, et al. Role of imaging in management of desmoid-type fibromatosis: a primer for radiologists. Radiographics. 2016; 36(3):767–782

Gounder MM, Mahoney MR, Van Tine BA, et al. Sorafenib for advanced and refractory desmoid tumors. N Engl J Med. 2018; 379(25):2417–2428

Park JS, Nakache YP, Katz J, et al. Conservative management of desmoid tumors is safe and effective. J Surg Res. 2016; 205(1):115–120

Sheth PJ, Del Moral S, Wilky BA, et al. Desmoid fibromatosis: MRI features of response to systemic therapy. Skeletal Radiol. 2016; 45(10):1365–1373

Turner B, Alghamdi M, Henning JW, et al. Surgical excision versus observation as initial management of desmoid tumors: a population based study. Eur J Surg Oncol. 2019; 45(4):699–703

Case 97

Robert D. Boutin

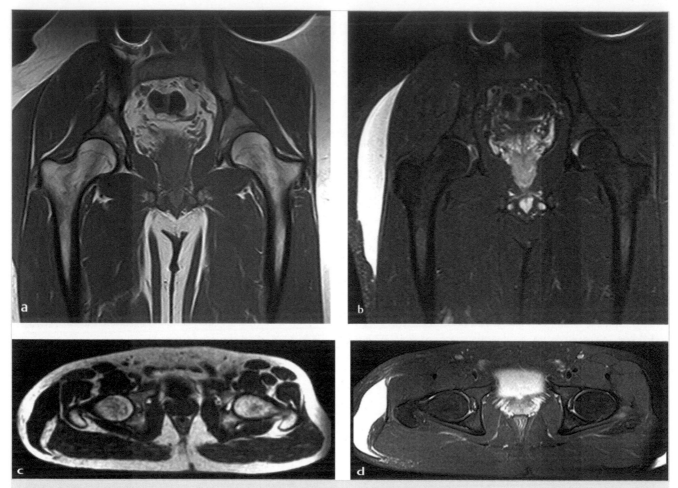

Fig. 97.1 Coronal T1-weighted (**a**), coronal fat-suppressed T2-weighted (**b**), axial T1-weighted (**c**), and axial fat-suppressed T2-weighted (**d**) images of the pelvis show a large, fusiform, peritrochanteric collection of homogeneous fluid-like signal intensity located superficial to the fascia at the interface with the subcutaneous fat layer.

■ Clinical History

Λ 39-year-old man with a history of a motor vehicle accident complaining of decreased cutaneous sensation and a mass lateral to the right hip (▶ Fig. 97.1).

■ Key Finding

Posttraumatic fluid-like collection in the deep subcutaneous tissue along the superficial aspect of the fascia.

■ Top 3 Differential Diagnoses

- **Morel–Lavallee lesion:** Morel–Lavallee lesions are the result of trauma with shearing forces superficial to the fascia. With such internal degloving injuries, a hemolymphatic collection is formed, most commonly in the back/flank, hip/thigh, and knee regions (classically located lateral to the greater trochanter of the hip).

  Imaging features evolve over time, as expected, with collections containing variable amounts of blood products and lymphatic fluid, often with globules of fat. Acute/subacute collections tend to appear more heterogeneous and have ill-defined margins with perilesional edema (resembling hematomas). Chronic collections become more homogeneous and often develop a fibrous pseudocapsule. Regardless of the age of the Morel–Lavallee lesion, they have an ovoid or fusiform shape, and do not have internal vascularity.
- **Bursitis:** Collections that appear fluid-like can occur superficial to the fascia in bursae. In the hip region, for example, there are numerous bursae that may be affected by inflammation/infection and repetitive microtrauma. This is seen most often in the setting of tendinopathy with peritendinitis in patients with greater trochanteric pain syndrome. Superimposed imaging findings of edema and fluid also are commonly observed immediately after percutaneous injections (e.g., corticosteroid injection).

  Infections involving the greater trochanteric bursa region are rare in the absence of overlying skin disruption (e.g., ulceration). In developing countries, however, massive trochanteric bursal fluid distension is a well-recognized complication of indolent infection with mycobacteria (e.g., tuberculosis).
- **Neoplasm:** Soft-tissue neoplasms can be in the differential diagnosis of a mass lesion located superficial to the fascia. The most common neoplasms associated with the fascia are nodular fasciitis (most commonly in the upper extremities of young adults) and fibromatosis.

  Neoplasms have vascularity and abnormal enhancement after contrast administration. Sarcomas are located most commonly deep to the fascia, but superficial neoplasms can occur. Sarcomas often appear heterogeneous, with areas of intralesional necrosis.

■ Diagnosis

Morel–Lavallee lesion.

✓ Pearls

- A wide variety of hemorrhagic, inflammatory, and neoplastic lesions can occur in the deep subcutaneous soft tissue abutting the fascia.
- A Morel-Lavallee lesion is a posttraumatic, fluid-like collection in the deep subcutaneous tissue along the superficial aspect of the fascia. The imaging appearance evolves according to the age of the injury.
- The imaging appearance of a Morel–Lavallee lesion is essentially pathognomonic when a characteristic appearance is observed in a classic location after high-energy trauma.

■ Suggested Readings

De Coninck T, Vanhoenacker F, Verstraete K. Imaging features of Morel-Lavallée lesions. J Belg Soc Radiol. 2017; 101 Suppl 2:15

Kirchgesner T, Tamigneaux C, Acid S, et al. Fasciae of the musculoskeletal system: MRI findings in trauma, infection and neoplastic diseases. Insights Imaging. 2019; 10(1):47

McKenzie GA, Niederhauser BD, Collins MS, Howe BM. CT characteristics of Morel-Lavallée lesions: an under-recognized but significant finding in acute trauma imaging. Skeletal Radiol. 2016; 45(8):1053–1060

McLean K, Popovic S. Morel-Lavallée lesion: AIRP best cases in radiologic-pathologic correlation. Radiographics. 2017; 37(1):190–196

Nickerson TP, Zielinski MD, Jenkins DH, Schiller HJ. The Mayo Clinic experience with Morel-Lavallée lesions: establishment of a practice management guideline. J Trauma Acute Care Surg. 2014; 76(2):493–497

Spain JA, Rheinboldt M, Parrish D, Rinker E. Morel-Lavallée injuries: a multimodality approach to imaging characteristics. Acad Radiol. 2017; 24(2):220–225

Case 98

Robert D. Boutin

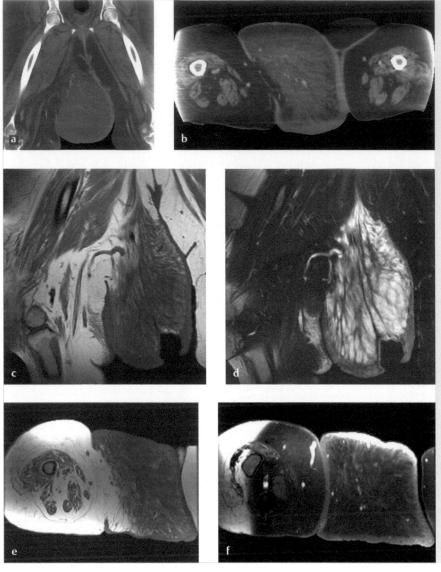

Fig. 98.1 Coronal (**a**) and axial (**b**) postcontrast CT images demonstrate a large pendulous mass arising from the inner aspect of the right thigh. This superficial mass has soft-tissue density (hyperdense compared to normal subcutaneous fat). A follow-up MRI shows skin thickening with ulceration of the huge mass on coronal T1-weighted (**c**) and fat-suppressed T2-weighted (**d**) images. The lesion is displayed as predominantly intermediate T1 and hyperintense T2 signal intensity, with edema outlining thickened "lace-like" bands of low-signal connective tissue (fibrosis) in the pendulous mass. Axial T1 (**e**) and postcontrast fat-suppressed T1-weighted (**f**) images show similar findings, with only mild nonfocal enhancement within this superficial mass at the medial aspect of the right thigh.

■ Clinical History

A 65-year-old morbidly obese woman with hypothyroidism and a chronically enlarging mass at the medial thigh region. "Solitary mass, without pain. Evaluate panniculus versus hernia versus neoplasm" (▶ Fig. 98.1).

■ Key Finding

Large, pendulous mass at the inner thigh in a morbidly obese patient.

■ Top 3 Differential Diagnoses

- **Massive localized lymphedema:** Massive localized lymphedema is an area of hypertrophic superficial soft tissue secondary to chronic obesity-induced lymphedema. In morbidly obese patients, progressive deposition of subcutaneous fat and retarded lymph drainage can result in gigantic pseudoneoplastic lesions, especially in areas of loose skin at the inner thigh, groin, and lower abdominal regions.

  On clinical examination, massive localized lymphedema may initially be confused with more common findings of a large panniculus, hernia, or neoplasm. Massive localized lymphedema, unlike typical lymphedema, is more localized and cannot be reversed by conservative management (e.g., compression stockings). Treatment focuses on surgical resection of the overgrown tissue, in addition to weight loss. If untreated, massive localized lymphedema may progress to angiosarcoma (~10% of cases; see below).

  On histologic evaluation of these masses, there is lymphatic proliferation with lymhangiectasia, thickening of fibrous connective tissue bands, and edema with capillary vascular proliferation. There are characteristically fibroblasts, but no lipoblasts that would be seen in a liposarcoma.

- **Well-differentiated liposarcoma:** Well-differentiated liposarcoma, also known as atypical lipoma, occurs much more commonly in the deep (subfascial) soft tissues than the superficial (subcutaneous) fat layer. In both locations, these lesions typically have well-defined margins that sharply demarcate the mass from the surrounding tissue; edema is not a prominent feature. With these lipomatous tumors, histology samples are positive for MDM2 gene amplification.

- **Angiosarcoma:** Angiosarcoma is a rare neoplasm (<2% of soft-tissue sarcomas) that generally has poor prognosis. Important risk factors are prior radiation therapy and chronic lymphedema, generally with a latency period of over 5 years. In patients with risk factors, angiosarcoma may be considered in the presence of a vascular tumor with an aggressive, infiltrative appearance (e.g., fungating mass in the subcutaneous fat with a background of diffuse lymphedema).

■ Diagnosis

Massive localized lymphedema.

✓ Pearls

- Massive localized lymphedema is a superficial pseudoneoplastic lesion associated with localized obstruction of lymphatic flow, most commonly at the inner thigh of morbidly obese patients.

- Unlike lymphedema and cellulitis, well-differentiated liposarcomas have well-defined margins that result in a sharp distinction between lipomatous and nonlipomatous tissue.

- Angiosarcoma is a rare, aggressive neoplasm that is associated with risk factors of chronic lymphedema or radiation therapy after a long latency period (many years).

■ Suggested Readings

Chopra K, Tadisina KK, Brewer M, Holton LH, Banda AK, Singh DP. Massive localized lymphedema revisited: a quickly rising complication of the obesity epidemic. Ann Plast Surg. 2015; 74(1):126–132

Co M, Lee A, Kwong A. Cutaneous angiosarcoma secondary to lymphoedema or radiation therapy - A systematic review. Clin Oncol (R Coll Radiol). 2019; 31(4):225–231

Gaballah AH, Jensen CT, Palmquist S, et al. Angiosarcoma: clinical and imaging features from head to toe. Br J Radiol. 2017; 90(1075):20170039

Maclellan RA, Zurakowski D, Grant FD, Greene AK. Massive localized lymphedema: a case-control study. J Am Coll Surg. 2017; 224(2):212–216

Petscavage-Thomas JM, Walker EA, Bernard SA, Bennett J. Imaging findings of adiposis dolorosa vs. massive localized lymphedema. Skeletal Radiol. 2015; 44(6): 839–847

Case 99

Robert D. Boutin

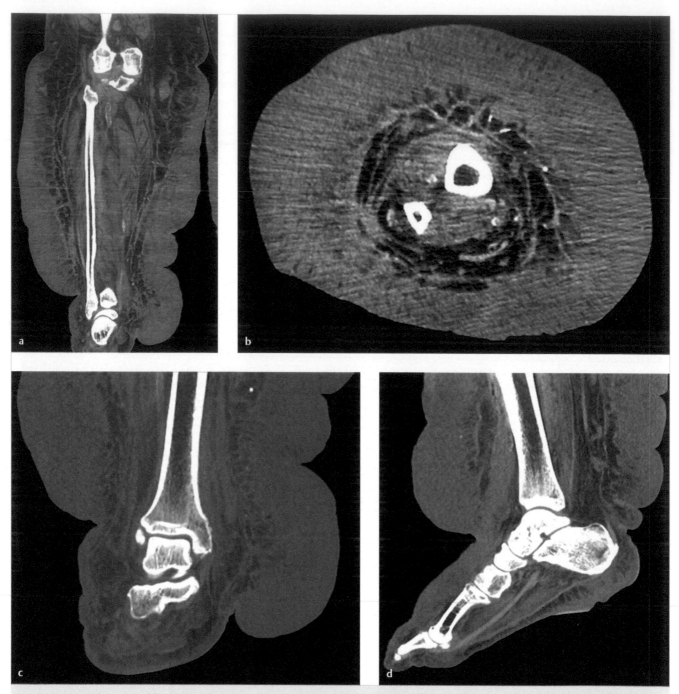

Fig. 99.1 Coronal **(a)** and axial **(b)** CT images of the leg show massive "elephant-like" thickening and increased density diffusely in the subcutaneous fat layer, with a "honeycomb" appearance of stranding in the deeper subcutis. Coronal **(c)** CT image of the ankle region shows soft-tissue thickening is most prominent adjacent to the medial malleolus; the corresponding sagittal **(d)** image shows sparing of the plantar aspect of the foot.

■ Clinical History

Adult patient who immigrated from Southeast Asia as a child presents with chronic swelling in the lower leg region (▶ Fig. 99.1).

■ Key Finding

Leg, ankle, and foot edema, with prominent thickening and increased density in the subcutaneous fat layer.

■ Top 3 Differential Diagnoses

- **Cellulitis:** Cellulitis can be defined as a bacterial infection (with or without purulence) involving the dermis and associated subcutaneous tissue, usually unilaterally and in a lower extremity (≥60%). A skin defect (e.g., fissure, wound, or penetrating trauma) is typically the portal of entry for infectious agents (most commonly *Staphylococcus aureus* and *Streptococcus pyogenes*).

  Imaging examinations generally show nonspecific, diffuse soft-tissue edema involving the subcutaneous fat layer, often with thickening, hyperemia, and stranding that appears infiltrative. Thus, cellulitis can be differentiated from most soft-tissue neoplasms, because cellulitis has poorly defined borders and lacks a discrete mass.

- **Vascular disorders:** Noninflammatory causes of soft-tissue edema include a wide array of vascular disorders that may be unilateral or bilateral, such as venous thrombosis, chronic venous insufficiency, or congestive heart failure.

  Imaging often begins with sonography in order to determine appropriate treatment (e.g., venous thrombosis versus infection). Deep vein thrombosis is classically associated with nonspecific subfascial edema (thrombophlebitis). Noninflammatory vascular disorders classically lack hyperemia, and therefore postcontrast enhancement is generally not observed (unlike cellulitis). With long-standing venous disease, subcutaneous fibrosis (termed lipodermatosclerosis) and soft-tissue ulceration may occur.

- **Lymphedema:** Lymphedema is defined as the accumulation of lymph in the extracellular space. Stagnant, protein-rich lymph initiates an inflammatory response that leads to soft-tissue thickening (adipocyte proliferation with fibrous tissue deposition) which can eventually cause elephantiasis (severe fibrosclerotic lymphedema).

  Although lymphedema can be congenital (primary), it is usually acquired (secondary). Worldwide, the most common cause of lymphedema is filariasis, which is a mosquito-borne, parasitic infection that infects an estimated 120 million people in 81 countries (according to the World Health Organization, lymphatic filariasis is the world's second leading cause of chronic disability). In industrialized countries, lymphedema is most commonly caused by cancer, surgery, and radiation therapy.

  Imaging may be used to confirm an appropriate diagnosis and assess treatment response. In acute and subacute settings, a characteristic appearance of "honeycombing" of subcutaneous fat lobules and thickening of the underlying fascia has been described, but it is not specific. Thickening of the subcutis in the leg region is typical, with progressive increase in fat density seen on CT as the condition becomes more severe.

  In patients with lymphatic filariasis, the edema characteristically begins and progresses most prominently adjacent to the medial malleolus (with sparing of the plantar aspect of the foot). With sonography, adult parasitic worms can easily be seen because of their size (7–10 cm in length) and rapid movement ("filarial dance sign").

■ Diagnosis

Lymphedema (secondary to filariasis).

✓ Pearls

- Cellulitis, vascular disease, and lymphedema are distinct conditions, but may co-exist in any given patient. Obesity is an important risk factor for all three conditions in industrialized countries.
- Cellulitis, vascular disease, and lymphedema have a wide array of causes; treatment is directed at the underlying cause.

- Lymphedema is most commonly secondary to filariasis infection in tropical/subtropical regions, but cancer patients (often after surgery or radiation) are most commonly affected in industrialized countries.

■ Suggested Readings

Dietrich CF, Chaubal N, Hoerauf A, et al. Review of dancing parasites in lymphatic filariasis. Ultrasound Int Open. 2019; 5(2):E65–E74

Fish JH, Lurie F. Evaluation of edema of the extremity. In: Current Management of Venous Diseases. Springer, Cham; 2018:51–63

Goel TC, Goel A. Chronic lymphedema-elephantiasis of lower extremity. In: Lymphatic Filariasis. Springer, Singapore; 2016:169–205

Hayeri MR, Ziai P, Shehata ML, Teytelboym OM, Huang BK. Soft-tissue infections and their imaging mimics: from cellulitis to necrotizing fasciitis. Radiographics. 2016; 36(6):1888–1910

Patel M, Lee SI, Akyea RK, et al. A systematic review showing the lack of diagnostic criteria and tools developed for lower-limb cellulitis. Br J Dermatol. 2019; 181 (6):1156–1165

Shin SU, Lee W, Park EA, Shin CI, Chung JW, Park JH. Comparison of characteristic CT findings of lymphedema, cellulitis, and generalized edema in lower leg swelling. Int J Cardiovasc Imaging. 2013; 29(2) Suppl 2:135–143

Case 100

Robert D. Boutin

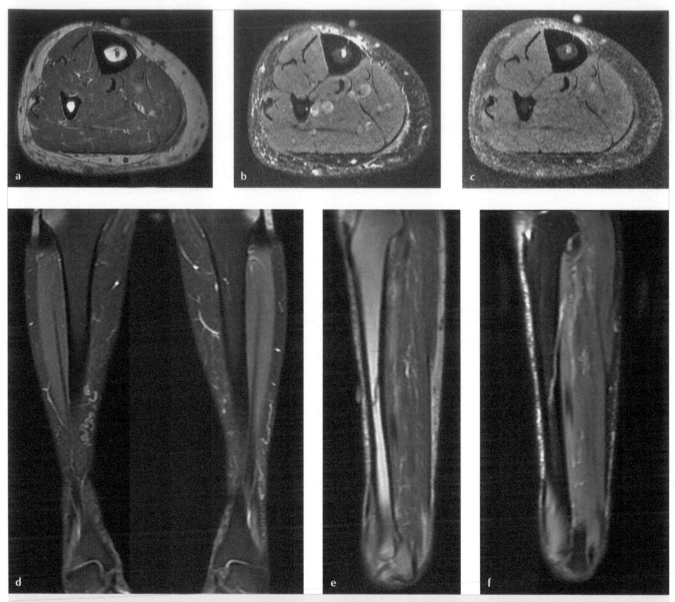

Fig. 100.1 Axial T1-weighted **(a)**, fat-suppressed T2 weighted **(b)**, postcontrast fat-suppressed T1-weighted **(c)** images of the leg demonstrate linear increased signal intensity traversing the tibial cortex (subjacent to a skin marker). Coronal fat-suppressed T2-weighted **(d)** image shows an area of tortuous varicose veins in the subcutaneous fat layer (anteromedial to the midshaft of the right tibia). Sagittal T1-weighted **(e)** and fat-suppressed T2-weighted **(f)** images show continuity between the pretibial varices and a prominent intraosseous vein in the tibial midshaft.

■ **Clinical History**

A 68-year-old man with a 3-month history of "extreme pain" at the mid tibia and a clinical concern for a "soft-tissue mass" (▶ Fig. 100.1).

■ Key Finding

Triad of key findings: Pretibial varices, linear cortical defect in mid tibia, and prominent nutrient vein within the mid tibia.

■ Top 3 Differential Diagnoses

- **Intraosseous venous drainage anomaly:** Varicose veins are often located in the legs, and they are commonly associated with venous valvular incompetence. Venous perforators (communications between superficial and deep venous systems of the lower extremity) may occur through bone and are increasingly recognized in the phlebology literature.

  Clinical diagnosis may be supplemented by duplex sonography in symptomatic patients (e.g., suspected thrombophlebitis). Treatment may be nonsurgical or surgical (e.g., compression stockings, sclerotherapy, ablation, phlebectomy). Of note, treatment may be influenced when an intraosseous venous drainage anomaly is present.

  An intraosseous venous drainage anomaly is diagnosed when pretibial varices are in continuity with both a tibial shaft cortical defect and a prominent intraosseous vein. Pertinent negatives include the absence of a neoplastic mass and bone marrow edema.

- **Angiomatous lesions:** Vascular masses may be considered in the presence of focally prominent vessels. Sonography and contrast-enhanced MRI may be helpful in assessing vascular hemodynamics and ruling out a soft-tissue neoplasm. Differential diagnosis can potentially include a wide array of benign and malignant vascular masses, including simple vascular malformations (e.g., venous malformation or arteriovenous malformation).

- **Stress fracture:** The tibial shaft is a classic site for fatigue-type stress fractures in athletes and military recruits. With repetitive microtrauma, a spectrum of tibial stress changes may occur, typically beginning with periosteal edema and endosteal bone edema on fat-suppressed, fluid-sensitive images. With progression of biomechanical overload, a tibial stress fracture line (or lines) is characteristically located at the anterior cortex. A pertinent negative is that stress fractures are not in continuity with focally prominent blood vessels.

■ Diagnosis

Intraosseous venous drainage anomaly.

✓ Pearls

- Varicose veins in the pretibial soft tissue may communicate with an intraosseous varix via a focal defect in the anterior cortex of the mid tibia, an entity referred to as an intraosseous venous drainage anomaly.

- Recognition of an intraosseous venous drainage anomaly is pivotal for appropriate diagnosis and treatment.

- The characteristic triad of imaging features with an intraosseous venous drainage anomaly allows for confident differentiation from vascular neoplasms and stress fractures in the leg.

■ Suggested Readings

Boutin RD, Sartoris DJ, Rose SC, et al. Intraosseous venous drainage anomaly in patients with pretibial varices: imaging findings. Radiology. 1997; 202(3):751–757

Jung SC, Lee W, Chung JW, et al. Unusual causes of varicose veins in the lower extremities: CT venographic and Doppler US findings. Radiographics. 2009; 29 (2):525–536

Kachlik D, Pechacek V, Hnatkova G, Hnatek L, Musil V, Baca V. The venous perforators of the lower limb - A new terminology. Phlebology. 2019; 34(10):650–668

Kwee RM, Kavanagh EC, Adriaensen ME. Intraosseous venous drainage of pretibial varices. Skeletal Radiol. 2013; 42(6):843–847

Ramelet AA, Crebassa V, D Alotto C, et al. Anomalous intraosseous venous drainage: bone perforators? Phlebology. 2017; 32(4):241–248

Rezaie ES, Maas M, van der Horst CMAM. Episodes of extreme lower leg pain caused by intraosseous varicose veins. BMJ Case Rep. 2018; 2018:bcr-2017

Case 101

Robert D. Boutin

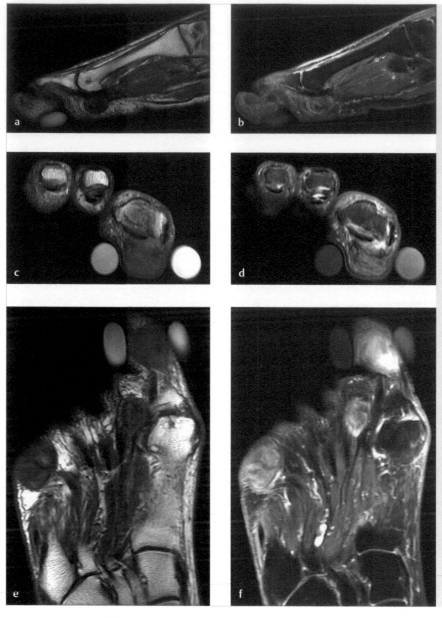

Fig. 101.1 Sagittal proton density-weighted (**a**), sagittal fat-suppressed T2-weighted (**b**), coronal T1-weighted (**c**), coronal fat-suppressed T2-weighted (**d**), and axial T1-weighted (**e**) images of the forefoot show nodular masses in the subcutaneous fat layer that are characterized by relatively low-signal intensity on all pulse sequences. After contrast administration, axial fat-suppressed T1-weighted (**f**) imaging shows enhancement of these lesions, most prominently at the largest lesion located plantar to the great toe. Markers on the skin bracket at the most symptomatic lesion.

■ Clinical History

A 75-year-old woman with slowly developing, firm, painless, subcutaneous lumps in her feet (▶ Fig. 101.1).

■ Key Finding

Multiple T2-hypointense masses in the subcutaneous fat layer of the foot.

■ Top 3 Differential Diagnoses

- **Rheumatoid nodules:** Rheumatoid arthritis is a chronic auto-immune disorder characterized by symmetric inflammatory disease that targets the synovium, but can also have many extra-articular manifestations.

  Extra-articular involvement is known to affect many organ systems, including bone (e.g., osteopenia), muscle (e.g., myositis), and subcutaneous tissues.

  The most common subcutaneous manifestation is the rheumatoid nodule (life-time prevalence, >20%). Rheumatoid nodules contain chronic inflammatory tissue and range in size from 0.2 to 5 cm. These nodules are often found in the subcutaneous fat layer at pressure points (e.g., superficial to the olecranon, calcaneus, and metatarsal heads). On MRI, these nodules have variable signal characteristics, but are often of intermediate-to-low signal intensity on T1 and T2 images, and show variable postcontrast enhancement. When cystic necrosis occurs in nodules, they display T2 hyperintensity and minimal enhancement.

  Rheumatoid nodules almost always occur in patients who are rheumatoid factor positive, which are more common in severe disease phenotypes. Rheumatoid nodules do not require treatment when asymptomatic, but injection or surgical excision may be appropriate for nodules that are painful, interfere with function, or erode the overlying skin.

- **Tophaceous gout:** Tophaceous gout (monosodium urate crystal deposition disease) most commonly affects the foot and other acral structures, often targeting joints, entheses, tendons, and other extra-articular soft tissues.

  Like rheumatoid nodules, gouty tophi on MRI often show nonspecific intermediate T1 signal and variable T2 signal intensity. T2 hypointensity is characteristically seen in the subcutaneous fat layer on nonfat-suppressed images of tophi containing calcification and reactive fibrous tissue.

- **Plantar fat pad lesions:** In most asymptomatic individuals, MRI shows intermediate-to-low signal intensity on T1 and T2 images in the fat pad under the 1st and 5th metatarsal heads (median size, 9 mm). The diminished signal in the subcutaneous fat layer presumably represents reactive fibrous tissue and can occur in areas of adventitial bursae secondary to mechanical stress. If these adventitial bursae become acutely inflamed, then T2 hyperintensity results.

■ Diagnosis

Rheumatoid nodules.

✓ Pearls

- Rheumatoid nodules typically occur in patients with known rheumatoid arthritis as firm masses in the subcutaneous fat layer over pressure points.
- Gout is regarded as the most common form of inflammatory arthritis in men, but it may present with extra-articular masses that are occasionally mistaken for neoplasms.
- In the plantar fat pads under the 1st and 5th metatarsal heads, decreased T2 signal is commonly asymptomatic, and corresponds to areas of fibrosis and adventitious bursae.

■ Suggested Readings

Ryu K, Takeshita H, Takubo Y, et al. Characteristic appearance of large subcutaneous gouty tophi in magnetic resonance imaging. Mod Rheumatol. 2005; 15(4):290–293

Studler U, Mengiardi B, Bode B, et al. Fibrosis and adventitious bursae in plantar fat pad of forefoot: MR imaging findings in asymptomatic volunteers and MR imaging-histologic comparison. Radiology. 2008; 246(3):863–870

Towiwat P, Chhana A, Dalbeth N. The anatomical pathology of gout: a systematic literature review. BMC Musculoskelet Disord. 2019; 20(1):140

Upadhyay N, Saifuddin A. The radiographic and MRI features of gout referred as suspected soft tissue sarcoma: a review of the literature and findings from 27 cases. Skeletal Radiol. 2015; 44(4):467–476

Xue Y, Cohen JM, Wright NA, Merola JF. Skin signs of rheumatoid arthritis and its therapy-induced cutaneous side effects. Am J Clin Dermatol. 2016; 17(2):147–162

Ziemer M, Müller AK, Hein G, Oelzner P, Elsner P. Incidence and classification of cutaneous manifestations in rheumatoid arthritis. J Dtsch Dermatol Ges. 2016; 14 (12):1237–1246

Case 102

Robert D. Boutin

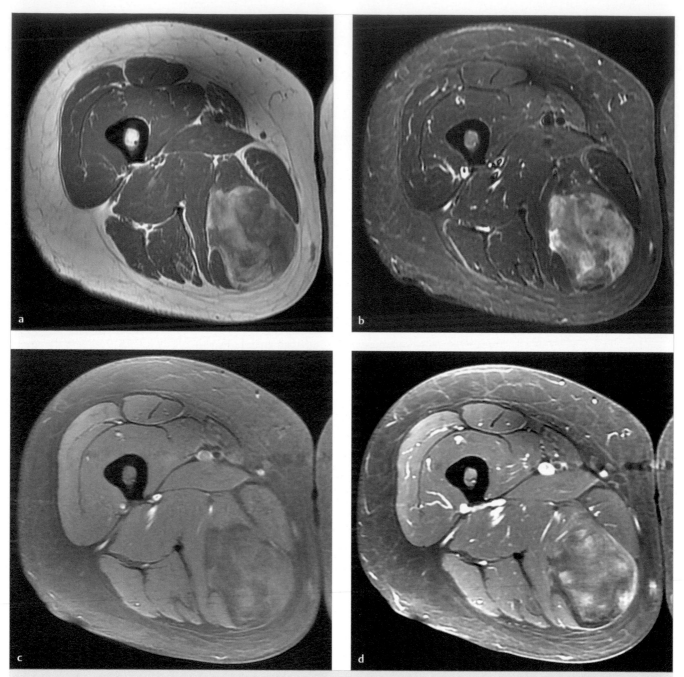

Fig. 102.1 Axial T1-weighted (**a**), axial fat-suppressed T2-weighted (**b**), axial fat-suppressed T1-weighted (**c**), and axial postcontrast fat-suppressed T1-weighted (**d**) images of the thigh demonstrate a soft-tissue mass in the posterior compartment that contains heterogeneous hyperintensity on T1 (only without fat suppression) and T2 pulse sequences. After contrast administration, there is heterogeneous enhancement of the mass.

■ Clinical History

A 39-year-old man with a slowly growing painless mass in the thigh (▶ Fig. 102.1).

■ Key Finding

Large subfascial soft-tissue mass with heterogeneous signal on T1, T2, and postcontrast images.

■ Top 3 Differential Diagnoses

- **Atypical lipoma:** The diagnosis of atypical lipoma/liposarcoma should be considered when a large, deep (subfascial), heterogeneous, enhancing mass contains some tissue that is isointense with fat.

  The histologic subtype of lipomatous tumor affects patient treatment and prognosis. Four specific histologic subtypes of liposarcoma include atypical lipoma (termed well-differentiated liposarcoma in the retroperitoneum) (~40–50%), myxoid/round cell liposarcoma (~30–40%), dedifferentiated liposarcoma (~10%), and pleomorphic liposarcoma (~5–10%). Notably, pleomorphic liposarcomas may not contain any conspicuous lipomatous tissue on imaging.

  Atypical lipoma is located most commonly in the lower extremity and trunk, usually in or between muscles (not located subcutaneously). However, the MRI appearance of benign lipomas and atypical lipomas overlap, and cytogenetic analysis of tissue for MDM2 is now used routinely at tertiary care centers for differentiating simple lipoma from atypical lipoma. With MRI, the likelihood of atypical lipoma/liposarcoma (compared to simple lipoma) increases with patient age, large tumor size (e.g., maximum diameter >10 cm), thick (>2 mm) septations, increased nonadipose tissue, and contrast enhancement. Atypical lipomas have no metastatic ability.

- **Myxoid liposarcoma:** Myxoid liposarcomas often contain a relatively small amount of macroscopic fat and show areas of high-T2 signal owing to the myxoid stroma. When a round cell component is also present, low-to-intermediate T1 and T2 signal contributes to heterogeneity of the mass on MRI. In some cases, myxoid liposarcomas contain little to no macroscopic fat.

  Myxoid liposarcomas with round cell component are more biologically aggressive, which influences use of neoadjuvant therapy. Unlike other sarcomas (which most commonly metastasize to the lungs), these sarcomas have a relatively high incidence of metastasis to extrapulmonary soft tissue.

- **Dedifferentiated liposarcoma:** Dedifferentiated liposarcoma occurs more commonly in the retroperitoneum than the extremities. They are defined by the presence of a biphasic combination of a well-differentiated liposarcoma and a nonadipocytic sarcoma (which is typically high grade, often resembling an undifferentiated pleomorphic sarcoma).

  Dedifferentiated liposarcoma is suggested by solid, nodular nonlipomatous components within a lipomatous mass; these nonlipomatous nodular components should be targeted for biopsy.

■ Diagnosis

Myxoid liposarcoma.

✓ Pearls

- Liposarcoma is regarded as the most common soft-tissue sarcoma (~35% of sarcomas), and it is most commonly seen in middle-aged to older adults.
- The diagnosis of liposarcoma should be considered when a large, deep (subfascial), heterogeneous, enhancing mass contains some tissue that is isointense with fat.

- Four specific histologic subtypes of liposarcoma are atypical lipoma (in the extremities), myxoid/round cell liposarcoma, dedifferentiated liposarcoma, and pleomorphic liposarcoma.

■ Suggested Readings

Fletcher CDM, Bridge JA, Hogendoorn PCW, et al, eds. World Health Organization Classification of Tumours of Soft Tissue and Bone, 4th edition. Lyon: IARC Press; 2013

Knebel C, Neumann J, Schwaiger BJ, et al. Differentiating atypical lipomatous tumors from lipomas with magnetic resonance imaging: a comparison with MDM2 gene amplification status. BMC Cancer. 2019; 19(1):309

Kuhn KJ, Cloutier JM, Boutin RD, Steffner R, Riley G. Soft tissue pathology for the radiologist: a tumor board primer with 2020 WHO classification update [published online ahead of print Aug 2, 2020]. Skeletal Radiol

Morag Y, Yablon C, Brigido MK, Jacobson J, Lucas D. Imaging appearance of well-differentiated liposarcomas with myxoid stroma. Skeletal Radiol. 2018; 47 (10):1371–1382

Rizer M, Singer AD, Edgar M, Jose J, Subhawong TK. The histological variants of liposarcoma: predictive MRI findings with prognostic implications, management, follow-up, and differential diagnosis. Skeletal Radiol. 2016; 45(9):1193–1204

Teniola O, Wang KY, Wang WL, Tseng WW, Amini B. Imaging of liposarcomas for clinicians: Characteristic features and differential considerations. J Surg Oncol. 2018; 117(6):1195–1203

Case 103

Robert D. Boutin

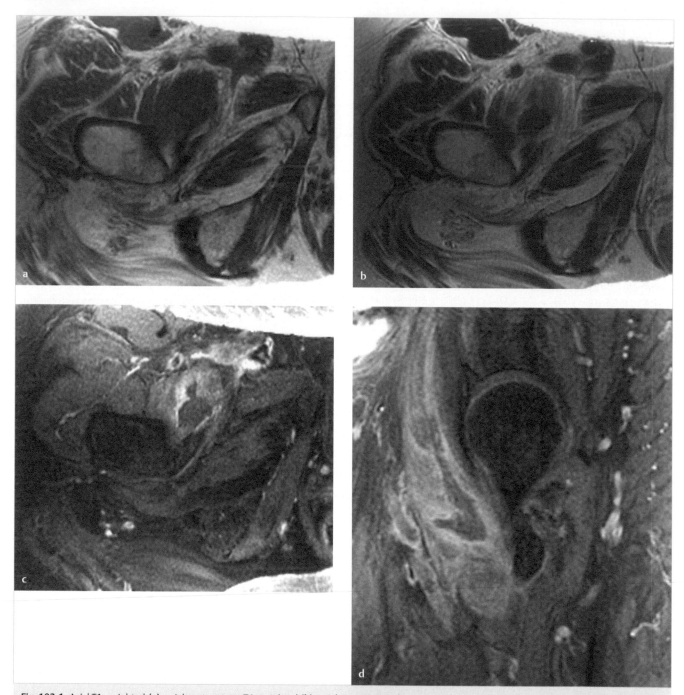

Fig. 103.1 Axial T1-weighted **(a)**, axial postcontrast T1-weighted **(b)**, axial postcontrast fat-suppressed T1-weighted **(c)**, and sagittal postcontrast, fat-suppressed T1-weighted **(d)** images of the right hip show a rim-enhancing lesion within the iliopsoas muscle.

■ Clinical History

An 85-year-old woman with a history of right hip and groin pain (▶ Fig. 103.1).

■ Key Finding

Rim-enhancing mass in the iliopsoas muscle.

■ Top 3 Differential Diagnoses

- **Hematoma:** Hemorrhage into the iliopsoas muscle may be primary (spontaneous) or secondary to numerous causes (e.g., anticoagulant therapy, bleeding diathesis, trauma).

  As with hematomas elsewhere, the imaging findings of an intramuscular hematoma in the iliopsoas evolve over time. Acutely, a fluid–fluid level with features of uncoagulated blood (hematocrit effect) may be seen on CT and MRI. On CT, acute hematomas classically show increased attenuation, while nonacute hematomas have nonspecific decreased attenuation (relative to muscle). On MRI, characteristic features of a hematoma can also include hyperintense T1 signal in subacute hematomas and a thin rim of hypointense T2 signal in a chronic hematoma. In many cases, however, the imaging features of a hematoma overlap with abscess and neoplasm.

  Given that the imaging features are nonspecific, correlation with clinical history and laboratory findings is important.

- **Abscess:** Iliopsoas abscess may be seen as a primary process (e.g., intramuscular seeding of a pathogen in an immunocompromised host) or secondary to contiguous spread of infection from an adjacent source (e.g., diverticulitis, appendicitis, perinephric abscess, vertebral discitis/osteomyelitis). Pathogens may include *Staphylococcus aureus*, enteric bacteria, or atypical organisms (e.g., *Mycobacterium tuberculosis*).

  Clinically, the classic triad of fever, back pain, and groin pain is both insensitive and nonspecific for iliopsoas abscess; the triad is present in a minority of patients. Femoral neuropathy and limp are also present in some patients. With laboratory evaluation, leukocytosis may be initially observed in only about half of all patients, but the erythrocyte sedimentation rate and C-reactive protein values are usually elevated.

  With CT and MRI, an abscess is typically seen as a fluid-like mass, with adjacent enhancing edema. Gas bubbles or air–fluid levels may also be present in a minority of cases.

- **Neoplasm:** The iliopsoas may be affected by a primary neoplasm (e.g., sarcoma) or metastasis.

  Muscle metastases are relatively rare, but the iliopsoas is one of the most commonly affected muscles. Muscle metastases are generally observed in late stage disease when other metastases are already present. Iliopsoas metastases can occur with a wide range of primary neoplasms, including lymphoma, melanoma, and various carcinomas (e.g., lung, breast, renal, colorectal).

  With imaging, findings often include a hypodense lesion on CT and a T2-hyperintense lesion on MRI. Postcontrast CT and MRI can show rim enhancement at the margin of a necrotic neoplasm that potentially mimics hematoma or abscess.

■ Diagnosis

Hematoma.

✓ Pearls

- The most common masses in the iliopsoas are hematomas, abscesses, and neoplasms.
- Imaging should be interpreted with knowledge of clinical and laboratory findings. Imaging features alone (in the absence of clinical/laboratory data) can be nonspecific for differentiating between the various causes of the iliopsoas disorders.
- CT and MRI are important for detecting iliopsoas disorders. When appropriate, CT can be used to guide diagnostic aspiration, biopsy, or drainage.

■ Suggested Readings

Alonso CD, Barclay S, Tao X, Auwaerter PG. Increasing incidence of iliopsoas abscesses with MRSA as a predominant pathogen. J Infect. 2011; 63(1):1–7

Lenchik L, Dovgan DJ, Kier R. CT of the iliopsoas compartment: value in differentiating tumor, abscess, and hematoma. AJR Am J Roentgenol. 1994; 162(1):83–86

Podger H, Kent M. Femoral nerve palsy associated with bilateral spontaneous iliopsoas haematomas: a complication of venous thromboembolism therapy. Age Ageing. 2016; 45(1):175–176

Singh AK, Gervais DA, Hahn PF, Mueller PR. Neoplastic iliopsoas masses in oncology patients: CT findings. Abdom Imaging. 2008; 33(4):493–497

Case 104

Robert D. Boutin and Jasjeet Bindra

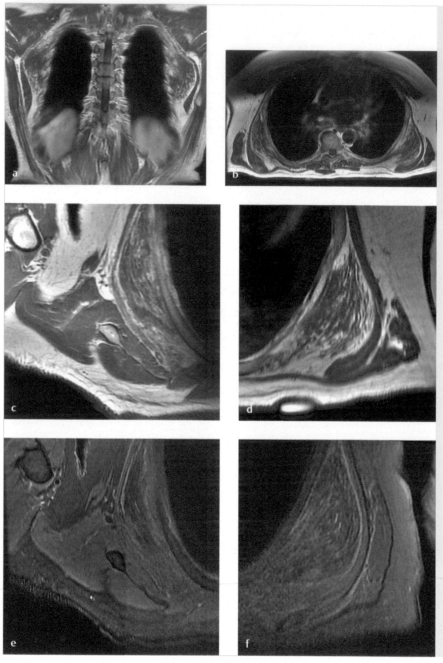

Fig. 104.1 Coronal T1-weighted (**a**) and axial T1-weighted (**b**) images of the chest with a large field of view show bilateral soft-tissue masses. Additional axial T1-weighted (**c, d**) and axial fat-suppressed T2-weighted (**e, f**) images with a small field of view were then performed. These images show the soft-tissue masses between the inferior pole of the scapula and the subjacent chest wall. These masses have a crescent-like shape, are relatively large (measuring 12 cm in transaxial long axis), and exert mass effect on the overlying serratus anterior muscles bilaterally. The masses are heterogeneous, with signal intensity that follows muscle intermixed with fatty striations.

■ Clinical History

A 70-year-old man with a 15-year history of pain and masses "the size of grapefruit" near the inferior angle of the scapulae bilaterally. He describes the masses as "popping out" when he adducts his arms across his body (▶ Fig. 104.1).

■ Key Finding

Infrascapular, soft-tissue mass containing diffuse streaks of fatty tissue–Roentgen classic.

■ Diagnosis

Elastofibroma dorsi: Elastofibroma dorsi is regarded as fibro-fatty pseudotumor that may arise from mechanical friction between the chest wall and the overlying scapula.

These lesions are typically observed as incidental findings during cross-sectional imaging of patients over the age of 60 years (e.g., ~2% of all chest CTs in older adults; ~25–50% are bilateral). On 18F-FDG positron emission tomography (PET)/CT scans, elastofibroma dorsi may also be incidentally detected, generally with mild-to-moderate standardized update values (SUVs) that should not be misinterpreted as representing malignancy.

The diagnosis of elastofibroma dorsi can be made with high-confidence in older adults with a typical fibrofatty soft-tissue mass in an infrascapular location, especially when bilateral lesions are present. Elastofibroma dorsi (i.e., elastofibromas adjacent to inferior scapular tip) represents approximately 95% of elastofibromas. Rare locations for elastofibromas include the greater trochanter, ischial tuberosity, and olecranon.

When elastofibromas cause prominent clinical symptoms (e.g., pain, stiffness, or snapping) and conservative management fails, the treatment of choice is often surgical excision.

✓ Pearls

- Elastofibroma dorsi is considered a reactive pseudotumor that may be incidental or associated with symptoms.
- Treatment of elastofibromas with surgical excision is usually only advocated for lesions causing persistent, prominent symptoms.

- Elastofibroma dorsi often has a pathognomonic imaging appearance of a fibrofatty, infrascapular mass in the soft tissues of an older adult, particularly when bilateral lesions are present.

■ Suggested Readings

Davidson T, Goshen E, Eshed I, Goldstein J, Chikman B, Ben-Haim S. Incidental detection of elastofibroma dorsi on PET-CT: initial findings and changes in tumor size and standardized uptake value on serial scans. Nucl Med Commun. 2016; 37 (8):837–842

Haihua R, Xiaobing W, Jie P, Xinxin H. Retrospective analysis of 73 cases of elastofibroma. Ann R Coll Surg Engl. 2020; 102(2):84–93

Olchowy C, de Delás-Vigo MA, Perez M, Ciriaco N, Oronoz RD. Triple elastofibromas located in the supra- and infrascapular regions-a case report. Skeletal Radiol 2018; 47(4):569–573

Tepe M, Polat MA, Calisir C, Inan U, Bayav M. Prevalence of elastofibroma dorsi on CT: Is it really an uncommon entity? Acta Orthop Traumatol Turc. 2019; 53 (3):195–198

Walker EA, Fenton ME, Salesky JS, Murphey MD. Magnetic resonance imaging of benign soft tissue neoplasms in adults. Radiol Clin North Am. 2011; 49(6):1197–1217, vi

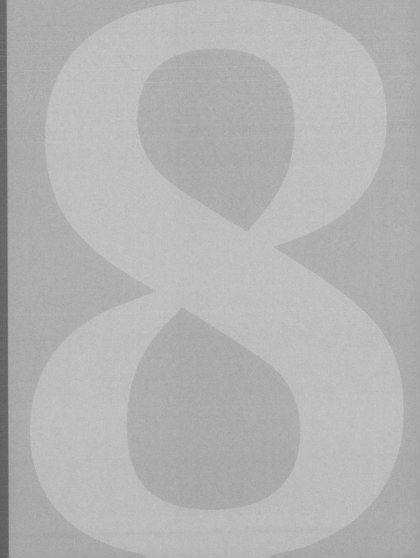

Part 8

Metabolic Musculoskeletal Conditions

Case 105

Jasjeet Bindra

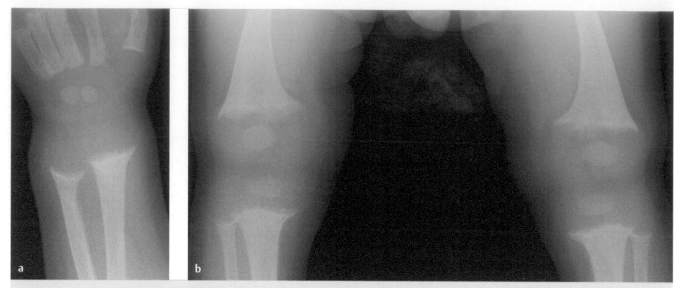

Fig. 105.1 PA radiograph of the wrist **(a)** shows fraying and cupping of distal metaphyses of radius and ulna. Frontal image of bilateral knees **(b)** demonstrates similar fraying of distal femoral, proximal tibial, and fibular metaphyses.

■ Clinical History

A 2-year-old male with failure to thrive (▶ Fig. 105.1).

■ Key Finding

Frayed metaphyses.

■ Top 3 Differential Diagnoses

- **Rickets:** Rickets is caused by deficiency of Vitamin D. It may be due to nutritional deficiency, malabsorption, anticonvulsant therapy, chronic liver disease, renal tubular insufficiency (Fanconi syndrome), or chronic renal disease. Vitamin D is essential for mineralization of osteoid. Failure of mineralization at growth plates leads to disorganized chondrocyte growth, and hypophosphatemia leads to impaired apoptosis of hypertrophic chondrocytes, which results in long cartilage cell columns and the radiographic findings of widening of growth plate and cupping and fraying of the metaphyses. Diaphyseal bowing, protrusio acetabuli, rachitic rosary (expansion of the anterior rib ends at costochondral junctions), and scoliosis can also be seen due to increased malleability of bones. Rachitic manifestations are most prominent at the sites of greatest growth, including the knee, distal tibia, proximal humerus, distal radius and ulna, and anterior ends of middle ribs.

- **Hypophosphatasia:** In hypophosphatasia, a rare genetic disorder, there is decreased mineralization of bone caused by deficiency of tissue nonspecific alkaline phosphatase. The skeletal findings, including metaphyseal fraying, resemble those of rickets.

- **Stress:** Excessive stress on growing physes and metaphyses can cause widening of the growth plate, sclerosis, and irregularity of metaphyses. This is seen in "gymnast wrists"—a chronic overuse injury seen in children who participate in gymnastics. Repetitive compressive forces can result in a chronic Salter–Harris 1 injury of distal radius.

■ Additional Diagnostic Considerations

- **Achondroplasia:** Achondroplasia is an autosomal dominant rhizomelic dwarfism with several characteristic skeletal abnormalities like metaphyseal irregularity, short and bowed extremities, narrowing of interpediculate distances caudally in spine, cranial enlargement, and short broad ribs.

- **Metaphyseal chondrodysplasia:** This is a group of disorders characterized by metaphyseal widening and flaring similar to rickets. Short stature, atlantoaxial instability, and platyspondyly are also commonly associated.

■ Diagnosis

Rickets.

✓ Pearls

- Rachitic manifestations are most prominent at the sites of greatest growth.
- Skeletal findings of hypophosphatasia resemble those of rickets and osteomalacia.

- "Gymnast wrists" present as physeal widening, metaphyseal irregularity, and sclerosis at wrists.

■ Suggested Readings

Chang CY, Rosenthal DI, Mitchell DM, Handa A, Kattapuram SV, Huang AJ. Imaging findings of metabolic bone disease. Radiographics. 2016; 36(6):1871–1887

Glass RB, Norton KI, Mitre SA, Kang E. Pediatric ribs: a spectrum of abnormalities. Radiographics. 2002; 22(1):87–104

Case 106

Eva Escobedo

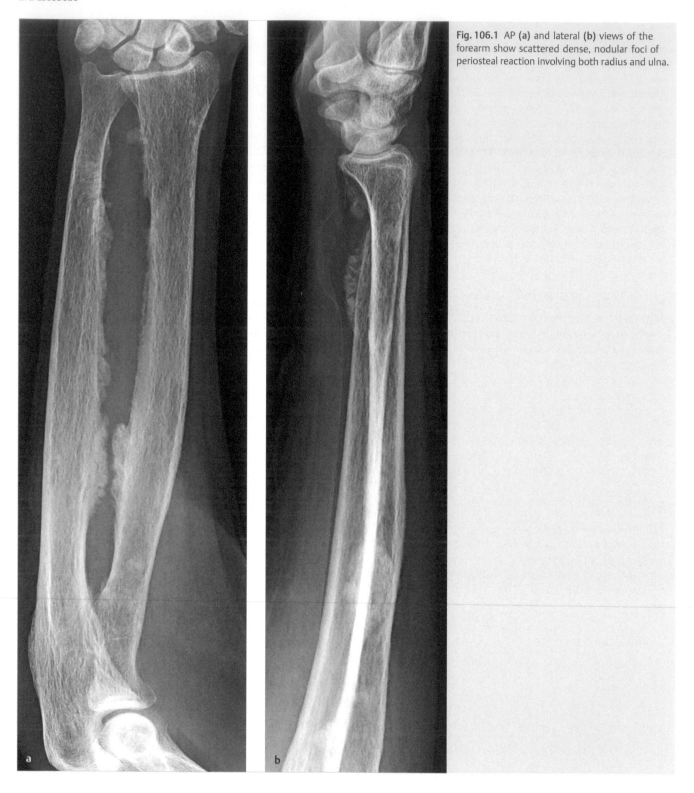

Fig. 106.1 AP (**a**) and lateral (**b**) views of the forearm show scattered dense, nodular foci of periosteal reaction involving both radius and ulna.

■ Clinical History

A 67-year-old male with inability to supinate forearm (▶ Fig. 106.1).

■ Key Finding

Generalized periosteal reaction.

■ Top 3 Differential Diagnoses

- **Hypertrophic osteoarthropathy (HOA):** The secondary form of HOA is much more common than primary (pachydermoperiostosis). The majority of cases are associated with intrathoracic disease, most commonly malignancy, but extrathoracic causes include cirrhosis, biliary disease, and inflammatory bowel disease. The common clinical presentation is clubbing and bone and joint pain. Radiographs show symmetric, solid, or layered periostitis involving the diaphysis of long bones, with tibia, fibula, radius, and ulna being most commonly affected. Advanced cases can affect all tubular bones and extend to the metaphysis and epiphysis. The exact mechanism is unclear, but neurogenic and humoral pathways have been proposed.
- **Thyroid acropachy:** Thyroid acropachy is a rare complication of autoimmune thyroid disease presenting with swelling of the hands and feet, clubbing of the digits, and often pretibial myxedema and exophthalmos. It can be seen after treatment of Grave's disease, and patients may be euthyroid or hypothyroid. Radiographs show a characteristic spiculated, feathery or lacy periosteal reaction, usually bilateral and symmetric, and involving the tubular bones of hands and feet. Long bone involvement is rare.
- **Voriconazole-induced periostitis:** This is a relatively recently described etiology of painful diffuse periostitis in posttransplant patients taking voriconazole, an antifungal medication, for prophylaxis or treatment of aspergillus infection. Radiographs show dense, focal, nodular, and irregular periostitis that can affect the tubular bones as well as clavicles, ribs, scapula, and pelvis. Symptoms resolve with discontinuation of the drug.

■ Additional Diagnostic Considerations

- **Pachydermoperiostosis (primary HOA):** This is a rare hereditary disease that presents in a similar fashion to secondary HOA. Skin thickening of the forehead and scalp may be additional components.
- **Venous stasis:** This is usually seen in the lower extremities, and may be associated with phleboliths, subcutaneous edema, and sometimes soft-tissue calcifications.
- **Hypervitaminosis A:** Common causes include high-dose dietary supplements and long-term use of retinoids for acne or cancer. Cortical thickening and ligament and tendon calcification may be other features.

■ Diagnosis

Voriconazole induced periostitis.

✓ Pearls

- Voriconazole-induced periostitis can be distinguished from HOA by more diffuse involvement (as opposed to predominantly long bone involvement), absence of clubbing, and elevated alkaline phosphatase. A clinical history of transplantation and voriconazole therapy is helpful.
- Thyroid acropachy can be distinguished from HOA by less involvement of the long bones, and a spiculated, fluffy, or lacy appearance of periosteal proliferation.
- The finding of generalized symmetric periostitis requires a search for underlying malignancy if other underlying causes are not recognized.

■ Suggested Readings

Chen L, Mulligan ME. Medication-induced periostitis in lung transplant patients: periostitis deformans revisited. Skeletal Radiol. 2011; 40(2):143–148

Yap FY, Skalski MR, Patel DB, et al. Hypertrophic osteoarthropathy: clinical and imaging features. Radiographics. 2017; 37(1):157–195

Case 107

Jasjeet Bindra

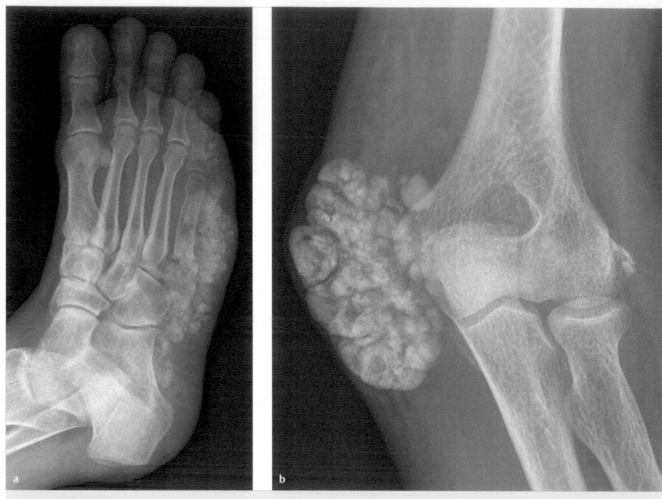

Fig. 107.1 Oblique view of the foot **(a)** shows a lobulated calcific mass along the lateral aspect. Oblique view of the elbow **(b)** reveals a similar lobulated calcific mass along the posteromedial side of the joint. The patient is on dialysis for chronic renal failure.

■ Clinical History

A 68-year-old female with enlarging masses at various sites (▶ Fig. 107.1).

■ Key Finding

Periarticular calcified mass.

■ Top 3 Differential Diagnoses

- **Calcinosis of renal failure:** The most frequent cause of periarticular calcified mass is chronic renal failure. This lesion is also called secondary tumoral calcinosis. There is no radiologic or histologic difference between these lesions and lesions of tumoral calcinosis. The diagnosis is made solely on clinical history, serum chemistry, and glomerular filtration rate. These calcium accumulations can be massive. Typically, other imaging features of renal osteodystrophy are present.
- **Tumoral calcinosis:** Tumoral calcinosis is a familial condition characterized by single or multiple painless, calcified masses. The patients are usually of African descent. It has a characteristic radiographic appearance of an amorphous, cystic, multilobulated, calcified mass in a periarticular location. Extensor surfaces are usually affected. These masses most commonly occur around hip, shoulder, and elbow. Fluid–fluid levels may be seen due to layering of calcium on CT, commonly termed "sedimentation sign."
- **Heterotopic ossification:** Heterotopic ossification is usually due to injury, cerebrospinal disorder, or burns. In cases of spinal cord injury, it is most commonly seen around hips. It primarily occurs in muscles but may be seen around ligaments or joint capsules. Faint calcifications are seen initially which evolve into well-defined ossification after 6 weeks or more. Maturation of ossification proceeds centrifugally with more mature bone seen at the periphery surrounding less mature bone in the center. Late lesions look like mature bone.

■ Additional Diagnostic Considerations

- **Gout:** Tophaceous gout may result from long-standing hyperuricemia. Calcified periarticular tophi are usually faintly radiopaque and commonly associated with underlying erosions of bone.
- **Synovial sarcoma:** Synovial sarcoma is a malignant mesenchymal neoplasm, which may show calcifications in one third of cases. Two thirds of synovial sarcomas occur in lower extremities and can involve periarticular regions. Radiologic appearance of this tumor is variable but can show dense calcification involving only a portion of the tumor.

■ Diagnosis

Calcinosis of renal failure.

✓ Pearls

- Calcinosis of renal failure is radiologically similar to tumoral calcinosis.
- Tumoral calcinosis has a characteristic amorphous, lobulated, calcific mass in a periarticular location.
- Late lesions of heterotopic ossification look like mature bone with cortex and medullary space.

■ Suggested Readings

Manaster BJ, May DA, Disler DG. Musculoskeletal Imaging, The Requisites. 4th ed. Philadelphia: Mosby Elsevier; 2013

Olsen KM, Chew FS. Tumoral calcinosis: pearls, polemics, and alternative possibilities. Radiographics. 2006; 26(3):871–885

Case 108

Jasjeet Bindra

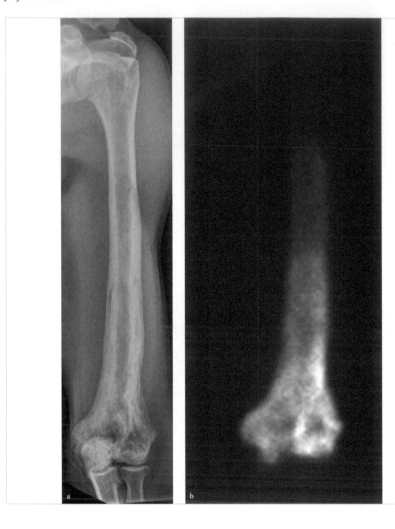

Fig. 108.1 AP view of the humerus **(a)** shows cortical and trabecular thickening, and sclerosis of mid to distal humerus. Limited view bone scan **(b)** reveals intense, increased radionuclide uptake in the mid to distal humerus, corresponding to the area of radiographic abnormality.

■ Clinical History

A 72-year-old male with incidental finding on humeral radiographs (▶ Fig. 108.1).

■ Key Finding

Long bone sclerosis.

■ Top 3 Differential Diagnoses

- **Fibrous dysplasia:** Fibrous dysplasia is a benign, noninherited bone disease that is characterized by replacement of normal lamellar cancellous bone by abnormal fibrous tissue. It is categorized as monostotic or polyostotic and may occur as a component of McCune–Albright syndrome or the rare Mazabraud syndrome. Classically, the lesions are intramedullary, expansile, and well-defined. There may be endosteal scalloping but a smooth cortical contour is always maintained. Lesions show varying degrees of hazy density. Some lesions may appear completely radiolucent or sclerotic. Amongst the long bones, the most common sites of involvement include femur, tibia, and humerus.
- **Paget's disease:** Paget's disease of the bone is a relatively common disorder that typically presents after 40 years of age. Classically, three phases have been described: lytic, mixed,

and blastic. The blastic phase manifests as osseous sclerosis, resulting in coarse trabecular, cortical thickening and bone enlargement. Although Paget's disease predominantly affects the axial skeleton, proximal long bones such as femur are frequently involved. Long bone involvement typically begins in a subchondral location.
- **Melorheostosis:** Melorheostosis (Leri disease) is a sporadic sclerosing skeletal dysplasia that typically manifests in late childhood or early adulthood. Patients may present with pain and stiffness of involved bones. It has a characteristic radiographic appearance consisting of cortical and medullary hyperostosis of a single bone or multiple adjacent bones with a flowing "dripping candle wax" appearance. Lower extremities are more commonly affected than upper extremities.

■ Additional Diagnostic Considerations

- **Erdheim–Chester disease:** Erdheim–Chester disease is a rare multisystem nonLangerhans cell histiocytosis. Radiographically, bilateral, symmetric, diaphyseal and metaphyseal involvement of long bones is seen with cortical thickening and narrowing of medullary cavity. The lower extremities are more commonly affected than the upper extremities. Bone infarcts and periostitis may also be seen.
- **Progressive diaphyseal dysplasia:** Progressive diaphyseal dysplasia is an autosomal dominant disorder that results in hyperostosis along the periosteal and endosteal surfaces of long bones. It usually manifests in childhood. Radiographically, there is bilateral, symmetric cortical thickening of the diaphysis of long bones. Tibia is the most commonly affected bone, and metaphyses and epiphyses are typically not involved.

■ Diagnosis

Paget's disease.

✓ Pearls

- Fibrous dysplasia lesions are intramedullary, expansile, and well-defined.
- Paget's disease of long bones begins in a subchondral location.

- Melorheostosis has a characteristic flowing "dripping candle wax" appearance.

■ Suggested Readings

Fitzpatrick KA, Taljanovic MS, Speer DP, et al. Imaging findings of fibrous dysplasia with histopathologic and intraoperative correlation. AJR Am J Roentgenol. 2004; 182(6):1389–1398

Ihde LL, Forrester DM, Gottsegen CJ, et al. Sclerosing bone dysplasias: review and differentiation from other causes of osteosclerosis. Radiographics. 2011; 31(7): 1865–1882

Case 109

Jasjeet Bindra

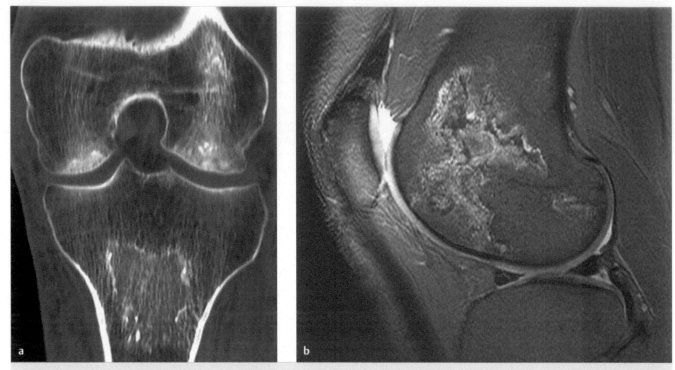

Fig. 109.1 Coronal reformatted CT image of the knee **(a)** shows multiple osseous areas of abnormality, with serpiginous sclerotic margins in distal femur and proximal tibia. Sagittal, fat-suppressed, proton density weighted MR image of the knee **(b)** demonstrates the typical appearance of a bone infarct with a "map-like" rim of low-signal intensity, with an inner rim of high-signal intensity (i.e., the double line sign) in the lateral femoral condyle.

■ Clinical History

A 45-year-old female with knee pain. Patient has been on long-term steroids (▶ Fig. 109.1).

■ Key Finding

Multiple bone infarcts.

■ Top 3 Differential Diagnoses

• **Sickle cell disease:** In sickle cell disease, osteonecrosis results from sickling of red blood cells in bone marrow, which causes stasis of blood. In young children, infarction usually occurs in the diaphysis of small bones of hands and feet, a condition called "hand-foot syndrome." Both in children and adults, long bones are commonly affected. Infarcts typically occur in medullary cavities and epiphyses. Osteonecrosis involving epiphyseal regions of long bones is generally termed avascular necrosis (AVN). Humeral and femoral heads are the most commonly involved sites. Acute infarcts cause osteolysis; later, lucency and sclerosis are seen in a patchy distribution. If cortical bone is infarcted, subperiosteal new bone may form, leading to "bone-within-bone" appearance. In AVN, crescent-shaped lucency in subchondral bone with subsequent collapse of articular surface may be seen. MRI appearance depends on the stage of the infarct. A serpiginous double line with inner hyperintense and outer hypointense margin on T2-weighted images may be seen. Other imaging findings of sickle cell disease like widening of diploic space, osteopenia with coarsened trabeculae, biconcave vertebral bodies, and extramedullary hematopoiesis can be seen.

• **Steroids:** Corticosteroid use is the most common nontraumatic cause of osteonecrosis. Most cases are due to systemically administered corticosteroids and/or high-dose daily therapy, particularly in patients with underlying comorbidities such as connective tissue diseases. The pathogenesis of steroid-induced osteonecrosis is likely multifactorial, including increased apoptotic activity of the cells, suppression of osteoclast/osteoblast generation in bone marrow, and prolongation of the lifespan of some osteoclasts.

• **Alcohol abuse:** Excessive alcohol use has been correlated with osteonecrosis. This may be due to fat emboli, increased marrow pressure, and increased cortisol levels. Other sequelae of excessive alcohol intake on imaging may include hepatic steatosis, cirrhosis, and portal hypertension.

■ Additional Diagnostic Considerations

• **Gaucher's disease:** It is a familial sphingolipid storage disorder. Accumulation of lipid-laden macrophages called Gaucher cells in the reticuloendothelial system, including the marrow, increases marrow pressure and leads to bone infarcts. Generalized osteoporosis, Erlenmeyer flask deformity of distal femur, and susceptibility both to fracture and osteomyelitis can also be seen. Any of these radiographic features seen in conjunction with hepatosplenomegaly should suggest the diagnosis of Gaucher's disease.

• **Systemic lupus erythematosus (SLE):** In SLE, the vasculitis may be additive to the steroid therapy in causing AVN.

■ Diagnosis

Steroid-induced osteonecrosis.

✓ Pearls

• In sickle cell anemia, imaging features of marrow hyperplasia, osteonecrosis, and osteomyelitis can be seen.
• Corticosteroid use is the most common nontraumatic cause of avascular necrosis.
• Other sequelae of alcohol abuse such as alcohol-related liver disease can help pinpoint the etiology in alcohol-associated bone infarcts.

■ Suggested Readings

Ejindu VC, Hine AL, Mashayekhi M, Shorvon PJ, Misra RR. Musculoskeletal manifestations of sickle cell disease. Radiographics. 2007; 27(4):1005–1021

Manaster BJ, May DA, Disler DG. Musculoskeletal Imaging, The Requisites. 4th ed. Philadelphia: Mosby Elsevier; 2013

Case 110

Jasjeet Bindra

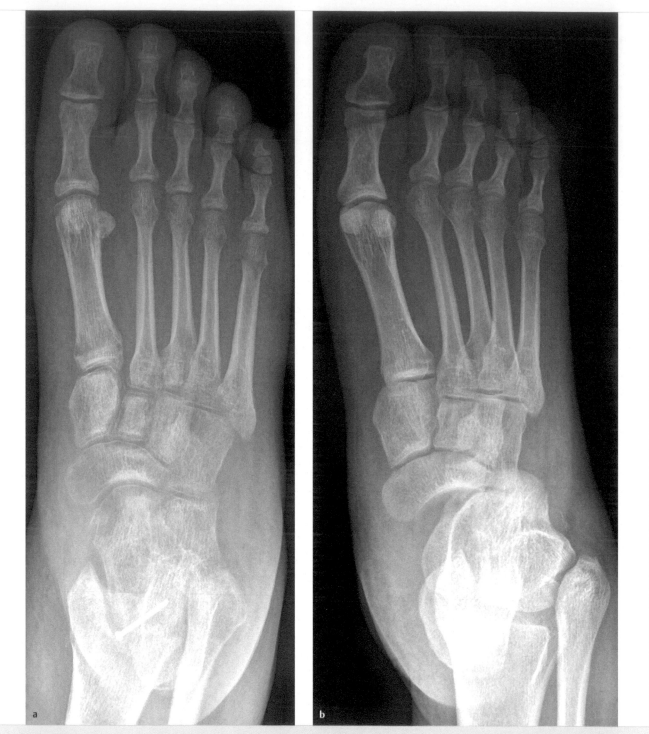

Fig. 110.1 Frontal radiograph of the foot (**a**) shows diffusely decreased bone density. Frontal image of the same foot (**b**) from 4 weeks ago demonstrates talar dislocation.

■ Clinical History

A 19-year-old female for follow-up appointment with orthopedic surgeon (▶ Fig. 110.1).

■ **Key Finding**

Osteoporosis.

■ **Top 3 Differential Diagnoses**

- **Primary osteoporosis:** Primary osteoporosis, most common form of osteoporosis, includes postmenopausal and senile osteoporosis. In women, after menopause, estrogen deficiency results in a period of accelerated bone loss. Age-related bone loss is believed to start in both men and women around the beginning of the fifth decade. Osteoporosis is defined as bone mineral density 2.5 or more standard deviations below that of a young healthy adult, as measured by dual energy X-ray absorptiometry, for postmenopausal women or men older than 50 years of age. Main radiographic features are increased radiolucency of bone and cortical thinning. Trabecular bone changes are most prominent in the axial skeleton and juxta-articular appendicular skeleton. Cortical changes include widening of the marrow canal, endosteal scalloping, and intracortical tunneling. Osteoporotic bones are prone to fractures with most common fracture locations being forearm, hip, and spine. Osteoporotic vertebral fractures rarely demonstrate a visible cortical break or significant callus formation.
- **Drug induced osteoporosis:** Steroid-associated osteoporosis is the most common form of secondary osteoporosis. Osteonecrosis, tendon rupture, and joint infections may be seen as associated findings. Osteoporosis is also seen with multiple other drugs such as heparin.
- **Regional osteoporosis:** Regional osteoporosis affects only a part of the skeleton, usually appendicular skeleton. It can be seen in a variety of conditions such as immobilization or disuse, reflex sympathetic dystrophy, and transient osteoporosis of large joints.

■ **Additional Diagnostic Consideration**

- **Hyperparathyroidism:** In hyperparathyroidism, subperiosteal resorption is the most characteristic radiographic feature such as at the radial side of middle phalanges and sacroiliac joints. Other findings including soft tissue calcifications, abnormal renal appearance (in renal osteodystrophy), and brown tumors can help guide the diagnosis.

■ **Diagnosis**

Disuse osteoporosis.

✓ **Pearls**

- Primary osteoporosis is postmenopausal or senile and is seen as increased bone radiolucency and cortical thinning.
- Steroid-induced osteoporosis may show osteonecrosis, tendon rupture, and joint infections as associated features.
- Subperiosteal resorption is the most characteristic radiographic feature of hyperparathyroidism.

■ **Suggested Readings**

Chang CY, Rosenthal DI, Mitchell DM, Handa A, Kattapuram SV, Huang AJ. Imaging findings of metabolic bone disease. Radiographics. 2016; 36(6):1871–1887

Guglielmi G, Muscarella S, Bazzocchi A. Integrated imaging approach to osteoporosis: state-of-the-art review and update. Radiographics. 2011; 31(5):1343–1364

Case 111

Jasjeet Bindra

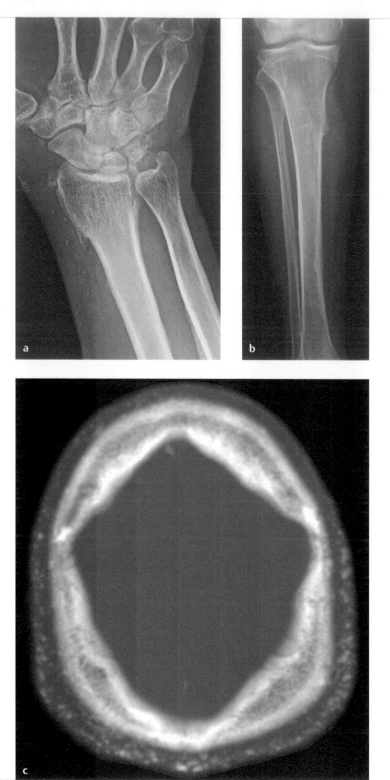

Fig. 111.1 PA view of the wrist and AP view of tibia and fibula (**a, b**) show multiple small soft-tissue calcifications. Axial CT image of the head (**c**) shows similar multiple small calcifications in the scalp.

■ Clinical History

A 40-year-old male with short stature (▶ Fig. 111.1).

■ Key Finding

Widespread soft tissue calcifications.

■ Top 3 Differential Diagnoses

- **Chronic renal failure:** Soft-tissue and vascular calcifications are commonly present in uremic patients secondary to disturbances in calcium and phosphate balance and hyperparathyroidism. Calcifications can present as calcinosis cutis, calciphylaxis, tumoral calcinosis, and calcifications of visceral organs. Calciphylaxis is a rare condition involving vascular calcifications and cutaneous necrosis. There is medial calcification and intimal fibrosis of the cutaneous arterioles combined with thrombotic occlusion, leading to ischemic skin necrosis. This condition is associated with high-mortality rate. The most frequent cause of a periarticular calcified mass is chronic renal failure. This lesion is also called secondary tumoral calcinosis. There is no radiologic or histologic difference between these lesions and lesions of tumoral calcinosis. The diagnosis is made solely on clinical history, serum chemistry, and glomerular filtration rate.
- **Dermatomyositis:** Calcifications seen in dermatomyositis are usually subcutaneous and nonspecific calcifications. "Sheet like" calcifications along fascial or muscle planes are less common but thought to be pathognomonic for the disease. Calcifications are more common in juvenile dermatomyositis than adult onset disease. Calcifications are also seen in other collagen vascular diseases like scleroderma and CREST syndrome.
- **Myocysticercosis:** Ovoid flecks of calcification resembling grains of rice in the soft tissues are characteristic of infection with pork tapeworm, Taenia Solium (cysticercosis). Infection which leads to extraintestinal disease (including myocysticercosis) usually occurs as a result of eating food or drinking water contaminated by human feces containing T. Solium eggs. Infective embryos hatch from the eggs, actively cross the intestinal mucosa, lodge into the capillaries of muscle and brain tissue, and then develop into larval cysts. When the parasite dies, an inflammatory response with perilesional edema ensues, followed by calcification. These calcifications parallel the long axis of muscles.

■ Additional Diagnostic Consideration

- **Pseudohypoparathyroidism (PHP):** Pseudohypoparathyroidism describes a group of disorders characterized by parathormone resistance at target organs, mainly the kidneys and skeleton. Somatic features include short stature and short digits. Soft-tissue calcifications and ossifications can be seen. The classic form of PHP is characterized by hypocalcemia, hyperphosphatemia, and elevated serum PTH levels. Pseudopseudohypoparathyroidism is clinically and radiologically the same as pseudohypoparathyroidism but serum levels of parathormone and calcium are normal.

■ Diagnosis

Pseudohypoparathyroidism.

✓ Pearls

- Secondary tumoral calcinosis is radiologically indistinguishable from primary tumoral calcinosis.
- "Sheet like" calcifications in soft tissues are pathognomonic of dermatomyositis.
- Calcifications resembling "grains of rice" are seen in myocysticercosis.

■ Suggested Readings

Blane CE, White SJ, Braunstein EM, Bowyer SL, Sullivan DB. Patterns of calcification in childhood dermatomyositis. AJR Am J Roentgenol. 1984; 142(2):397–400

Olsen KM, Chew FS. Tumoral calcinosis: pearls, polemics, and alternative possibilities. Radiographics. 2006; 26(3):871–885

Case 112

M. Jason Akers and Jasjeet Bindra

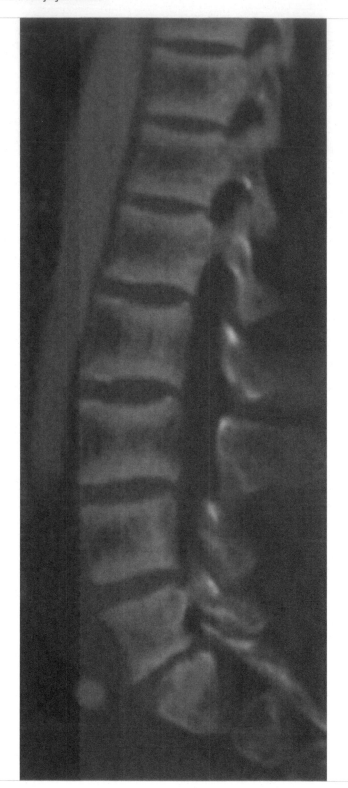

Fig. 112.1 Sagittal reformation CT image of lumbar spine shows superior and inferior endplate sclerosis at all levels in the visualized spine. There is relative lucency within the central vertebral bodies between the areas of endplate sclerosis, with an indistinct transition between the areas of sclerosis and the central areas of lucency.

■ Clinical History

A 33-year-old male with back pain (▶ Fig. 112.1).

■ Key Finding

"Rugger jersey" appearance of the spine.

■ Top 3 Differential Diagnoses

- **Renal osteodystrophy:** Renal osteodystrophy represents a constellation of musculoskeletal abnormalities that occur in chronic renal failure, including secondary hyperparathyroidism, osteoporosis, osteosclerosis, osteomalacia, and soft-tissue and vascular calcifications. Osteosclerosis is common and results from an increased amount of abnormal osteoid. A classic site for osteosclerosis is the vertebral body endplates. The "rugger jersey" appearance of the spine is created by the relative lucency of the central aspect of the vertebral bodies between the sclerotic endplates. The striate pattern is reminiscent of rugby players' alternating color horizontally striped shirts. The margins between the sclerotic and lucent portions of the vertebral body are smudgy, rather than sharp. Look for extraskeletal evidence of chronic renal failure, including surgical clips in the abdomen from nephrectomy or renal transplant and dialysis catheters in the chest.
- **Osteopetrosis:** Osteopetrosis represents a group of hereditary disorders characterized by abnormal osteoclastic activity, resulting in dense bones. The "sandwich" appearance of the vertebral bodies is classic for osteopetrosis. The appearance is similar to the "rugger jersey" spine of renal osteodystrophy, with the difference being a sharp margin between the sclerotic endplates and more lucent bone centrally. The classic "bone-in-bone" appearance occurs within the pelvis and long bones.
- **Paget's disease:** Paget's disease occurs in middle-aged and elderly patients and is characterized by excessive and abnormal bone remodeling. Most cases are polyostotic and the majority of cases involve the pelvis, spine, skull, femur, or tibia. The more common appearance of Paget's disease in the spine is the "picture frame" vertebral body caused by overall increased density, with sclerosis most marked at the periphery and a relatively lucent center. As in other bones, the classic features of Paget's disease in the spine are bony (vertebral) enlargement, coarsened trabeculae, and overall increased bone density.

■ Diagnosis

Renal osteodystrophy.

✓ Pearls

- The "rugger jersey" appearance of the vertebral bodies in renal osteodystrophy has smudgy margins.
- The "sandwich" vertebrae in osteopetrosis have sharp interfaces between sclerotic and lucent bone.
- Paget's disease is characterized by bony enlargement, coarsened trabeculae, and increased bone density.

■ Suggested Readings

Chew F. Musculoskeletal Imaging A Teaching File. 3rd ed. Philadelphia, PA: Elsevier Saunders; 2005

Lim CY, Ong KO. Various musculoskeletal manifestations of chronic renal insufficiency. Clin Radiol. 2013; 68(7):e397–e411

Martell BS, Dyer RB. The rugger jersey spine. Abdom Imaging. 2015; 40(8):3342–3343

Wittenberg A. The rugger jersey spine sign. Radiology. 2004; 230(2):491–492

Case 113

Jennifer Chang

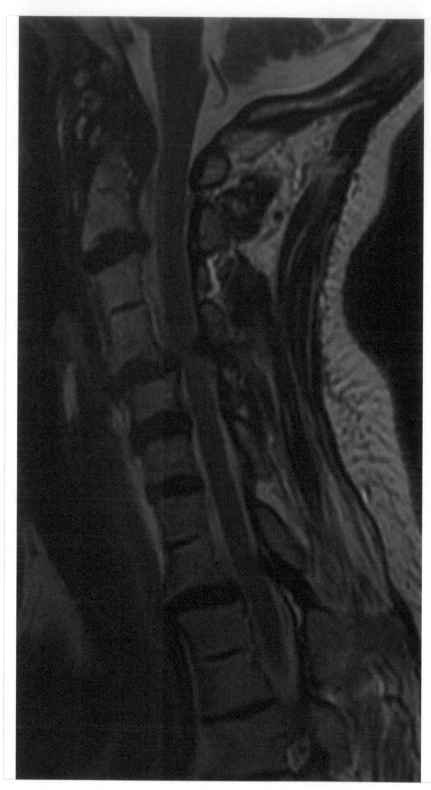

Fig. 113.1 Sagittal T2-weighted MR image of the cervical spine demonstrates near complete fusion of the C3–4, C7–T1, and T1–T2 disc space and elongation of the fused vertebral bodies.

■ **Clinical History**

A 73-year-old female with neck pain (▶ Fig. 113.1).

■ Key Finding

Vertebral body fusion.

■ Top 3 Differential Diagnoses

- **Developmental:** A derivative of the notochord, vertebral bodies form from the cells of the sclerotome and any deviation in the normal development results in congenital anomalies which can be in a variety of configurations, including hemivertebrae, resulting in scoliosis, block vertebrae, or congenital vertebral fusion. Block vertebra results from a failure of the segmentation process, can be complete or partial, and occurs in the cervical or lumbar spine.
- **Juvenile Inflammatory arthritis (JIA):** JIA is a polyarticular arthritis which can involve the cervical spine, particularly at C2–C3 and C3–C4, resulting is ankylosis, as well as decreased height and width of the vertebral bodies secondary to early epiphyseal closure. Initial symptoms include cervical pain and torticollis, and loss of mobility and extension can be progressive secondary to cervical fusion.
- **Postoperative:** Anterior cervical discectomy is approached from the front, with removal of the intervertebral disc and placement of bone graft or implant, and subsequent plate and screw fixation. Evaluation on radiographs should include instrument positioning and failure, including infection, which can appear as bony resorption, destruction surrounding the implant, and hardware fracture.

■ Additional Diagnostic Considerations

- **Klippel–Feil syndrome (KFS):** Congenital malformation defined by segmentation anomalies at one or multiple levels of the cervical spine with associated fusion. Originally described as a clinical triad of a short neck, low posterior hairline, and restricted cervical motion, KFS is classified into three subtypes based on the level and extent of vertebral fusion. In KFS, the vertebral bodies are narrowed in the AP dimension and there can be associated scoliosis or Sprengel deformity, a deformity related to abnormal scapular positioning.
- **Postinfectious:** Discitis and osteomyelitis of the spine can result in narrowing of the disc space and collapse of the adjacent vertebral bodies, resulting later in intervertebral body fusion. MRI findings of spodylodiscitis include increased T2 signal in the disc space and adjacent endplates, with corresponding T1-hypointensity, and associated enhancement.

■ Diagnosis

Klippel–Feil syndrome.

✓ Pearl

A "waist" can be seen at the level of intervertebral disc between fused segments, in cases of congenital vertebral fusion/block vertebra; this is not seen in acquired vertebral fusion.

■ Suggested Readings

Cohen PA, Job-Deslandre CH, Lalande G, Adamsbaum C. Overview of the radiology of juvenile idiopathic arthritis (JIA). Eur J Radiol. 2000; 33(2):94–101

Haque S, Bilal Shafi BB, Kaleem M. Imaging of torticollis in children. Radiographics. 2012; 32(2):557–571

Young PM, Berquist TH, Bancroft LW, Peterson JJ. Complications of spinal instrumentation. Radiographics. 2007; 27(3):775–789

Case 114

Jennifer Chang

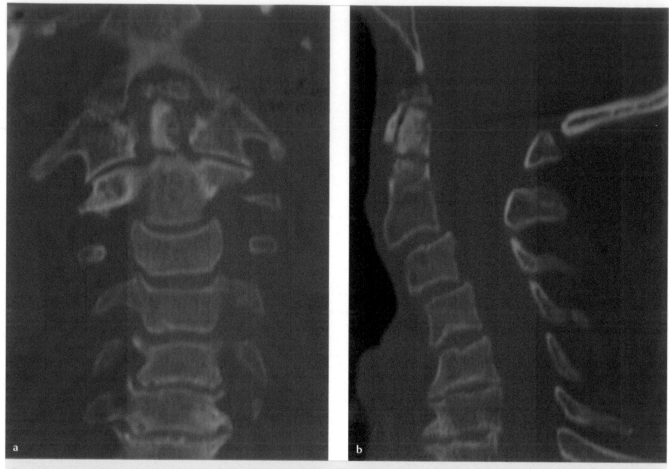

Fig. 114.1 Coronal **(a)** and sagittal **(b)** CT images of the cervical spine demonstrate a lucency consistent with a fracture through the odontoid.

■ Clinical History

An 86-year-old male with ground level fall (▶ Fig. 114.1).

■ Key Finding

Odontoid fracture.

■ Top 3 Differential Diagnoses

- **Type 1:** Based on the Anderson and D'Alonzo classification, Type 1 odontoid fractures are stable fractures involving the dens above the transverse ligament, where it is attached to C1, and are rare. The mechanism involves avulsion of the alar ligament with avulsion of the tip of the dens.
- **Type 2:** Type 2 fractures are transverse fractures through the base of the dens and are the most common type of odontoid fractures. These fractures have a tendency for nonunion due to poor blood supply. Greater than 6 mm displacement is a risk factor for nonunion. This is also the most significant factor in determination for surgery. Treatment usually involves C1–C2 posterior fusion.
- **Type 3:** Type 3 fractures are the second most common type of odontoid fractures and involve the body of the axis and occasionally the facets of C1–C2. These fractures are considered unstable and can be treated surgically or with halo immobilization.

■ Additional Diagnostic Considerations

- **Os odontoideum:** Os odontoideum is a smooth, well-corticated, ossific density at the superior aspect of a hypoplastic dens, whose etiology has been debated to be congenital or traumatic. It can also be seen with a hypertrophied anterior arch of C1. Surgery is reserved for symptomatic or unstable cases.
- **Persistent ossiculum terminale:** A small, smooth, well-corticated ossicle at the tip of the dens is a normal anatomic variant. It is due to the failure of fusion of the secondary ossification center of the dens, which is supposed to fuse around the age of 12.

■ Diagnosis

Type 2 odontoid fracture.

✓ Pearls

- Fractures are best seen on open mouth, odontoid views on radiographs, and posterior displacement should be evaluated on lateral views.
- Type 2 odontoid fractures are common in elderly secondary to falls; however, they are also seen in children secondary to blunt trauma due to large head to spine ratio.
- In contrast to fractures, which are irregular and lucent, developmental variants and anomalies have smooth and well-corticated margins.

■ Suggested Reading

O'Brien WT, Sr, Shen P, Lee P. The dens: normal development, developmental variants and anomalies, and traumatic injuries. J Clin Imaging Sci. 2015 (e-pub ahead of print) DOI: 10.4103/2156-7514.159565

Case 115

Jennifer Chang

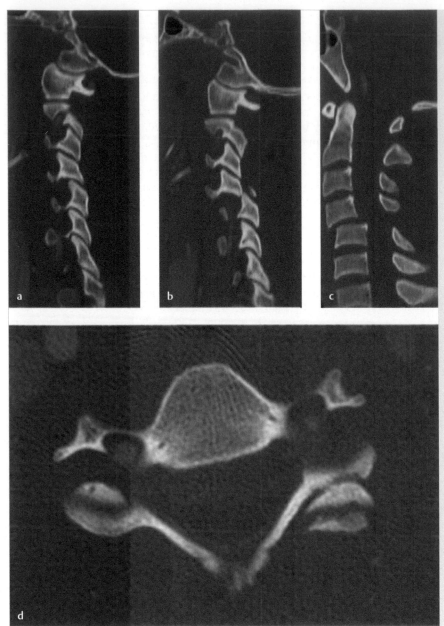

Fig. 115.1 Sagittal CT image of the cervical spine on the left **(a)** demonstrates mild subluxation of the C4–C5 facet joint, whereas there is a dislocation of the C4 inferior articular facet on the C5 superior articular facet on the right **(b)**. Sagittal CT image of the cervical spine in the midline **(c)** demonstrates anterolisthesis of C4 on C5, and axial CT at the same level **(d)** demonstrates a "reverse hamburger sign."

■ Clinical History

A 32-year-old patient's status postrollover motor vehicle crash (▶ Fig. 115.1).

■ Key Finding

Hyperflexion injury.

■ Top 3 Differential Diagnoses

- **Bilateral facet dislocation:** In an unstable injury associated with spinal cord injury, there is dislocation of the inferior articular facets over the lower vertebra's superior articular facets anteriorly, with translation of the vertebral body as well. Findings are best seen on sagittal CT reconstructions, but axial views can also demonstrate a "reverse hamburger" sign. There is also associated disruption of the anterior and posterior longitudinal ligaments. Facets are considered subluxed if there is more than 2 mm of diastasis, or there is less than 50% coverage of the articular surfaces.
- **Compression fracture:** Also termed wedge fractures, these result from axial loading or can be secondary to insufficiency in osteoporotic patients. There is height loss involving the anterior vertebral body, with fracture of the superior endplate seen, as increased density secondary to impaction. This injury generally involves the mid to lower cervical spine.
- **Flexion teardrop fracture:** The mechanism includes flexion and compression usually from motor vehicle accidents or diving, and this is an unstable injury associated with neurologic deficits and occasional paraplegia. There is a teardrop fracture fragment from the anterior inferior aspect of the vertebral body, widening of the interspinous processes, decreased height of the vertebral body, and posterior displacement of the vertebral body into the spinal canal.

■ Additional Diagnostic Considerations

- **Sprain:** Soft-tissue injury without evidence of fracture is seen as edema within the posterior soft tissues. These findings are best demonstrated on STIR or fat-suppressed, T2-weighted sequences with abnormal signal in the posterior soft tissues. Occasionally, bone contusions in the form of edema within the vertebral bodies can also be seen.
- **Unilateral facet dislocation:** In a hyperflexion injury with rotation, there is unilateral displacement of the inferior articular facet over the lower vertebra's superior articular facet, which is also termed jumped or perched facet. Lateral views demonstrate a "bow-tie" sign of the locked facet and, often, there is widening of the interspinous distance.

■ Diagnosis

Unilateral facet dislocation.

✓ Pearl

- Consider CT angiography (CTA) in cases of unilateral (more common) and bilateral facet dislocations, as there is increased incidence of vertebral artery injury.

■ Suggested Readings

Dreizin D, Letzing M, Sliker CW, et al. Multidetector CT of blunt cervical spine trauma in adults. Radiographics. 2014; 34(7):1842–1865

Kim KS, Chen HH, Russell EJ, Rogers LF. Flexion teardrop fracture of the cervical spine: radiographic characteristics. AJR Am J Roentgenol. 1989; 152(2):319–326

Case 116

Jennifer Chang

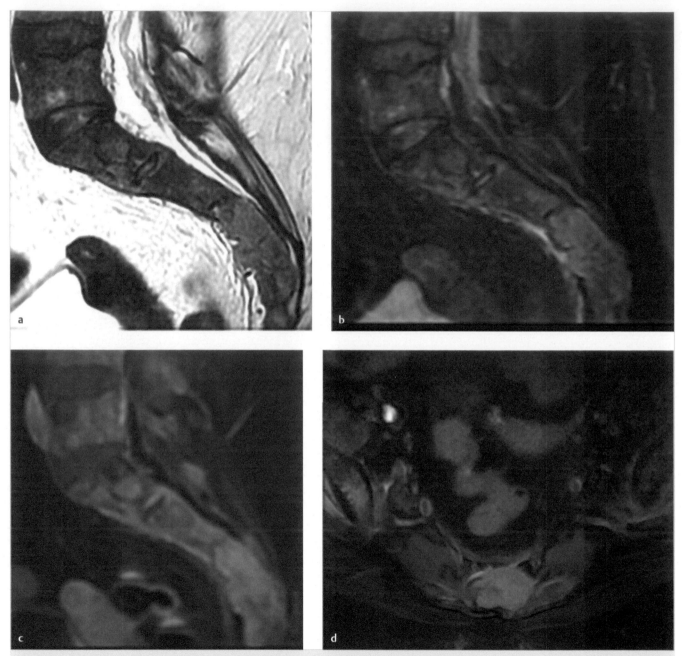

Fig. 116.1 Sagittal T2-weighted STIR, and postcontrast T1 weighted MR images **(a–c)**, and axial, fat-suppressed, T2-weighted MR image **(d)** of sacrum demonstrate a midline sacral lesion extending beyond the bony margins with enhancement.

■ **Clinical History**

A 53-year-old female with chronic back pain (▸ Fig. 116.1).

■ Key Finding

Midline sacral lesion.

■ Top 3 Differential Diagnoses

- **Chordoma:** This is the most common primary malignant sacral tumor. It is more common in males and occurs in the 4th to 7th decades of life. Chordomas arise from malignant degeneration of notochordal remnants and are most commonly found in the sacrococcygeal region and then in the clivus. They are lytic lesions with internal calcifications and soft-tissue component with low-T1 and increased T2 signal on MRI.
- **Metastasis:** The most common causes include lung, breast, and kidney malignancies, which are generally lytic. Common blastic metastatic lesions include breast or prostate carcinoma. Adjacent spread to the sacrum can also be seen with bladder, rectal, or uterine cancers.
- **Myeloma:** Myeloma is a malignant clonal neoplasm which results in overproduction of monoclonal immunoglobulins, and distribution of disease follows red marrow, including the vertebrae, ribs, skull, and pelvis. Plasmacytoma is a single myelomatous lesion with common sites of involvement including the vertebrae or pelvis. Radiographs demonstrate well-circumscribed lytic or "punched out" lucency.

■ Additional Diagnostic Considerations

- **Ewing sarcoma:** It is a malignant aggressive bone tumor with bony destruction and moth-eaten or permeative pattern with associated soft-tissue component. It is seen in children and young adults. There is intermediate T1 and low-to-intermediate signal on T2-weighted images with diffuse or peripheral nodular contrast enhancement on MRI.
- **Giant cell tumor (GCT) of bone:** The second most common primary sacral neoplasm after chordoma, GCTs are destructive, lytic, and expansile lesions which are generally eccentric in location, however, they can involve the entire sacrum as well as the sacroiliac joints. They are heterogeneous on T2- and T1-weighted images secondary to internal hemorrhage and necrosis and are very vascular lesions.

■ Diagnosis

Metastasis from breast cancer.

✓ Pearls

- If multiple lesions are seen within the spine in addition to the sacrum, top differentials include metastasis or multiple myeloma.
- Chordomas lie in the midline, whether in sacrum or clivus, unlike chondrosarcomas, which tend to lie eccentrically.

■ Suggested Reading

Diel J, Ortiz O, Losada RA, Price DB, Hayt MW, Katz DS. The sacrum: pathologic spectrum, multimodality imaging, and subspecialty approach. Radiographics. 2001; 21(1):83–104

Case 117

Jennifer Chang

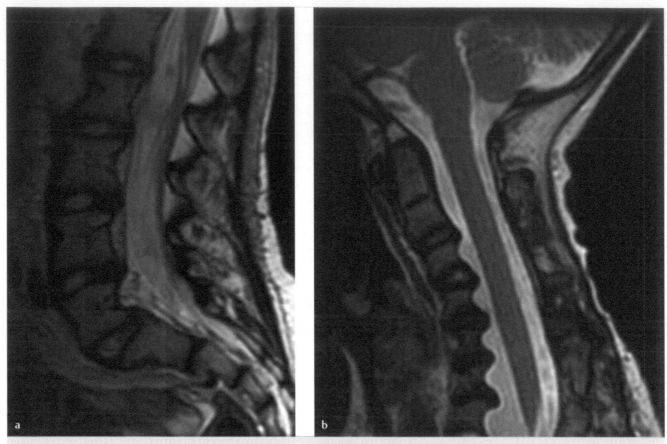

Fig. 117.1 Sagittal T2-weighted MR images of the lumbar **(a)** and cervical **(b)** spine demonstrate scalloping of the posterior aspects of the vertebral bodies.

■ Clinical History

A 30-year-old male, history withheld (▶ Fig. 117.1).

■ Key Finding

Posterior vertebral body scalloping.

■ Top 3 Differential Diagnoses

- **Increased spinal pressure:** Intraspinal masses, such as ependymoma, especially myxopapillary ependymoma, schwannoma, neurofibroma, lipoma, dermoid, and arachnoid cysts, can result in increased spinal pressure and exaggeration of the normal concavity or scalloping of the posterior wall of the vertebral bodies. Secondary findings of intraspinal masses can also include widening of the interpediculate distance. Cases of uncontrolled hydrocephalus have also been reported to result in posterior scalloping.
- **Dural ectasia:** There are few inherited disorders which can exhibit dural ectasia such as neurofibromatosis (NF) type 1, Marfan's syndrome, and Ehlers–Danlos syndrome. Dilatation of the thecal sac is postulated to be a result of pulsatile pressure of the cerebrospinal fluid on a defective dural wall, which mostly affects the lumbrosacral spinal region. Dural ectasia in NF-1 can also be secondary to neurofibromas or the presence of meningocele, most common in the thoracic spine.
- **Congenital disorders:** Spinal findings in achondroplasia, a skeletal dysplasia resulting in dwarfism, include posterior vertebral scalloping, gibbus deformity, kyphosis, hypoplastic vertebral bodies, canal stenosis on the basis of shortened pedicles, as well as progressive decrease in interpedicular distance in the lumbar spine. Mucopolysaccharidoses such as Hurler and Morquio syndrome are also associated with dural ectasia.

■ Additional Diagnostic Consideration

- **Acromegaly:** A feature sometimes seen in these patients, posterior scalloping, is thought to be the result of hypertrophy of soft tissue in the spinal canal and increased bone resorption.

■ Diagnosis

Dural ectasia from neurofibromatosis type 1.

✓ Pearls

- Presence of spinal manifestations including scoliosis, thoracic meningoceles, neurofibromas, and dural ectasia should suggest the diagnosis of NF-1.
- Although hypoplastic vertebral bodies and dural ectasia are seen in both achondroplasia and mucopolysaccharidoses, there is no narrowing of the spinal canal in mucopolysaccharidoses.

■ Suggested Readings

Ho NC, Hadley DW, Jain PK, Francomano CA. Case 47: dural ectasia associated with Marfan syndrome. Radiology. 2002; 223(3):767–771

Wakely SL. The posterior vertebral scalloping sign. Radiology. 2006; 239(2):607–609

Case 118

Jennifer Chang

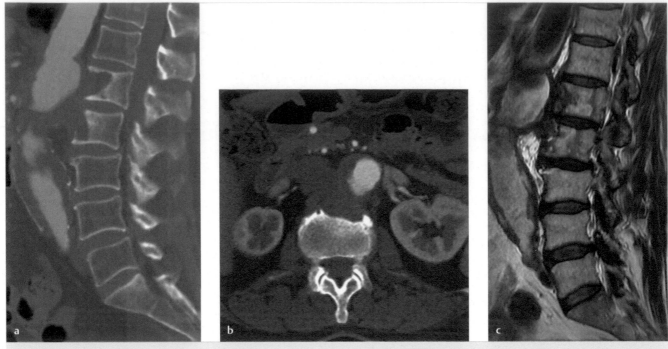

Fig. 118.1 CT images in the sagittal (**a**) and axial (**b**) plane, as well as T2-weighted MR image (**c**) of lumbar spine demonstrate anterior scalloping of the L1 and L2 vertebral bodies.

■ Clinical History

A 68-year-old male with ill-defined abdominal pain (▶ Fig. 118.1).

■ Key Finding

Anterior vertebral body scalloping.

■ Top 3 Differential Diagnoses

- **Lymphadenopathy:** Anterior scalloping of the vertebral bodies commonly results from mass lesions in the retroperitoneal space or mediastinum, with resorption of the bone secondary to pressure. Hodgkin's lymphoma is a common cause of lymphadenopathy among patients between the ages of 20 to 40 years, and can result in anterior scalloping, with osteolytic and/or osteosclerotic (ivory vertebra) lesions. Adjacent paravertebral soft tissue and bony extension can also occur in Hodgkin's lymphoma.
- **Tuberculous spondylitis:** Also known as "Pott's disease," infection by tuberculosis affects the thoracolumbar spine. The extension of abscess beneath the anterior longitudinal ligament, or "subligamentous" spread, results in irregularity of the anterior margin of the vertebral body, preservation of the disc space, and paraspinal collections, in which calcifications are highly suggestive of tuberculosis (TB) infection. Progressive vertebral collapse can lead to anterior wedging, focal kyphosis, and gibbus deformity.
- **Aortic aneurysm:** The pulsatile pressure in aortic aneurysms may result in erosion of the anterior vertebral bodies, which lie adjacent to the aorta. Imaging reveals focal dilatation of aorta. Calcifications from atheromatous disease may be present in the aortic wall.

■ Additional Diagnostic Consideration

- **Down syndrome:** Other vertebral anomalies in Down syndrome include atlanto-axial and atlanto-occipital instability, scoliosis, spondylolisthesis, and squared or block vertebral bodies.

■ Diagnosis

Aortic aneurysm.

✓ Pearls

- In the evaluation of Pott's disease, MRI should address the question of cord compression or epidural involvement. Postcontrast images can demonstrate subligamentous or dural enhancement.
- In TB, disc space can be preserved until later stages of disease. Calcifications in paraspinal collections are highly suggestive of TB.

■ Suggested Readings

Jung NY, Jee WH, Ha KY, Park CK, Byun JY. Discrimination of tuberculous spondylitis from pyogenic spondylitis on MRI. AJR Am J Roentgenol. 2004; 182(6):1405–1410

Rivas-Garcia A, Sarria-Estrada S, Torrents-Odin C, Casas-Gomila L, Franquet E. Imaging findings of Pott's disease. Eur Spine J. 2013; 22 Suppl 4:567–578

Case 119

M. Jason Akers and Jasjeet Bindra

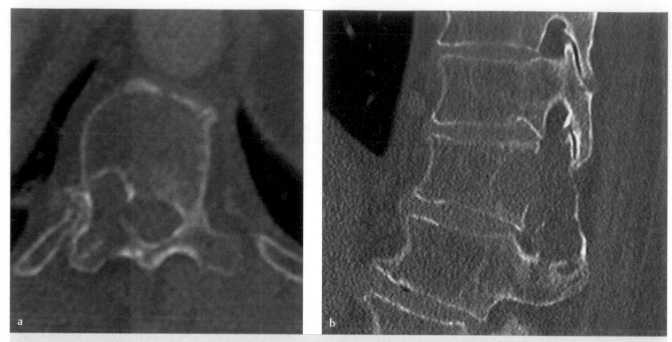

Fig. 119.1 Axial CT image **(a)** of thoracic spine shows a mildly expansile lytic lesion involving the right posterior T11 vertebral body and pedicle. Sagittal reformatted CT image at the same level **(b)** shows the full extent of the lesion.

■ Clinical History

A 64-year-old female with increasing back pain (▶ Fig. 119.1)

■ **Key Finding**

Lytic lesion of posterior elements of spine.

■ **Top 3 Differential Diagnoses**

- **Aneurysmal bone cyst (ABC):** ABC is a benign expansile neoplasm containing thin-walled, blood-filled cavities thought to occur as a result of trauma. They can be isolated or associated with other tumors. ABCs are usually seen in children and young adults, and commonly occur in long bone metaphyses and the posterior elements of the spine. In the spine, ABCs are classically centered in the pedicle and extend into the vertebral body. The pedicle appears absent on AP radiographs of the spine. Cortical thinning and focal cortical destruction are common. There may also be extension into the epidural space, causing canal stenosis. Fluid–fluid levels result from hemorrhage within the lesion.
- **Osteoblastoma:** Osteoblastoma is a benign osteoid forming tumor thought to be a larger version (>1.5 cm) of osteoid osteoma. As much as 40% occur in the spine and originate in the posterior elements, often extending into the vertebral body. They present as expansile lesions with narrow zones of transition and variable mineralization. The matrix is better visualized on CT than radiographs. There may be an ABC component with fluid–fluid levels. Tumors can incite an inflammatory response with associated peritumoral edema that extends beyond the margins of the lesion.
- **Infection (tuberculosis [TB]):** TB causes granulomatous infection of the spine and adjacent soft tissues. Isolated posterior element involvement can occur particularly in the thoracic spine. Patients usually have prominent epidural and paraspinal disease, with large paraspinal abscesses dissecting over multiple levels. Tuberculous spondylitis is more likely to spare intervertebral discs while causing prominent bony destruction.

■ **Additional Diagnostic Considerations**

- **Metastases:** Metastases usually occur in older patients, and involve the posterior vertebral body first, with extension into the posterior elements. Metastases most commonly spread to the spine hematogenously. Lytic metastases tend to be less expansile and more permeative in appearance, occurring as a destructive lesion with an associated soft-tissue mass. Multiple vertebral levels are commonly involved.
- **Langerhans cell histiocytosis (LCH):** LCH is a disease occurring in children which is characterized by abnormal histiocyte proliferation, producing granulomatous skeletal lesions. The classic presentation in the spine is vertebra plana with preservation of the disc space. LCH can also present as an aggressive lytic lesion with soft-tissue mass and extension into the spinal canal. Other sites of involvement include the skull with a beveled edge appearance, mandible, long bones, ribs, and pelvis.

■ **Diagnosis**

Metastatic lesion.

✓ **Pearls**

- ABCs are benign expansile lytic lesions that contain fluid–fluid levels due to internal hemorrhage.
- Osteoblastoma has an osteoid matrix and typically has peritumoral edema that extends beyond the lesion.
- Posterior element involvement of the thoracic spine with paraspinal abscesses suggests TB spondylitis.
- Lytic metastases typically occur in older patients, appear permeative/destructive, and affect multiple levels.

■ **Suggested Readings**

DiCaprio MR, Murphy MJ, Camp RL. Aneurysmal bone cyst of the spine with familial incidence. Spine. 2000; 25(12):1589–1592

Long SS, Yablon CM, Eisenberg RL. Bone marrow signal alteration in the spine and sacrum. AJR Am J Roentgenol. 2010; 195(3):W178:200

Shaikh MI, Saifuddin A, Pringle J, Natali C, Sherazi Z. Spinal osteoblastoma: CT and MR imaging with pathological correlation. Skeletal Radiol. 1999; 28(1):33–40

Case 120

Jennifer Chang

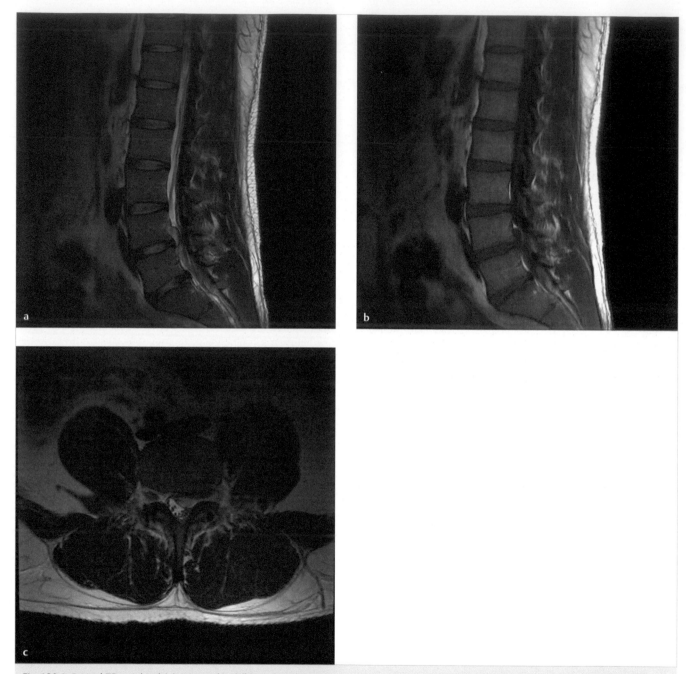

Fig. 120.1 Sagittal T2 weighted **(a)**, T1-weighted **(b)**, and axial T2-weighted **(c)** images of the lumbar spine demonstrate a T1-hypointense and T2-hyperintense epidural mass in the left subarticular zone along the posterior inferior aspect of the L4 vertebral body.

■ **Clinical History**

A 27-year-old male with left leg sciatica (▶ Fig. 120.1).

■ Key Finding

Epidural mass.

■ Top 3 Differential Diagnoses

- **Hematoma:** Presentation can be related to spinal cord or cauda equina compression. MRI signal characteristics of a hematoma follow evolution of hemorrhage, and signal will vary depending on the stage of evolution; in the subacute phase, it can be T1-hyperintense and T2-hypointense. If a gradient echo (GRE) sequence is performed, there can be blooming secondary to blood products. While there is no enhancement, peripheral enhancement of the adjacent dura can be noted. Etiologies include spontaneous (coagulopathy or anticoagulation medication), trauma, or iatrogenic causes.
- **Disc:** Degenerative disc disease results due to loss of water content within the discs and is extremely common. The pathophysiology is multifactorial, resulting from a combination of mechanical stresses, age, genetic predisposition, trauma, and inflammation. A degenerated disc can herniate into the anterior epidural space through a perforation of the annulus fibrosis. Once in the anterior epidural space, it can migrate and lose contact with its parent disc (sequestration).
- **Abscess:** Risk factors for an epidural abscess include predisposing conditions such as diabetes, alcoholism, HIV, recent surgery, or IV drug abuse. Spread can be through hematogenous dissemination or contiguous spread in the epidural space, with Staphylococcus aureus being the most common organism. MRI with contrast should be performed which demonstrates T2 hyperintensity, homogeneous enhancement in more phelgmonous collections, or peripheral enhancement if an organized fluid collection with pus is present.

■ Additional Diagnostic Considerations

- **Metastasis:** Metastases are the most common vertebral tumors. They are generally varied in size and multiple; also, they can have associated compression fractures with soft-tissue component which extends into the epidural space. Osteolytic lesions are more common than osteoblastic metastases.
- **Arteriovenous malformation:** This rare spinal vascular lesion is a fistulous connection between the epidural venous plexus and epidural arterial arcade, often in the ventral epidural space. Patients can present with progressive myelopathy or radiculopathy. MRI can demonstrate T2 hyperintensity in the spinal cord and dilatation of the perimedullary veins. Definitive diagnosis is made with conventional angiogram.
- **Epidural lipomatosis:** This condition can occur with chronic steroid use, obesity, or Cushing's syndrome. Lipomatous tissue in epidural space circumferentially surrounds the dural sac and follows the signal characteristics of fat, with T1 and T2 hyperintesity, which suppresses on STIR or T2, fat-suppressed images. Epidural fat thickness greater than 7 mm is diagnostic of epidural lipomatosis

■ Diagnosis

Disc extrusion.

✓ Pearls

- Windowing on noncontrast CT can allow you to see acute epidural hematomas, which can demonstrate biconvex shape with well-defined margins and distal tapering.
- A herniated disc is usually seen in the anterior epidural space; migration to the posterior epidural space is rare.

■ Suggested Readings

Gala FB, Aswani Y. Imaging in spinal posterior epidural space lesions: a pictorial essay. Indian J Radiol Imaging. 2016; 26(3):299–315

Kiyosue H, Tanoue S, Okahara M, Hori Y, Kashiwagi J, Mori H. Spinal ventral epidural arteriovenous fistulas of the lumbar spine: angioarchitecture and endovascular treatment. Neuroradiology. 2013; 55(3):327–336

Modic MT, Ross JS. Lumbar degenerative disk disease. Radiology. 2007; 245(1): 43–61

Case 121

Jennifer Chang and Jasjeet Bindra

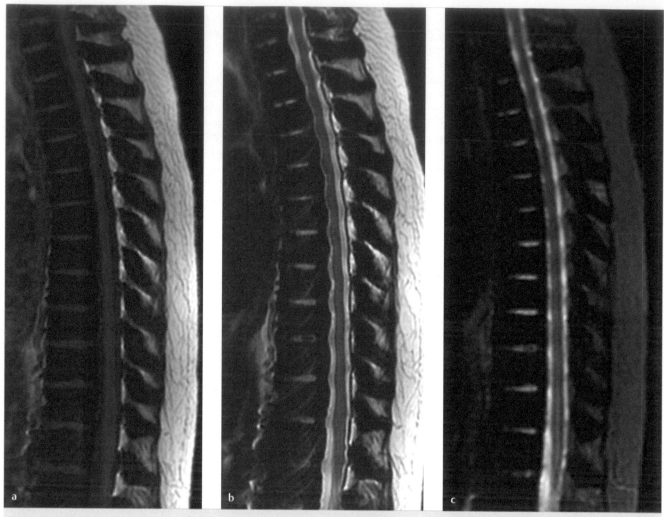

Fig. 121.1 Sagittal T1-weighted **(a)**, T2-weighted **(b)**, and STIR **(c)** images of the thoracic spine demonstrate diffuse hypointensity of the marrow signal on all sequences.

■ Clinical History

A 27-year-old female with acute on chronic back pain (▶ Fig. 121.1).

■ Key Finding

Diffuse marrow T1- and T2-low signal.

■ Top 3 Differential Diagnoses

- **Hemosiderosis:** Synonymous with secondary hemochromatosis, it is a description of abnormal extracellular iron deposition within the reticuloendothelial cells of the spleen, bone marrow, and liver, which results in diffuse marrow hypointensity on T1- and T2-weighted images in spine. Etiology involves multiple blood transfusions.
- **Myelofibrosis:** Myelofibrosis is characterized by replacement of bone marrow by connective tissue and progressive fibrosis. Other features found in myelofibrosis include extramedullary hematopoiesis, splenomegaly, hepatomegaly and anemia. On bone scan, it can cause a "superscan" appearance with intense symmetric activity in the bones, especially in the acute phases. Patients are generally older with a mean age of 60 years, have an indolent course, and have a poor prognosis. There is an association with chemotherapy or radiation therapy.
- **AIDS (acquired immunodeficiency syndrome):** Patients with HIV infection can have diffuse marrow hypointensity on T1- and T2-weighted images. This is considered to be due to abnormally increased iron within the bone marrow secondary to anemia from chronic disease in which the release of iron from macrophages is impaired. Patients with AIDS have other associated musculoskeletal complications, including infections such as pyomyositis, arthritis, osteonecrosis, osteoporosis, and neoplasms such as lymphoma or Kaposi sarcoma.

■ Additional Diagnostic Consideration

- **Gaucher disease:** In this most common lysosomal storage disease, there is deficiency of glucocerebrosidase, resulting in buildup of glucocerebrosides in the reticuloendothelial system. There is infiltration of the bone marrow by Gaucher cells, resulting in low-signal on T1- and T2-weighed sequences. Other bony changes include osteopenia, osteonecrosis, pathologic fractures, and lytic lesions.

■ Diagnosis

Thalassemia major hemosiderosis.

✓ Pearls

- With advancing age, generally over 40 years, the vertebral bone marrow becomes increasingly replaced with fatty marrow. In an adult, where there is a predominance of yellow marrow in spine, marrow signal should be evaluated on T1-weighted sequences and should be hyperintense relative to the disc.
- With diffuse abnormalities, extensive replacement of the vertebral marrow may create the impression of a normal study, and careful comparison of T1-weighted signal to adjacent discs or muscle is required to make the diagnosis.

■ Suggested Readings

Booth TC, Chhaya NC, Bell JR, Holloway BJ. Update on imaging of non-infectious musculoskeletal complications of HIV infection. Skeletal Radiol. 2012; 41(11):1349–1363

Hanrahan CJ, Shah LM. MRI of spinal bone marrow: part 2, T1-weighted imaging-based differential diagnosis. AJR Am J Roentgenol. 2011; 197(6):1309–1321

Simpson WL, Hermann G, Balwani M. Imaging of Gaucher disease. World J Radiol. 2014; 6(9):657–668

Case 122

Jennifer Chang and Jasjeet Bindra

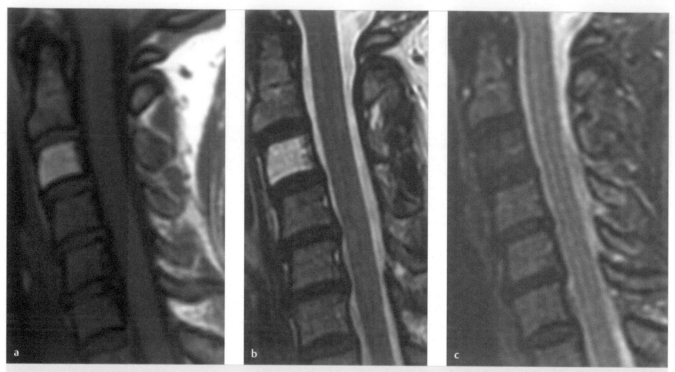

Fig. 122.1 Sagittal T1-weighted **(a)**, T2 weighted **(b)**, and STIR **(c)** images of the cervical spine demonstrate T1 and T2 hyperintensity of the C3 vertebral body, and which is hypointense on STIR-weighted images.

■ Clinical History

A 45-year-old female with left neck pain (▶ Fig. 122.1).

■ Key Finding

Focal T1 signal increase in vertebral body.

■ Top 3 Differential Diagnoses

- **Hemangioma:** Common benign lesions in the spine, they demonstrate T1 and T2 hyperintensity on MRI secondary to their fat content, and on CT, they have a corduroy or polka dot-appearance due to coarsened trabeculae. There can be significant enhancement secondary to the vascularity of these lesions.
- **Modic change:** Type 2 Modic change in degenerative disc disease demonstrates T1 hyperintensity, and T2 hyperintensity secondary to fatty yellow marrow replacement. Type 1 Modic changes refer to acute degenerative changes in the subchondral bone marrow, including edema and inflammation, and demonstrate T1 hypointensity and T2 hyperintensity. Type 3 Modic changes are bony sclerosis of the endplates with T1 and T2 hypointensity on MRI.

- **Paget's disease:** A disease resulting in abnormal remodeling of the bone, it affects patients older than 40 years and frequently involves the spine, pelvis, skull, and proximal long bones. There are three stages of disease, including a lytic phase with mainly osteoclastic activity, mixed phase with osteoblastic and osteoclastic activity, and late sclerotic or blastic phase. In the spine, Paget's disease demonstrates flattening of the anterior margin of the vertebral body, or squaring, and cortical thickening and sclerosis involving the vertebral body margins, giving a "picture frame" appearance on radiographs and an "ivory vertebra" in the blastic phase. On MRI, the most common pattern has signal characteristics similar to that of fat, with T1 hyperintensity presumably corresponding to long-standing disease.

■ Additional Diagnostic Considerations

- **Melanoma:** Metastases from melanoma can spread to the spine, and the paramagnetic effects of melanin or associated hemorrhage result in T1 hyperintensity of these circumscribed lesions.
- **Lipoma:** Intraosseous lipomas are rare lesions, most commonly found in the lower extremity rather than the spine, which can have associated calcification.

- **Focal fatty marrow:** A normal variant, these are focal regions of T1 and T2 hyperintensity which suppress on STIR or fat-suppressed, T2 sequences.

■ Diagnosis

Hemangioma.

✓ Pearls

- Vertebral hemangiomas are characterized by increased T1- and T2-weighted signal intensity corresponding to fat content.
- Modic type 2 discogenic degenerative end plate changes exhibit hyperintense T1-weighted signal intensity

- T1 hyperintense bone marrow lesions are usually benign except melanoma.

■ Suggested Readings

Shah LM, Hanrahan CJ. MRI of spinal bone marrow: part I, techniques and normal age-related appearances. AJR Am J Roentgenol. 2011; 197(6):1298–1308

Theodorou DJ, Theodorou SJ, Kakitsubata Y. Imaging of Paget disease of bone and its musculoskeletal complications: review. AJR Am J Roentgenol. 2011; 196(6) Suppl:S64–S75

Case 123

Jennifer Chang

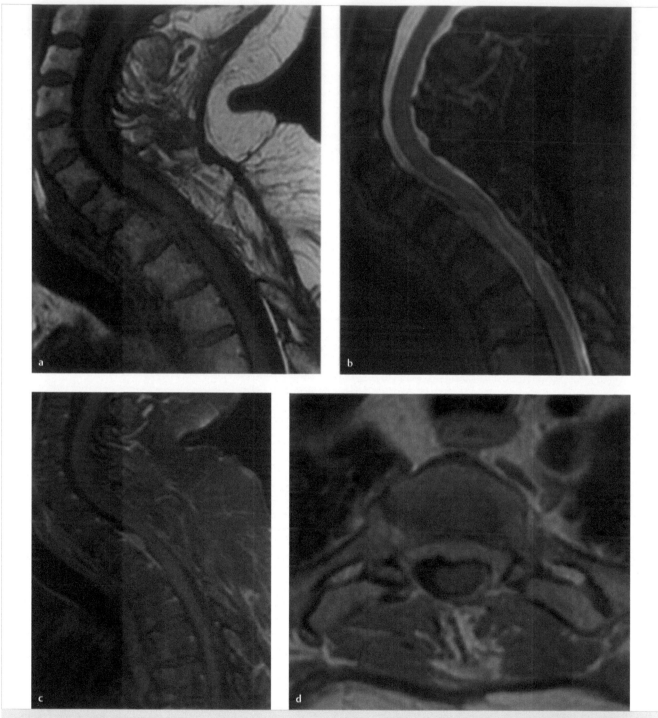

Fig. 123.1 Sagittal T2-weighted **(a)**, fat-suppressed, T2 weighted **(b)**, postcontrast sagittal **(c)**, and axial fat-suppressed, T1-weighted **(d)** images of the cervicothoracic spine demonstrate an intradural, extramedullary mass with enhancement along the ventral aspect of the thecal sac at the T1–T2 level.

■ **Clinical History**

A 70-year-old woman with neck pain (▶ Fig. 123.1).

■ Key Finding

Intradural, extramedullary mass.

■ Top 3 Differential Diagnoses

- **Meningioma:** Meningiomasmost commonly occur in the thoracic spine. They are the second most common intradural, extramedullary mass lesion, which comprise 25% of all spinal cord tumors. Their radiologic appearance is similar to those found intracranially with T1 and T2 isointensity, homogeneous enhancement, and dural tail. In the spine, they are more common in the elderly population and have a greater prevalence in females.
- **Nerve Sheath tumor:** Neurofibromas or schwannomas are benign peripheral nerve sheath tumors which are well-circumscribed masses with low-to-intermediate signal intensity on T1 and hyperintensity on T2, and demonstrate enhancement; definitive diagnosis between neurofibroma and schwannoma cannot be reliably made radiologically. Malignant peripheral nerve sheath tumors have poor prognosis, arise from degeneration of neurofibromas, and involve the paravertebral soft tissues.
- **Metastasis:** Although they are uncommon lesions in the intradural space, primary tumors which can metastasize here include lung, breast, gastrointestinal (GI), prostate, and melanoma. Drop metastases can occur from glioblastoma, astrocytoma, and ependymoma. In the pediatric population, drop metastases can occur from posterior fossa medulloblastoma, choroid plexus tumors, and germ cell tumors. In these cases, total spine MRI, including fat-saturated, T1-weighted images of the lumbar spine, should be included.

■ Additional Diagnostic Consideration

- **Paraganglioma:** A rare lesion usually found in the cauda equina and filum terminale, they are of neuroendocrine origin and are hypervascular tumors. They can be associated with multiple flow voids and have intense enhancement on post-contrast images.

■ Diagnosis

Meningioma.

✓ Pearls

- Neurofibromas are central in relation to the nerve, demonstrate fusiform enlargement, and exhibit the "target sign" on T2-weighted images where there is central hypointensity and peripheral hyperintensity with central enhancement; schwannomas are eccentric in relation to the nerve and can have cystic degeneration.
- Neurofibromas are associated with neurofibromatosis type 1, and schwannomas are associated with neurofibromatosis type 2.

■ Suggested Readings

Abul-Kasim K, Thurnher MM, McKeever P, Sundgren PC. Intradural spinal tumors: current classification and MRI features. Neuroradiology. 2008; 50(4):301–314

Beall DP, Googe DJ, Emery RL, et al. Extramedullary intradural spinal tumors: a pictorial review. Curr Probl Diagn Radiol. 2007; 36(5):185–198

Case 124

Jennifer Chang

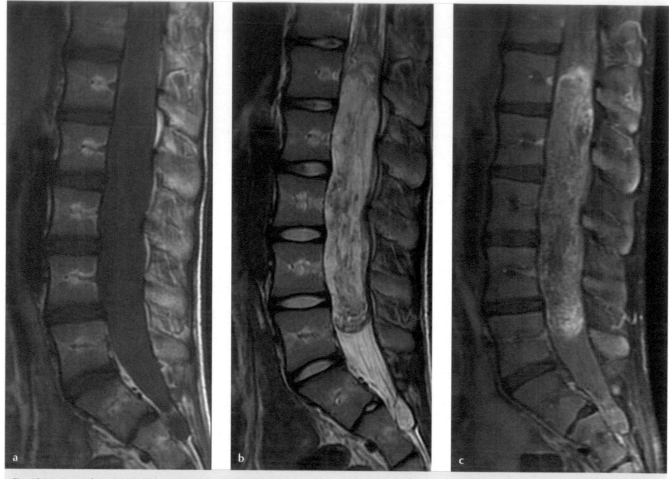

Fig. 124.1 Sagittal T1-weighted **(a)**, T2-weighted **(b)**, and postcontrast, fat-suppressed, T1-weighted **(c)** images of the lumbar spine demonstrate an intradural heterogeneously enhancing mass in the lumbar thecal sac.

■ Clinical History

A 13-year-old male with right leg pain for 1 year (▶ Fig. 124.1).

■ **Key Finding**

Intradural, intramedullary spinal cord mass.

■ **Top 3 Differential Diagnoses**

- **Hemangioblastoma:** Although mostly intramedullary lesions, hemangioblastomas can also involve the intradural space, most commonly involving the thoracic cord. They are well-defined vascular masses with associated, dilated tortuous feeding arteries and draining pial veins, which are manifested by enlarged flow voids. As in the posterior fossa, they can have a cyst with mural nodule appearance, of which the nodule enhances avidly. There can also be associated edema within the cord, hemosiderin cap sign from hemorrhage, and cord expansion.

- **Glial neoplasm:** These encompass ependymomas and astrocytomas, which are the most common intramedullary lesions. Ependymomas are more common in adults and are usually seen in the cervical spine, whereas astrocytomas are more common in children, and are also usually seen in the cervical and upper thoracic region.

- **Metastasis:** Metastases are rare lesions in this location, and most of them are solitary, with lung and breast being most common types of metastases. There can be associated cord expansion, cord edema, and enhancement.

■ **Additional Diagnostic Considerations**

- **Paraganglioma:** These hypervascular tumors can demonstrate a "salt and pepper" appearance with multiple flow voids and intense enhancement; also, they can have associated hemorrhage with a hemosiderin cap sign. WHO grade 1 lesions of neuroendocrine origin, they are generally found along the cauda equina or filum terminale.

- **Lymphoma:** Rarely found in the spinal cord, these have been reportedly found in the cervical cord and are solitary. In

contradistinction to their intracranial counterparts, these lesions have demonstrated T2 hyperintensity with contrast enhancement.

- **PNET** (primitive neuroectodermal) tumors in the spine are usually drop metastases from a primary intracranial tumor, with abnormal enhancement along the leptomeninges; however, rare cases have been reported in the spinal cord and along the cauda equina.

■ **Diagnosis**

Myxopapillary ependymoma.

✓ **Pearls**

- Myxopapillary ependymomas are associated with von Hippel–Lindau syndrome

- Myxopapililaryependymomas are the most common tumors of the conus medullaris, cauda equina, and filum terminale,

which comprise 30% of ependymomas. They are more common in males, and MRI findings include T2 hyperintensity with patchy enhancement.

■ **Suggested Readings**

Abul-Kasim K, Thurnher MM, McKeever P, Sundgren PC. Intradural spinal tumors: current classification and MRI features. Neuroradiology. 2008; 50(4):301–314

Case 125

Jennifer Chang

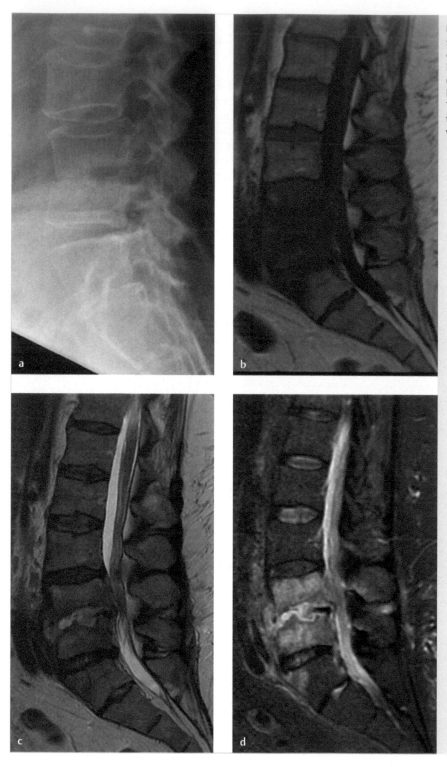

Fig. 125.1 Lateral radiograph **(a)** of the lumbar spine demonstrates focal kyphosis at L4–5 with decreased intervertebral disc space and endplate irregularity. Sagittal T1 weighted **(b)**, T2-weighted **(c)**, and STIR-weighted **(d)** sequences of the lumbar spine demonstrate marrow replacement, T2 hyperintensity within the disc space, destruction of the endplates, and edema within the vertebral bodies.

■ Clinical History

A 55-year-old man with severe lumbar pain, radiating into left hip and left lower extremity for several weeks (▶ Fig. 125.1).

■ Key Finding

End plate irregularity

■ Top 3 Differential Diagnoses

- **Degenerative disc disease:** Degenerative disc disease is the most commonly found entity in the spine. There is overall loss of hydration of the disc, with narrowing of the disc space. Changes to the marrow within the adjacent vertebral body endplates have been described by Modic. Endplate lesions called Schmorl nodes result from herniation of the intervertebral disc into the endplate.
- **Discitis:** Infection of the endplates is usually secondary to hematogenous spread of systemic infection, such as urinary tract infection or pneumonia, and can also occur in the postoperative setting. Risk factors include IV drug use, alcoholism, immunosuppression, and diabetes. The vertebral body endplate is affected by septic emboli, and infection spreads directly to the disc in adults, whereas in children, the nutrient vessels entering the nucleus pulposus allow for direct

infection. In both age groups, staphylococcus aureus is the most common organism. Radiologic hallmarks include bony destruction of the endplates, T2 hyperintensity of the disc, and abnormal enhancement of the disc and adjacent bone marrow. There can also be T1 hypointensity of the endplates with loss of normal marrow signal.

- **Neurogenic spondyloarthropathy:** Also known as Charcot spine, it is an uncommon destructive process which results from neurosensory deficits, such as in those with traumatic spinal cord injury. The lumbar spine and thoracolumbar junction is usually involved with sclerosis or osteolysis involving the endplates but can also include the facet joints. Osseous fragmentation, hypertrophic endplate osteophytes, soft-tissue calcifications, and spondylolisthesis are also usually present.

■ Additional Diagnostic Considerations

- **Dialysis spondyloarthropathy:** Destructive spondyloarthropathy is a known complication in patients with renal disease on chronic hemodialysis, with imaging findings in the spine including erosions of subchondral bone as well as bony sclerosis of the adjacent vertebral endplates. A more common site of involvement is the lower cervical spine.
- **Synovitis, acne, pustulosis, hyperostosis, and osteitis (SAPHO) syndrome:** This rare disorder is considered a type of seronegative spondyloarthropathy. It is characterized by skin conditions and osteoarticular lesions which can include

synovitis, hyperostosis, and osteitis, with multiple skeletal sites involved, including the anterior chest wall, spine, and long bones. Some regard chronic recurrent multifocal osteomyelitis (CRMO) to be a pediatric form of this syndrome.

- **Scheuermann's disease:** Classically criteria require three or more consecutive wedged thoracic vertebral bodies, resulting in kyphosis, especially in adolescent patients. Often times, disc space narrowing and endplate irregularity with Schmorl nodes are also seen.

■ Diagnosis

Discitis.

✓ Pearls

- Classic imaging appearance of Charcot spine involves anterior and posterior elements, whereas osteomyelitis usually only involves one vertebral column.
- Lack of T2 hyperintensity within the disc in a long-term dialysis patient can suggest destructive spondyloarthropathy and help exclude infection.

■ Suggested Readings

Earwaker JW, Cotten A. SAPHO: syndrome or concept? Imaging findings. Skeletal Radiol. 2003; 32(6):311–327

Ledbetter LN, Salzman KL, Sanders RK, Shah LM. Spinal Neuroarthropathy: pathophysiology, clinical and imaging features, and differential diagnosis. Radiographics. 2016; 36(3):783–799

Ledermann HP, Schweitzer ME, Morrison WB, Carrino JA. MR imaging findings in spinal infections: rules or myths? Radiology. 2003; 228(2):506–514

Theodorou DJ, Theodorou SJ, Resnick D. Imaging in dialysis spondyloarthropathy. Semin Dial. 2002; 15(4):290–296

Part 10

Pediatric or Developmental Musculoskeletal Conditions

Case 126

Rebecca Stein-Wexler

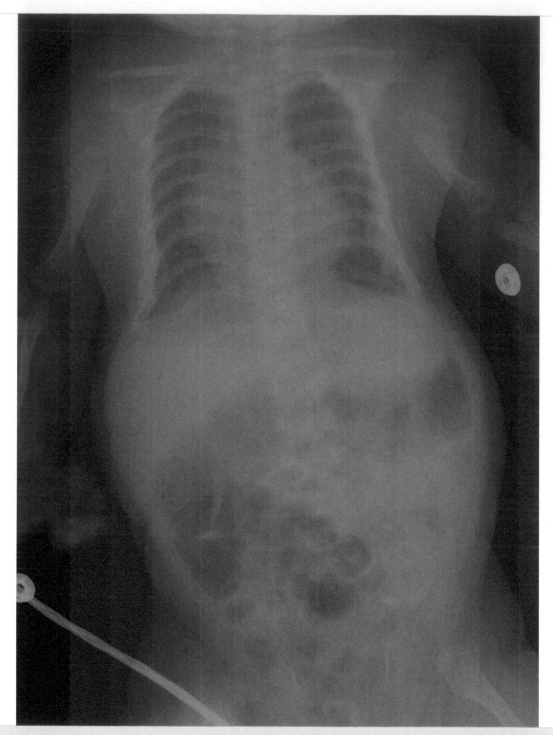

Fig. 126.1 Frontal radiograph shows unusually short ribs. The spine is normal, but humeri are short and thick. The cardiothymic silhouette appears enlarged.

■ Clinical History

A 2-month-old with short extremities and a heart murmur
(► Fig. 126.1).

■ Key Finding

Short rib skeletal dysplasia.

■ Top 3 Differential Diagnoses

- **Asphyxiating thoracic dystrophy (Jeune syndrome):** In this syndrome, the thorax is long and bell-shaped, with short, horizontal ribs that flare anteriorly. This configuration results in early respiratory compromise. Dysplastic acetabula resembling an upside-down trident is often seen. There is associated mild acromelic (distal) limb shortening, but long bones are not bowed. A normal spine and trident acetabula help differentiate this condition from thanatophoric dysplasia.
- **Ellis-van Creveld syndrome (chondroectodermal dysplasia):** Hair, nail, and teeth abnormalities are clinical hallmarks of this syndrome. There is progressive mesomelic (middle–tibial and radial) and acromelic (distal) limb shortening. The fibulae are markedly shortened. Radiographic features also include short ribs, fused capitate and hamate, cone-shaped epiphyses, and postaxial polydactyly. The femoral heads ossify prematurely, and the pelvis is abnormal, with flared iliac wings and a trident acetabulum. Congenital heart disease, typically atrial septal defect or atrioventricular cushion defect, is the major cause of morbidity.
- **Short rib polydactyly:** In this condition, the ribs are extremely short. Polydactyly may be either preaxial or postaxial. The pelvis and spine appear fairly normal, and long bones are normal. However, there may be cleft palate, hypoplastic epiglottis, cystic kidneys, and fetal hydrops.

■ Additional Diagnostic Considerations

- **Thanatophoric dysplasia:** Thanatophoric dysplasia is the most common lethal skeletal dysplasia which is uniformly fatal in the neonatal period. The ribs are very short, and as a result, the thorax is narrow. Lung hypoplasia causes respiratory failure. Patients with this disproportionate dwarfism have severe platyspondyly but wide intervertebral disks, leading to normal trunk length. The head is disproportionately large, and some patients have cloverleaf skull. Iliac bones are small. There is rhizomelic (proximal) limb shortening. Long bones are bowed and short. The femurs have a characteristic "telephone receiver" appearance.
- **Holt–Oram syndrome:** Like Ellis-van Creveld, this condition is characterized by cardiac disease (usually an atrial or ventricular septal defect) and limb abnormalities. However, the ribs are normal. The thumb is usually duplicated, hypoplastic, or triphalangeal. The radius is often hypoplastic, and there may be other anomalies of the shoulder and upper extremity.

■ Diagnosis

Ellis-van Creveld syndrome.

✓ Pearls

- Jeune syndrome (asphyxiating thoracic dysplasia) demonstrates a bell-shaped thorax, trident acetabula, and normal spine.
- Patients with Ellis-van Creveld have cardiac disease as well as progressive limb shortening, short ribs, and postaxial polydactyly.
- Bones in patients with short rib polydactyly are otherwise normal.

■ Suggested Readings

Glass RB, Norton KI, Mitre SA, Kang E. Pediatric ribs: a spectrum of abnormalities. Radiographics. 2002; 22(1):87–104

Miller E, Blaser S, Shannon P, Widjaja E. Brain and bone abnormalities of thanatophoric dwarfism. AJR Am J Roentgenol. 2009; 192(1):48–51

Panda A, Gamanagatti S, Jana M, Gupta AK. Skeletal dysplasias: a radiographic approach and review of common non-lethal skeletal dysplasias. World J Radiol. 2014; 6(10):808–825

Parnell SE, Phillips GS. Neonatal skeletal dysplasias. Pediatr Radiol. 2012; 42 Suppl 1: S150–S157

Case 127

Rebecca Stein-Wexler

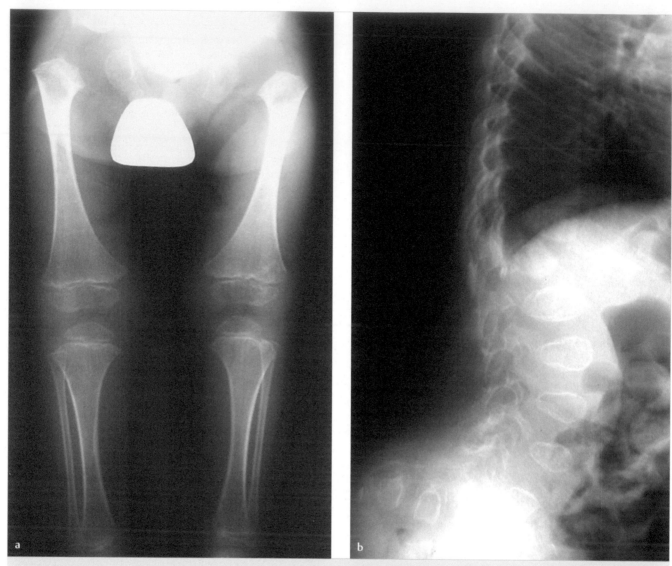

Fig. 127.1 Radiograph of the lower extremities **(a)** shows that ossification of the femoral heads is severely delayed, and ossification of the other visualized epiphyses is mildly delayed; the long bones are relatively short. Lateral view of the spine **(b)** shows that the L1 is short and triangular; the other vertebral bodies are pear-shaped.

■ Clinical History

A 4-year-old boy with hip pain and short stature (► Fig. 127.1).

■ Key Finding

Abnormal epiphyses.

■ Top 3 Differential Diagnoses

- **Spondyloepiphyseal dysplasia (SED):** SED "congenita" manifests at birth with absent calcaneal, knee, and pubic bone ossification, pear-shaped vertebrae, and short, broad iliac wings. Severe platyspondyly develops, with thin intervertebral disks. SED "tarda" usually manifests at age 5 to 10 years with platyspondyly (including hump-shaped posterior vertebral bodies), small pelvis, and mild-to-moderately small, irregular epiphyses.
- **Chondrodysplasia punctate:** There are two common subtypes, both characterized by stippled epiphyses at birth. The autosomal recessive form shows symmetrical rhizomelic shortening, stippling in the large joints, and sometimes stippling of laryngeal and tracheal cartilage. Coronal clefts are seen in vertebrae. The hands and feet are normal. The X-linked dominant type, "Conradi–Hunermann," shows occasional and asymmetrical limb shortening and involvement of the hands and feet as well as large joints. The larynx and trachea are normal, but vertebral bodies and endplates are stippled, leading to eventual kyphoscoliosis. Stippling resolves over time, and the patients have a normal lifespan. Mental retardation is a feature of the lethal form but not Conradi–Hunermann.
- **Spondyloepimetaphyseal dysplasia:** This dysplasia resembles multiple epiphyseal dysplasia, but there is concomitant metaphyseal involvement.

■ Additional Diagnostic Considerations

- **Multiple epiphyseal dysplasia:** This genetically heterogeneous disorder presents after age 2 to 4 years. Bilateral and symmetrical, delayed and fragmented epiphyses of long bones and distal extremities are characteristic. Pronounced wedging of distal tibial epiphysis may trigger the diagnosis. The spine resembles Scheuermann disease, with endplate irregularities, slight anterior wedging, and numerous Schmorl nodes.
- **Morquio syndrome:** A mucopolysaccharidosis, Morquio syndrome is characterized by delayed ossification of femoral heads, irregular epiphyses, and secondary metaphyseal widening. Other bones are involved as well, notably the spine, where there is platyspondyly with anterior beaking of the midportion of vertebral bodies. The bases of the 2nd through 5th metacarpals are pointed and clustered together. Ribs have a paddle appearance.

■ Diagnosis

Spondyloepiphyseal dysplasia.

✓ Pearls

- SED tarda manifests during childhood with mild-to-moderately small, irregular epiphyses and platyspondyly with hump-shaped posterior vertebral bodies.
- A wedged, slightly small distal tibial epiphysis is a clue to the diagnosis of multiple epiphyseal dysplasia.
- With Morquio syndrome, ossification of the femoral heads is delayed, and there are multiple irregular epiphyses; as far as Hurler syndrome is concerned, there is anterior vertebral body beaking.
- The autosomal recessive type of chondrodysplasia punctata has stippled epiphyses of large joints and less involvement of the axial skeleton, whereas with Conradi-Hunermann, the spine, hands, and feet may be affected as well.

■ Suggested Readings

Panda A, Gamanagatti S, Jana M, Gupta AK. Skeletal dysplasias: A radiographic approach and review of common non-lethal skeletal dysplasias. World J Radiol. 2014; 6(10):808–825

Parnell SE, Phillips GS. Neonatal skeletal dysplasias. Pediatr Radiol. 2012; 42 Suppl 1: S150–S157

Case 128

Rebecca Stein-Wexler

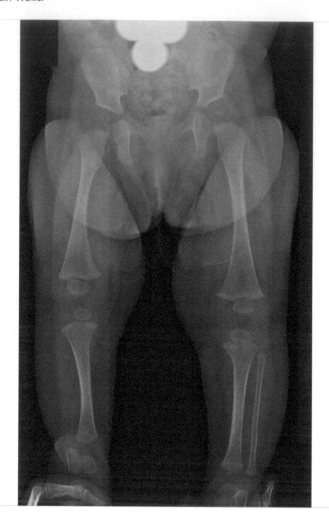

Fig. 128.1 Frontal radiograph of the lower extremities shows that the right fibula is absent, and the right tibia is relatively short. The femur is hypoplastic.

■ Clinical History

A 6-month-old with a short right lower extremity (▶ Fig. 128.1).

■ Key Finding

Limb deficiency.

■ Top 3 Differential Diagnoses

- **Longitudinal deficiency of the fibula:** In this condition, the fibula may be partly or completely absent, or it may simply be mildly hypoplastic. The anomaly is often accompanied by proximal focal femoral deficiency, coxa vara, clubfoot, and absent lateral rays. The remainder of the skeleton is usually normal. Perhaps counter-intuitively, femoral abnormalities are more common with a hypoplastic fibula than with one that is completely absent. A cartilaginous fibular anlage is often present, which tethers growth of the tibia. If the hip and/or femur are clearly abnormal as well, the diagnosis may be made in utero. If the fibula is absent or markedly hypoplastic, X-ray diagnosis is straightforward. The tibia is often bowed, short, and thick. However, subtle cases are diagnosed by an abnormally high-distal fibular physis (above the proximal tibial physis). Treatment is directed at establishing a usable weight-bearing lower extremity which often involves amputation. Longitudinal deficiency of the tibia is much less common than that of the fibula.
- **Longitudinal deficiency of the radius:** This sporadic condition usually consists of complete absence of the radius. However, the deficiency may be more limited and is occasionally manifested only by absence or hypoplasia of the thumb. As many as 1/3rd of patients are otherwise normal, but 1/3rd also have a syndrome such as thrombocytopenia-absent radius (TAR), VACTERL, or Holt–Oram. As many as 1/3rd have nonsyndromic-associated bone anomalies, with the likelihood of this increasing with the severity of deficiency. The radius is partly or (more often) completely absent, and the thumb is hypoplastic or absent. The ulna is short and bowed. If the radius is partially present, it may be fused with the ulna, and the radial head is often congenitally dislocated. The hand may be at a right angle to the forearm (radial clubhand).
- **Proximal focal femoral deficiency (PFFD):** This nonhereditary malformation ranges from mild dysgenesis of the proximal femur to near complete absence of the bone. Usually isolated and unilateral, it may be part of caudal regression syndrome. The tibia and fibula may be hypoplastic as well. The condition is classified according to the presence of the femoral head, connection between the femoral head and the shaft (bony, cartilaginous, or absent), and extent of acetabular dysplasia. US and MRI assess nonossified structures.

■ Additional Diagnostic Consideration

- **Longitudinal deficiency of the ulna:** At least part of the ulna is usually present in this disorder, which is more common in boys, usually on the right, and infrequently bilateral. Anomalies of the hand, wrist, and elbow bones are more severe than with radial deficiency. Carpal bones and digits are often missing or fused. Clubhand alignment is uncommon. Remote bony anomalies are common, including scoliosis, phocomelia, and PFFD. Other organ systems are usually normal. X-rays usually show a hypoplastic ulna, with ossification sometimes delayed until age of 2 years. The radius appears bowed and short. The radial head may be normal, dislocated, or fused to the humerus. The rays are often deficient or fused.

■ Diagnosis

Longitudinal deficiency of the fibula.

✓ Pearls

- Mild cases of fibular longitudinal deficiency are diagnosed by an unusually high-distal fibular physis.
- As many as 1/3rd of patients with longitudinal deficiency of the radius have an accompanying syndrome.
- US and MRI are useful for evaluating nonossified cartilaginous structures in PFFD.

■ Suggested Readings

Birch JG, Lincoln TL, Mack PW, et al. Congenital fibular deficiency: a review of 30 years' experience at one institution. J Bone Joint Surg Am. 2011; 93:1144–1151

Stein-Wexler R. The elbow and forearm: Congenital and developmental conditions. In: Stein-Wexler R, Wootton-Gorges SL, Ozonoff MB, eds. Pediatric Orthopedic Imaging. Berlin Heidelberg: Springer; 2015

Case 129

Rebecca Stein-Wexler

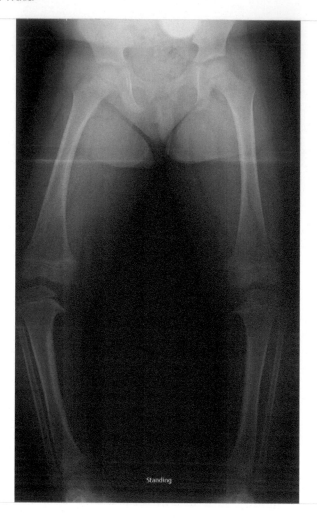

Fig. 129.1 Standing view of both lower extremities shows bilateral genu varus, worse on the right. The metaphyses are broad, slightly flared, and dense. There is beaking and depression of the proximal tibial medial metaphyses.

■ Clinical History

A 3-year-old girl with bowed legs (▶ Fig. 129.1).

■ Key Finding

Genu varum.

■ Top 3 Differential Diagnoses

- **Physiological bowing:** Tibial bowing is a common normal developmental finding until the age of 2 years, but it does increase the risk of developing pathological tibia vara. It results from either intrauterine molding or delayed transition to normal mild genu valgus. Measurement depends on the tibiofemoral angle, which is the angle subtended by lines drawn longitudinally to the diaphyses. In infants, up to 16 to 20 degrees of varus angulation at the knee is normal, but by the age of around 3 years, this should change to 10 degrees valgus. Images show prominent but nonfragmented medial proximal tibial beaks. Distal femoral and proximal tibial medial epiphyses are wedge-shaped. Medial cortical thickening of femurs and tibias resolve as the bones straighten.
- **Blount disease (tibia vara):** Obesity or early walking stresses the posteromedial proximal tibial metaphysis, leading to deformity of the epiphysis and physeal damage due to shearing stress. Like developmental bowing, this condition is more common in African Americans. Infantile Blount disease presents before the age of 4 years, whereas juvenile and adolescent forms manifest in older children, likely constituting later presentations of the same disease. Infantile Blount is defined by a tibial metaphyseal/diaphyseal angle of at least 16 degrees. Early cases show only metaphyseal beaking, but as disease progresses, the metaphysis becomes more irregular, depressed, and possibly fragmented. The tibia may subluxate laterally. Conservative treatment with orthoses is effective in mild cases of infantile Blount. Severe or delayed disease may be treated with realignment wedge osteotomy. MRI is primarily employed to evaluate formation of a medial physeal bar which, if present, mandates more complex surgery.
- **Rickets:** Cartilage accumulates due to deficient growth plate cartilage and osteoid mineralization, leading to growth failure and osseous deformity. Nutritional vitamin D deficiency and X-linked hypophosphatemia are the most common underlying metabolic abnormalities. The growth plate widens due to disorganized, excessive cartilage. The metaphyses and metaphyseal equivalents of rapidly growing bones are most severely affected: wrist, knees, and anterior ribs. Insufficiency fractures, periosteal new bone, and bowing are seen in the diaphyses. Lower extremity bowing develops as children begin to stand. In addition to bowing, X-rays show physeal widening and metaphyseal flaring, cupping, and fraying.

■ Additional Diagnostic Consideration

- **Syndromic bowing:** Metaphyseal chondrodysplasia, osteogenesis imperfecta, neurofibromatosis, and other syndromes may cause genu varum due to a variety of mechanisms.

■ Diagnosis

Blount disease.

✓ Pearls

- Genu varus up to 16 to 20 degrees is normal in children younger than 2 years of age.
- Pathological tibia vara shows excess bowing in children under the age of 2 years or bowing that persists beyond the age of 2 years.
- In Blount disease, metaphyseal beaking progresses to irregularity and, sometimes, fragmentation with lateral subluxation of the tibia.
- Rickets, commonly due to nutritional vitamin D deficiency or X-linked hypophosphatemia, shows physeal widening, metaphyseal cupping and fraying along with insufficiency fractures and diaphyseal bowing.

■ Suggested Readings

Cheema JI, Grissom LE, Harcke HT. Radiographic characteristics of lower-extremity bowing in children. Radiographics. 2003; 23(4):871–880

Ho-Fung V, Jaimes C, Delgado J, Davidson RS, Jaramillo D. MRI evaluation of the knee in children with infantile Blount disease: tibial and extra-tibial findings. Pediatr Radiol. 2013; 43(10):1316–1326

Shore RM, Chesney RW. Rickets: Part I. Pediatr Radiol. 2013; 43(2):140–151

Shore RM, Chesney RW. Rickets: Part II. Pediatr Radiol. 2013; 43(2):152–172

Case 130

Wonsuk Kim

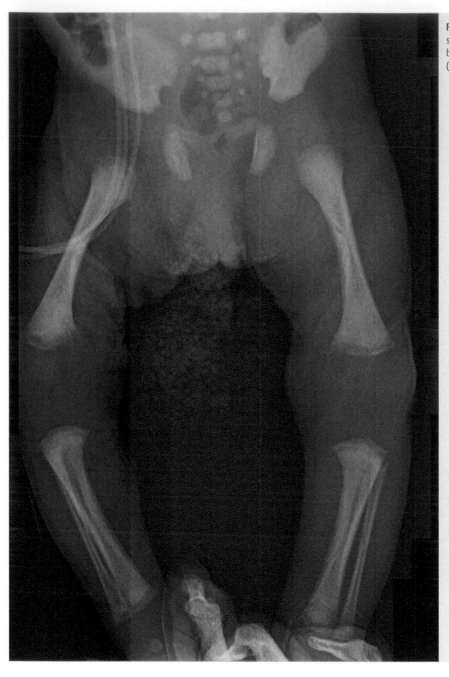

Fig. 130.1 AP radiograph of lower extremity shows symmetric transverse lucent metaphyseal bands adjacent to dense subphyseal bands. (Image courtesy of Rebecca Stein-Wexler.)

■ Clinical History

A newborn girl with mucocutaneous lesions (▶ Fig. 130.1).

■ Key Finding

Lucent metaphyses.

■ Top 3 Differential Diagnoses

- **Leukemia:** Acute leukemia is the most common pediatric malignancy, and acute lymphoblastic leukemia (ALL) comprises the majority of cases. Radiographic abnormalities are seen in up to 2/3rd of patients at diagnosis. Metaphyseal lucencies are the most common finding and occur at sites of fastest growth, such as the knees, ankles, and wrists. Other findings include periosteal reaction, focal osteolytic lesions, osteopenia, and fractures. Compression fractures of the spine are common.
- **Osteomyelitis:** Acute osteomyelitis is a significant cause of bone pathology in children, especially those under 5 years of age. Most cases occur due to hematogenous spread and involve the metaphyses. Scintigraphy and MRI are more sensitive than radiographs for early diagnosis. After about 10 days, radiographic findings such as ill-defined metaphyseal lucencies and periosteal bone formation may be seen.
- **Neuroblastoma:** Neuroblastoma commonly metastasizes to bone. Children with skeletal metastases may complain of bone pain and arthritis-like symptoms. Radiographic appearance resembles that of other small, round blue cell tumors such as Ewing sarcoma and leukemia. There may be periosteal reaction, one or more lytic foci, lucent horizontal metaphyseal lines, and pathological fractures. MRI, positron emission tomographic (PET) CT, and metaiodobenzylguanidine (MIBG) scans help assess for metastases.

■ Additional Diagnostic Considerations

- **TORSCH:** TORSCH (toxoplasmosis, rubella, syphilis, cytomegalovirus [CMV], herpes) infections are acquired transplacentally and often affect the metaphyses. Syphilis and others may cause symmetrical lucent metaphyseal bands adjacent to a subphyseal dense band. Wimberger sign—symmetrical focal destruction of the medial proximal tibial metaphyses—is seen in about 50% of cases of congenital syphilis as well. Rubella classically leads to a "celery stalk" appearance with longitudinally arrayed linear striations extending from the epiphyses into the metaphyses. Other TORSCH infections may cause similar findings.
- **Rickets:** Rickets is caused by vitamin D deficiency and leads to decreased mineralization of physeal cartilage. X-ray findings of physeal widening, loss of the zone of provisional calcification, metaphyseal fraying, and metaphyseal cupping are most evident at the fastest growing long bones (wrist and knee).
- **Scurvy:** This lethal but treatable disease is caused by vitamin C deficiency. Radiographic findings include prominent zones of provisional calcification in the metaphyses ("white lines" of Frankel) with subjacent lines of demineralization ("scurvy lines") and physeal widening.

■ Diagnosis

Congenital syphilis.

✓ Pearls

- Metaphyseal lucent bands are commonly seen with leukemia.
- TORSCH infections may manifest metaphyseal lucency with a "celery-stalk" appearance.
- Bony metastases are common in neuroblastoma and may show periosteal reaction, metaphyseal lucencies, lucent foci in other locations as well, and pathological fractures.

■ Suggested Readings

Blickman JG, van Die CE, de Rooy JW. Current imaging concepts in pediatric osteomyelitis. Eur Radiol. 2004; 14 Suppl 4:L55–L64

Mostoufi-Moab S, Halton J. Bone morbidity in childhood leukemia: epidemiology, mechanisms, diagnosis, and treatment. Curr Osteoporos Rep. 2014; 12(3): 300–312

Ranson M. Imaging of pediatric musculoskeletal infection. Semin Musculoskelet Radiol. 2009; 13(3):277–299

Case 131

Rebecca Stein-Wexler

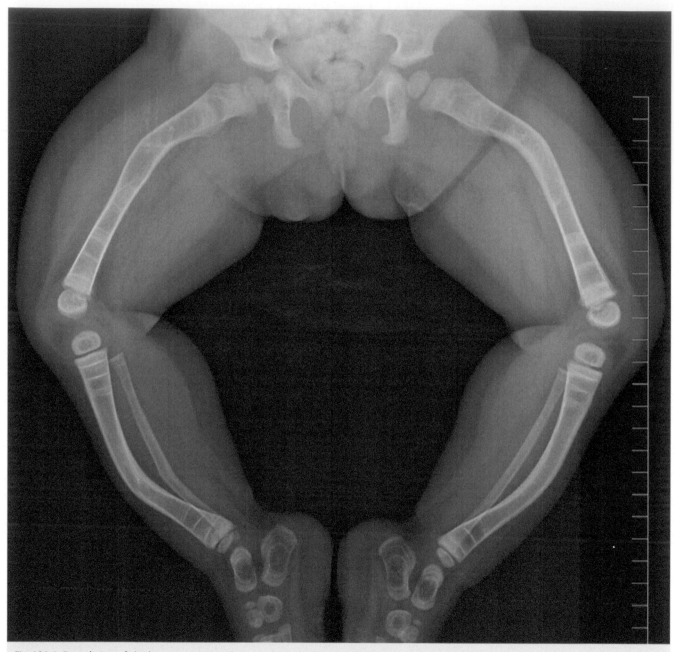

Fig. 131.1 Frontal view of the lower extremities shows multiple dense metaphyseal lines, along with bowing and osteoporosis.

■ Clinical History

A 2-year-old girl with a chronic disease (▶ Fig. 131.1).

■ Key Finding

Dense metaphyses.

■ Top 3 Differential Diagnoses

- **Physiological dense metaphyses:** In healthy young children between the age of 2 to 6 years, increased metaphyseal density may be seen during periods of prolonged exposure to sunlight, especially common after winter. The exact mechanism is unknown, but this phenomenon may result from overproduction of endogenous vitamin D. Clues to diagnosis are that (1) at the knee, the proximal end of the fibula appears normal, with no dense band, and (2) the dense band is no more dense than the diaphyseal or metaphyseal cortex.
- **Lead toxicity (plumbism):** Lead toxicity is most common between the ages of 1 and 3 years. It results from inhalation of lead dust or ingestion of contaminated water or fragments of lead paint. When serum lead levels exceed 50 micrograms/dL, excess lead impairs osteoclast function, leading to failure of bone resorption in the zone of provisional calcification. Bilateral, symmetrical, dense metaphyseal bands develop, which are typically denser than the cortex of the adjacent metaphysis or diaphysis. Such a band at the proximal end of the fibula is useful for diagnosis, since this area should be normal with physiological dense metaphyses. If high-lead levels persist, growth deformities, such as Erlenmeyer flask deformity, may develop. Other heavy metals have a similar effect. Although radiological findings are suggestive, diagnosis rests on laboratory tests.
- **Treated leukemia:** After treatment for leukemia, the metaphyses may appear dense. However, children with leukemia more often demonstrate lucent metaphyses.

■ Additional Diagnostic Considerations

- **Healing rickets:** Although patients with active rickets have frayed, flared, and cupped metaphyses with widening of the physis, healing bone shows dense juxtaphyseal metaphyseal bands. This is most pronounced in the metaphyses or metaphyseal equivalents of rapidly growing bones: the wrists, knees, and anterior ribs.
- **Bisphosphonate therapy:** Bisphosphanates treat patients with osteoporosis, usually due to osteogenesis imperfecta, steroid treatment, and neuromuscular disorders. These drugs increase bone density by inhibiting osteoclast-mediated bone resorption. Cyclical therapy leads to thin, dense metaphyseal lines that parallel the physis in long bones ("zebra stripes") and a "bone within bone" appearance of the spine and flat bones.
- **Syphilis:** In utero infection with *Treponema pallidum* may lead to bone abnormalities that manifest during the first 2 months of life. A dense sclerotic band may be positioned between the physis and the abnormally lucent metaphysis. About 50% of patients demonstrate the Wimberger sign, focal osteolysis of the medial proximal tibial metaphysis. Pathological fractures and periosteal new bone formation may be present as well. Patients may have a rash, hepatosplenomegaly, anemia, ascites, and nephrotic syndrome.

■ Diagnosis

Bisphosphonate therapy for underlying osteogenesis imperfecta.

✓ Pearls

- Physiological dense metaphyses appear no denser than adjacent cortex and spare the proximal fibula.
- Although active rickets is characterized by wide, frayed metaphysis, during the treatment phase, the metaphyses may appear dense.
- If lead levels exceed 50 micrograms/dL, dense metaphyseal bands may develop.
- Infants with syphilis may show a dense band between the physis and the abnormally lucent metaphysis.

■ Suggested Readings

Raber SA. The dense metaphyseal band sign. Radiology. 1999; 211(3):773–774

States LJ. Imaging of metabolic bone disease and marrow disorders in children. Radiol Clin North Am. 2001; 39(4):749–772

Case 132

Rebecca Stein-Wexler

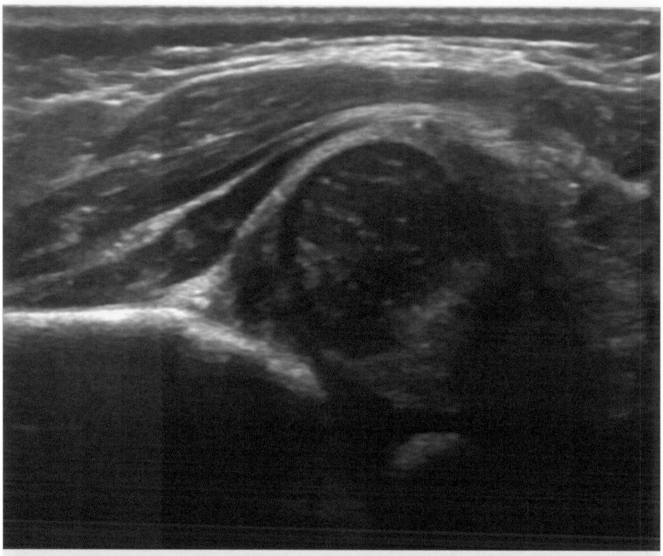

Fig. 132.1 Coronal flexion ultrasound of the left hip shows the acetabulum is shallow, and the femoral head is widely subluxated.

■ Clinical History

A 4-week-old breech baby with hip click (▶ Fig. 132.1).

■ Key Finding

Dislocated hip.

■ Top 3 Differential Diagnoses

- **Developmental dysplasia of the hip (DDH):** DDH is most common in infants who are female, first-born, and/or with breech presentation or a family history of DDH or joint laxity. The Barlow maneuver attempts to displace the femoral head by pistoning the flexed hip. The Ortolani maneuver attempts to reduce a displaced hip by flexion and abduction. US is used for diagnosis until age 6 months, when ossification of the femoral head causes too much acoustic shadowing. The coronal view best depicts acetabular contour, with an "alpha angle" of 60 degrees or more considered normal. Transverse flexion views best depict femoral head motion within the acetabulum. In older children, the acetabulum and femoral head position are assessed on X-rays. Pavlik harness treatment is usually successful. Occasionally, casting is needed. Refractory DDH may be treated with acetabuloplasty to improve acetabular angle and coverage, along with femoral osteotomy to improve the position of the femoral head. Limited CT or MRI is then employed to assess hip position.

- **Neuromuscular disorder:** The hip may subluxate and eventually dislocate in patients with cerebral palsy (CP) and other spastic neuromuscular conditions. With hyperactive adductor and iliopsoas muscles leading to persistent hip adduction, the acetabulum becomes oblique and shallow. Severe subluxation is common by the age of 7 years in patients with spastic CP. However, lateral coverage of the femoral head may be reduced for other reasons, such as disparity in size between the acetabulum (small) and femoral head (large), pelvic obliquity, adduction contracture, or femoral neck valgus/anteversion.
- **Trauma:** A traumatic hemarthrosis may lead to posterolateral subluxation or, rarely, dislocation of the hip. In cases where the femoral head has not ossified, a Salter I fracture with lateral displacement of the distal fragment may mimic femoral head dislocation. This may be seen with nonaccidental trauma. Severe trauma, such as motor vehicle collision, may cause posterior dislocation of the femoral head.

■ Additional Diagnostic Consideration

- **Teratologic hip dysplasia:** The incidence of hip dysplasia is increased with many skeletal dysplasias and syndromes. For example, as many as 5% of ambulatory children with Trisomy

21 have recurrent hip subluxation or dislocation. Patients with Ehlers–Danlos syndrome and Larsen syndrome also have an increased incidence of hip dislocation.

■ Diagnosis

Developmental dysplasia of the hip.

✓ Pearls

- DDH is most common in girls, first-borns, and among those with breech presentation and/or a family history of ligamentous laxity.
- Hip US is most useful until the age of 6 months.
- Patients with spastic CP have increased incidence of hip dislocation due to persistent hip adduction.

- Before the femoral head ossifies, Salter I fracture of the proximal femoral physis with lateral displacement of the metaphysis, which may occur with nonaccidental trauma, mimics DDH.

■ Suggested Readings

Grissom LE. The pelvis and hip: Congenital and developmental conditions. In: Stein-Wexler R, Wootton-Gorges SL, Ozonoff MB, eds. Pediatric Orthopedic Imaging. Berlin Heidelberg: Springer; 2015

Hägglund G, Lauge-Pedersen H, Wagner P. Characteristics of children with hip displacement in cerebral palsy. BMC Musculoskelet Disord. 2007; 8:101

Harcke HT. The role of ultrasound in diagnosis and management of developmental dysplasia of the hip. Pediatr Radiol. 1995; 25(3):225–227

Case 133

Robert J. Wood and Sandra L. Wootton-Gorges

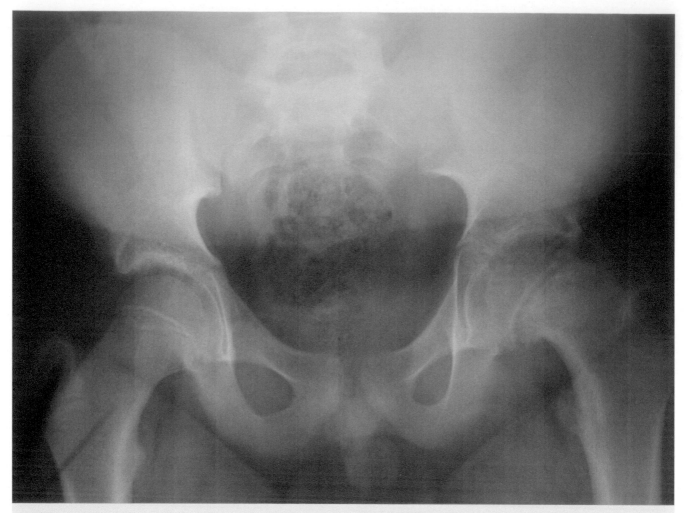

Fig. 133.1 Frontal view of the pelvis shows the left proximal femoral physis is wide, and the femoral head is posteromedially positioned with respect to the metaphysis. (Image courtesy of Rebecca Stein-Wexler.)

■ Clinical History

A 13-year-old boy with left hip pain (▶ Fig. 133.1).

■ Key Finding

Physeal widening.

■ Top 3 Differential Diagnoses

- **Salter–Harris type I fracture:** This relatively uncommon fracture results from a shearing force that parallels the growth plate. It is most often seen in children younger than 5 years of age. Although transient displacement is common, the fracture usually reduces spontaneously before imaging, making diagnosis difficult. Comparison with the contralateral side may be helpful.
- **Slipped capital femoral epiphysis (SCFE):** This Salter–Harris I shearing fracture of the capital femoral physis is the most common hip problem of adolescence. It is more common in boys, African–Americans, and in overweight patients with mildly delayed skeletal maturation. Children with endocrinopathies, especially those with hypothyroidism or undergoing growth hormone therapy, are more likely to develop SCFE. SCFE is bilateral at presentation in about 10%, but up to 1/3rd will eventually develop SCFE in the contralateral hip. Patients present with limp and hip or knee pain. Those with "stable" SCFE can walk, whereas those with "unstable" SCFE cannot. The frontal neutral view shows physeal widening, a relatively short-appearing femoral head (due to rotation), and no femoral head projecting lateral to Klein's line (drawn along the lateral femoral neck). The frog lateral view shows posteromedial offset of the femoral head with respect to the femoral neck. Sclerotic reactive bone, with posteromedial buttressing at the femoral neck, may be seen in subacute cases. Complications include chondrolysis, premature arthritis, pistol-grip deformity resulting in femoral-acetabular impingement, and limb-length discrepancy due to premature physeal closure.
- **Rickets:** Rickets causes deficient resorption of the zone of provisional calcification. The disease results from lack of calcium absorption or overexcretion of phosphate. Patients may manifest bowing deformity or increased risk of fractures, including SCFE. X-rays may show fraying and cupping of the long bone metaphyses (most prominent at the knees and wrists), physeal widening, osteopenia with coarse trabeculae, bowing deformity, and insufficiency fractures. Flared and irregular anterior rib ends may result in the "rachitic rosary." The metaphyseal fraying resolves with treatment, and metaphyses become unusually dense.

■ Additional Diagnostic Consideration

- **Osteomyelitis:** *Staphylococcus aureus* is the most common pathogen for bone infection. From age 18 months until skeletal maturity, the metaphysis is most often affected due to localized sluggish blood flow. Radiographs may demonstrate cortical fraying and periosteal reaction, moth-eaten lucency of the bone, and associated soft-tissue swelling. Sometimes the physis becomes widened. MRI shows low-T1- and high T2 signal within bone when radiographs are still normal.

■ Diagnosis

Slipped capital femoral epiphysis.

✓ Pearls

- SCFE is a Salter I fracture of the capital femoral physis.
- Offset of the femoral head with respect to the neck is best diagnosed on a frog lateral view.
- Rickets demonstrates metaphyseal fraying and cupping along with bowing deformity.
- Osteomyelitis most often affects the metaphysis and demonstrates periostitis, moth-eaten lucency, and soft-tissue swelling.

■ Suggested Readings

Aronsson DD, Loder RT, Breur GJ, Weinstein SL. Slipped capital femoral epiphysis: current concepts. J Am Acad Orthop Surg. 2006; 14(12):666–679

Gill KG. Pediatric hip: pearls and pitfalls. Semin Musculoskelet Radiol. 2013; 17(3): 328–338

Jarrett DY, Matheney T, Kleinman PK. Imaging SCFE: diagnosis, treatment and complications. Pediatr Radiol. 2013; 43 Suppl 1:S71–S82

Case 134

Wonsuk Kim

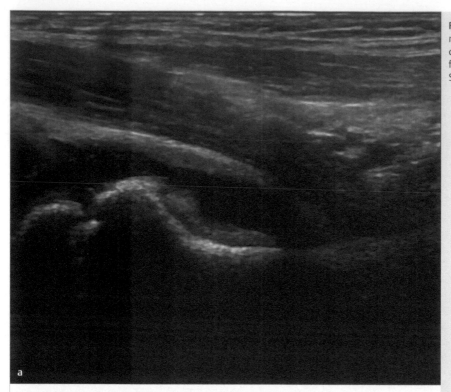

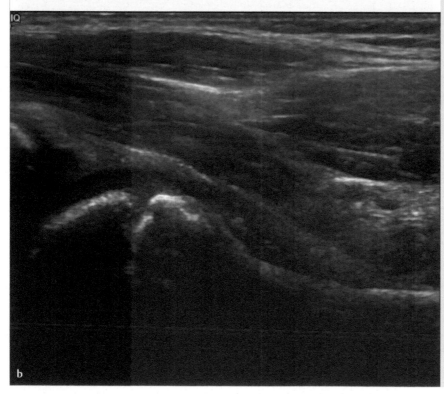

Fig. 134.1 Oblique sagittal ultrasound of the right hip (a) shows that the joint capsule is distended by anechoic fluid. Normal left hip (b) for comparison. (Images courtesy of Rebecca Stein-Wexler.)

■ **Clinical History**

A 3-year-old boy with right hip pain that developed after an upper respiratory infection (▶ Fig. 134.1).

■ Key Finding

Hip effusion.

■ Top 3 Differential Diagnoses

- **Toxic synovitis:** Toxic synovitis is the most common atraumatic cause of hip pain in young children. Most patients are between 3 and 8 years of age, and many cases are preceded by an upper respiratory infection. Joint fluid is present, which is better demonstrated with US than radiography. Treatment is supportive, and symptoms should resolve within 2 weeks. Avascular necrosis may develop in 1 to 2% of cases.
- **Septic arthritis:** This usually affects the hip or knee of young children. Common causative organisms are Gram positive cocci, especially *Staphylococcus aureus* and various *Streptococci*. Septic arthritis is an orthopedic emergency, as delay in diagnosis may lead to articular cartilage destruction, osteonecrosis,

impaired growth, and deformity. US is useful for diagnosing joint effusions prior to arthrocentesis. MRI findings of bone marrow edema, soft-tissue edema, and decreased femoral head enhancement are more prevalent in septic arthritis than toxic synovitis. Contrast-enhanced MRI demonstrates drainable fluid collections and appropriate sites for bone biopsy. Osteomyelitis may accompany septic arthritis.
- **Trauma:** Joint effusions in the setting of trauma often result from fracture. However, patients with septic arthritis or toxic synovitis may present with a history of trauma, so these diagnoses must also be entertained.

■ Additional Diagnostic Considerations

- **Juvenile idiopathic arthritis (JIA):** JIA is a clinical diagnosis with varied manifestations. It encompasses all arthritides of unknown origin in patients less than 16 years of age and that last more than 6 weeks. Depending on disease stage, X-rays may show joint effusion, soft-tissue swelling, osteopenia, joint space narrowing, and erosions. MRI may show synovial thickening, joint effusion, marrow edema, erosions, and cartilage thinning.
- **Hemophilia:** Hemophilia may be associated with recurrent bleeding into the joints with subsequent development of arthropathy. Arthropathy typically develops in the 1st and 2nd decades. The knee, ankle, elbow, and shoulder are most commonly affected. Radiographic findings in the acute phase

include hemorrhagic joint effusion (hemarthrosis). On MRI, the hypertrophied synovial membrane appears dark on all sequences secondary to susceptibility artifact from hemosiderin. Erosions may eventually develop.
- **Pigmented villonodular synovitis (PVNS):** PVNS represents the diffuse, intra-articular form of a spectrum of benign proliferative disorders that may affect the synovium, bursae, and tendon sheaths. PVNS occurs most often in the knee (80%), followed by hip, ankle, shoulder, and elbow. Peak presentation is in the 3rd and 4th decades. Radiographs may be normal or show periarticular soft-tissue swelling or erosions of the joint. MRI may show diffuse or nodular synovial thickening, with susceptibility artifact from hemosiderin.

■ Diagnosis

Toxic synovitis.

✓ Pearls

- Toxic synovitis is the most common atraumatic cause of hip pain in young children.
- Septic arthritis is a surgical emergency, as bacterial enzymes rapidly destroy joint cartilage.

- Trauma commonly precedes the onset of other causes of hip pain and may be a concomitant diagnosis.

■ Suggested Readings

Damasio MB, Malattia C, Martini A, Tomà P. Synovial and inflammatory diseases in childhood: role of new imaging modalities in the assessment of patients with juvenile idiopathic arthritis. Pediatr Radiol. 2010; 40(6):985–998

Jaramillo D, Dormans JP, Delgado J, Laor T, St Geme JW III. Hematogenous osteomyelitis in infants and children: imaging of a changing disease. Radiology. 2017; 283(3): 629–643

Llauger J, Palmer J, Rosón N, Bagué S, Camins A, Cremades R. Nonseptic monoarthritis: imaging features with clinical and histopathologic correlation. Radiographics. 2000; 20(Spec No):S263–S278

Case 135

Rebecca Stein-Wexler

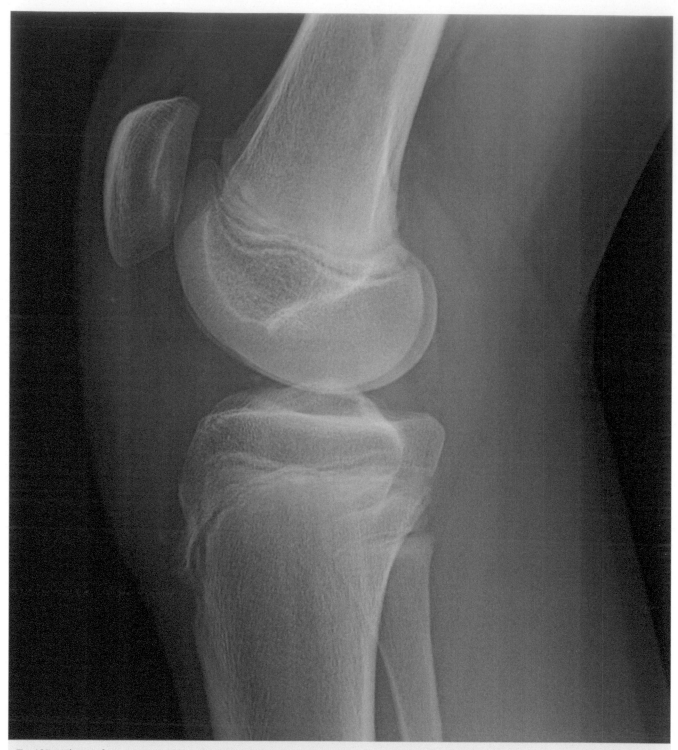

Fig. 135.1 There is fragmentation of the tibial tuberosity, and the infrapatellar tendon is very thick and ill-defined.

■ Clinical History

A 14-year-old male athlete with unilateral knee pain
(▶ Fig. 135.1).

■ Key Finding

Infrapatellar soft-tissue swelling.

■ Top 3 Differential Diagnoses

- **Osgood–Schlatter disease:** This traction "apophysitis" typically occurs in adolescent boys during growth spurts. Patella alta and valgus alignment at the knee predispose to the condition. Repetitive tensile force causes microfracture and avulsion of tibial tuberosity cartilage. If the tibial tuberosity has ossified, X-rays show one or more adjacent ossific densities, soft-tissue swelling, and edema of the distal patellar tendon and Hoffa's fat pad. If the fracture goes through cartilage only, ossific fragments will be seen after 3 to 4 weeks. Up to 50% of cases are bilateral. This benign, self-limited disorder heals with nonsteroidal anti-inflammatory drugs (NSAIDs) and physical therapy.
- **Sindig–Larsen–Johannsen disease:** Repetitive microtrauma causes this inferior patellar pole traction injury, usually in children between the ages of 10 to 14 years who are approaching skeletal maturity. Radiographs show, at least, one bone fragment near the lower pole of the patella and, possibly, patella alta. MRI shows abnormal signal in the lower pole of the patella, thickening of the patellar tendon, and edema in Hoffa's fat pad. Most lesions heal with NSAIDs and physical therapy.
- **Patellar sleeve fracture:** This acute avulsion injury affects children between the ages of 8 and 12 years after forceful contraction of the quadriceps muscle. Fracture of the cartilaginous lower pole of the patella results in a high-riding patella. The only radiographic evidence of this fracture may be a tiny sliver of bone at a variable distance from the patella's lower pole. MRI delineates the full extent of injury.

■ Additional Diagnostic Considerations

- **Proximal tibial transverse metaphyseal fracture:** This common and sometimes subtle fracture is often sustained in young children between the ages of 2 to 5 years while jumping on a trampoline. Slight cortical buckling and/or a subtle transverse lucency suggest the diagnosis.
- **Tibial tuberosity fracture:** The tibial tuberosity is prone to fracture during adolescence, as the physeal cartilage in this area matures to bone. Active knee extension and vigorous quadriceps contraction (jumping) cause this uncommon injury. This fracture is more common in those with prior Osgood–Schlatter. The avulsed bone is typically either displaced cephalad or hinged upward. Surgical fixation is usually needed.

■ Diagnosis

Osgood–Schlatter disease.

✓ Pearls

- Osgood–Schlatter disease shows patellar tendon thickening, edema in Hoffa's fat pad, and variable fragments adjacent to the tibial tuberosity.
- As children approach skeletal maturity, repetitive microtrauma may cause avulsion of the lower pole of the patella or Sindig–Larsen–Johannsen disease.
- The tiny infrapatellar sliver of bone that may be seen with patellar sleeve fractures greatly underestimates extent of disease, and MRI is generally needed for accurate diagnosis.

■ Suggested Readings

Kjellin I. The lower extremity: acquired disorders. In: Stein-Wexler R, Wootton-Gorges SL, Ozonoff MB eds. Pediatric Orthopedic Imaging. Berlin Heidelberg: Springer; 2015

Merrow AC, Reiter MP, Zbojniewicz AM, Laor T. Avulsion fractures of the pediatric knee. Pediatr Radiol. 2014; 44(11):1436–1445, quiz 1433–1436

Sanchez R, Strouse PJ. The knee: MR imaging of uniquely pediatric disorders. Magn Reson Imaging Clin N Am. 2009; 17(3):521–537, vii

Case 136

Rebecca Stein-Wexler

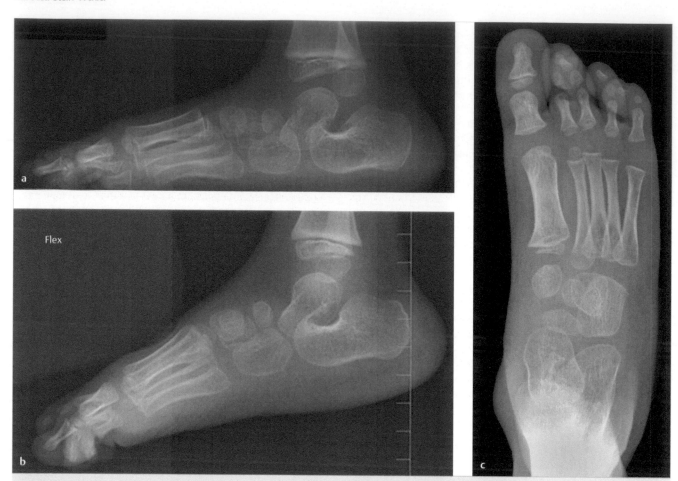

Fig. 136.1 Lateral weight-bearing view of the foot (**a**) shows the talus is vertical, almost parallel to the tibia, and the navicular is dorsally displaced; there is also pes planus. With plantar flexion (**b**), there is no significant improvement. Frontal weight-bearing view (**c**) shows that the talus is mildly deviated into valgus alignment.

■ **Clinical History**

Child with a foot deformity (▶ Fig. 136.1).

■ **Key Finding**

Foot deformity.

■ **Top 3 Differential Diagnoses**

- **Planovalgus foot (flatfoot):** This familial, acquired, flexible deformity is characterized by flattening of the plantar arch. It is usually asymptomatic. The condition is very common, especially in young children. However, by the age of 10 years, the incidence is similar to that in adults. Imaging is usually only performed if the condition is painful, in order to exclude other etiologies such as tarsal coalition. Ligamentous laxity allows the calcaneal position to deviate toward the midline (hindfoot valgus). The calcaneus is more horizontal than normal when viewed on a lateral weight-bearing X-ray. In addition, the Meary line, which is drawn along the long axis of the talus and first metatarsal, is convex downward. With severe cases, the talus may be directed inferiorly, more parallel to the long axis of the tibia than normal. However, it articulates normally with the navicular. Planovalgus foot may develop in patients with cerebral palsy and other neuromuscular disorders, but in that case, the foot is usually stiffer than with familial flatfoot.

- **Clubfoot (equinovarus):** The congenital form of this disorder may be inherited but may also result from muscle imbalance, connective tissue abnormalities, and intrauterine positioning. Older patients may develop clubfoot due to myelomeningocele, arthyrogryposis, and a variety of syndromes. Patients show plantar flexion at the ankle, hindfootvarus, and forefoot inversion and adduction. On X-rays, the talus is often small and deformed. The calcaneus is usually in equinus (more parallel to the tibial long axis than normal). The calcaneus is parallel to the talus and often superimposed. The navicular is displaced medially, and the forefoot is adducted. Inversion of the foot causes the metatarsal bases to be superimposed on each other on the frontal view and leads to a ladder-like appearance on the lateral view. The lateral metatarsals may be thick and sclerotic due to abnormal weight-bearing on the lateral side of the foot and stress reaction/fractures.

- **Congenital vertical talus:** This rare condition is usually bilateral and is syndromic in at least ½ of the cases. Nonsyndromic cases may result from abnormal rotational development of the foot and/or muscle imbalance. The tibialis posterior and peroneus longus tendons are positioned more anteriorly than normal and may function as dorsiflexors, and the Achilles tendon is short. As a result, the talus is severely plantar flexed, almost paralleling the tibial long axis. Unlike planovalgus foot, the navicular is dorsally dislocated, so it lies on the talar neck. The navicular aligns normally with the tarsal bones, but the talus does not. The calcaneus is laterally deviated into severe valgus, and like the talus, it is in equinus, which is almost parallel to the long axis of the tibia. There is marked plantar flexion, resulting in rocker-bottom deformity.

■ **Diagnosis**

Congenital vertical talus.

✓ **Pearls**

- With flatfoot deformity, the calcaneus is more horizontal than usual and deviated into valgus; in severe cases, the talar axis may align somewhat with the long axis of the tibia.
- Clubfoot is characterized by deviation of the calcaneus laterally, so it is parallel to the talus, along with forefoot adduction and foot inversion, so the metatarsals overlap too much on the frontal view but not enough on the lateral (ladder configuration).

- In congenital vertical talus, the talus is in equinus, and the calcaneus is deviated laterally into severe valgus.
- An important difference between flatfoot and congenital vertical talus is that the talus and navicular are aligned with the former, whereas with the latter, the navicular is dorsally dislocated.

■ **Suggested Readings**

Hammer MR, Pai DR. The foot and ankle: Congenital and developmental conditions. In: Stein-Wexler R, Wootton-Gorges SL, Ozonoff MB, eds. Pediatric Orthopedic Imaging. Berlin Heidelberg: Springer; 2015

Harty MP. Imaging of pediatric foot disorders. Radiol Clin North Am. 2001; 39(4): 733–748

Case 137

Jennifer L. Nicholas

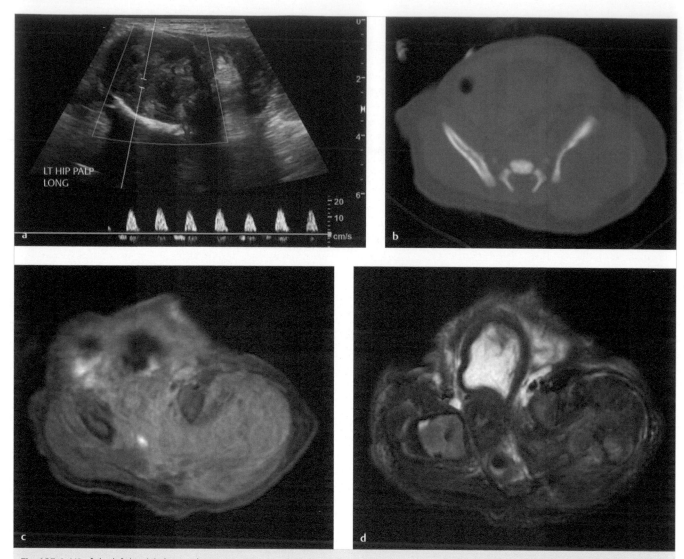

Fig. 137.1 US of the left hip **(a)** shows a heterogenous, vascular mass in the subcutaneous soft tissues that appears predominantly well defined. Axial CT **(b)** shows the mass is not calcified, and the adjacent iliac wing is thinned. Axial fat-suppressed gadolinium-enhanced T1 weighted MR image **(c)** shows a heterogeneous, partly necrotic, moderately enhancing mass whose periphery appears partly well circumscribed but that infiltrates the gluteus musculature and the pelvic sidewall. Axial T2-W fat-suppressed MRI **(d)** shows the mass is heterogeneous but predominantly hypointense. (Images courtesy of Rebecca Stein-Wexler.)

▪ Clinical History

A 2-day-old girl with a large left buttock mass (▶ Fig. 137.1).

■ **Key Finding**

Soft tissue mass in an infant.

■ **Top 3 Differential Diagnoses**

- **Infantile hemangioma**: Infantile hemangioma is the most common tumor of infancy, affecting up to10% of Caucasian children. Many are noted within the first month of life. There may be an associated cutaneous lesion, such as a pale spot, telangiectatic or macular red stain, or bruise-like pseudoechymotic patch. About 60% occur in the craniofacial region, 25% on the trunk, and 15% on the extremities. About 80% are solitary. At US, these high flow lesions usually appear solid, well defined, hypoechoic, and hypervascular, with homogeneous flow. MRI appearance varies with lesion phase. Multiple cutaneous hemangiomas may be a harbinger of hemangiomas elsewhere (usually the liver) and should prompt further imaging. Infantile hemangiomas typically proliferate in the first year of life and involute by age 5 years.
- **Infantile myofibroma**: This benign, nodular soft tissue tumor also occurs in muscle, bones, and viscera. Although rare, it is the most common fibrous tumor of infancy. Most infantile myofibromas present by age 2 years. The tumors may be solitary or multifocal (myofibromatosis). US appearance ranges from homogeneous and slightly hyperechoic to nearly anechoic with a thick rim. Many of these lesions regress without intervention. Treatment if needed is surgical excision.
- **Fibrous hamartoma of infancy**: Most fibrous hamartomas of infancy present as solitary painless nodules. Some have overlying skin changes, including altered pigmentation, eccrine gland hyperplasia, or hair. Most occur within the first year of life, and about ¼ are present at birth. The lesions are usually located in the subcutaneous soft tissues and lower dermis of the axilla, upper arm, upper trunk, inguinal region, and external genital area. US shows a heterogeneously hyperechoic mass with a "serpentine" pattern and ill-defined or lobulated margin without substantial blood flow. Fibrous hamartomas sometimes regress spontaneously, but the treatment of choice is local excision.

■ **Additional Diagnostic Considerations**

- **Infantile fibrosarcoma**: This large, rapidly growing tumor is the most common malignant soft tissue mass in infants and is usually encountered in the extremities. US typically shows a heterogeneous, infiltrative, hypervascular lesion. MRI appearance is nonspecific. The prognosis is better in children than in adults.
- **Neuroblastoma metastasis**: Neuroblastoma metastases are usually, solid, vascular lesions. They are primarily hyperechoic and may contain calcifications. Calcifications are readily recognized at CT.

■ **Diagnosis**

Infantile fibrosarcoma.

✓ **Pearls**

- Infantile hemangiomas should be well-defined and compressible and show high velocity flow.
- US appearance of infantile myofibromas varies from homogeneous and slightly echogenic to almost anechoic with a thick rim.
- Fibrous hamartoma of infancy should be in the subcutaneous soft tissues and lower dermis and is generally heterogeneously hyperechoic with a "serpentine" pattern.
- Infantile fibrosarcomas grow rapidly, are heterogeneous, and are poorly defined.

■ **Suggested Readings**

Dickey GE, Sotelo-Avila C. Fibrous hamartoma of infancy: current review. Pediatr Dev Pathol. 1999; 2(3):236–243

Lee S, Choi YH, Cheon JE, Kim MJ, Lee MJ, Koh MJ. Ultrasonographic features of fibrous hamartoma of infancy. Skeletal Radiol. 2014; 43(5):649–653

North PE. Pediatric vascular tumors and malformations. Surg Pathol Clin. 2010; 3(3): 455–494

Schurr P, Moulsdale W. Infantile myofibroma: a case report and review of the literature. Adv Neonatal Care. 2008; 8(1):13–20

Case 138

Rebecca Stein-Wexler

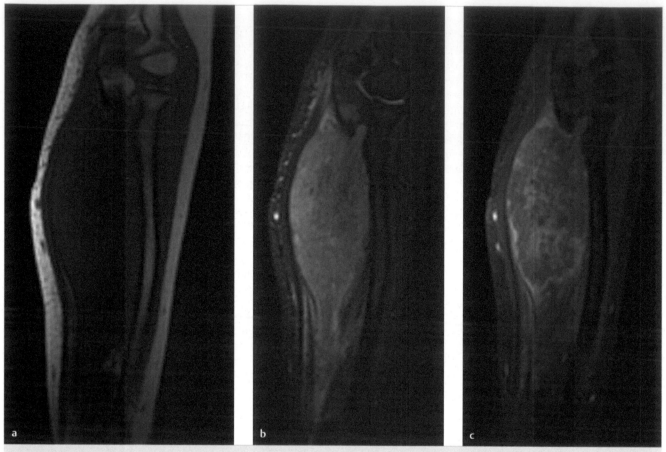

Fig. 138.1 Coronal T1-weighted MR image of the forearm **(a)** shows there is a solid mass that involves the flexor musculature; it is isointense to muscle. Coronal T2-weighted, fat-suppressed image **(b)** shows it is mildly heterogeneous but predominantly hyperintense, and there is mild adjacent soft-tissue edema. T1-weighted, fat-suppressed, contrast-enhanced image **(c)** shows heterogeneous enhancement.

▪ Clinical History

A 10-year-old boy who noticed a forearm mass 1 month ago; it continued to grow despite antibiotic therapy (▶ Fig. 138.1).

■ Key Finding

Large soft-tissue mass in an older child.

■ Top 3 Differential Diagnoses

- **Rhabdomyosarcoma (RMS):** Most pediatric soft-tissue masses are benign, but large size (>10 cm), deep, nonfascial location, older age, and heterogeneous noncircumscribed appearance increase the likelihood of malignancy. RMS is the most common pediatric soft-tissue sarcoma overall. However, infantile sarcoma (in infants) and synovial cell sarcoma (in older children) are more common in the extremities. Extremity RMS usually affects older children. Despite the name, it occurs in a variety of tissues, not just muscle. Extremity RMS is usually of the alveolar subtype, which has a worse prognosis than botryoid, and affects the head/neck and genitourinary tract. Radiographs and US show a nonspecific soft-tissue mass without calcification, which enhances intensely but heterogeneously at CT and MRI. It is dark on T1 and bright on T2, and there may be areas of necrosis. CT/MRI appearance is nonspecific but useful for evaluating disease extent. Complete surgical resection significantly improves prognosis.
- **Lymphoma:** Lymphoma can involve almost any organ in the body and should be considered in the differential diagnosis of any puzzling lesion. When localized to the soft tissues, it is usually of the nonHodgkin variety. Soft-tissue lymphoma may represent primary disease or result from contiguous or distant spread. The mass crosses fascial planes, engulfing more often than displacing vessels. Mass effect on vessels may cause distal soft-tissue swelling. Soft-tissue lymphoma is homogeneously hypoechoic on US and homogeneous on CT; intermediate signal on T1-weighted MRI and intermediate-to-hyperintense on T2-weighted. Both CT and MRI commonly show soft-tissue stranding and enhancement due to infiltration. Adjacent nodal stations may demonstrate confluent lymphadenopathy, which is unusual in other soft-tissue sarcomas. Chemotherapy and radiation therapy are the mainstays of treatment.
- **Synovial sarcoma:** This highly malignant tumor arises from primitive mesenchyme. Often misdiagnosed as a benign lesion, it may appear small and encapsulated at diagnosis. The mass may have been present for months to years. Although it is usually found within 7 cm of a joint, it does not arise from synovial tissue. Synovial sarcoma most often occurs at the hands, feet, or knee. About 1/3rd calcify and another 1/3rd demonstrate "triple signal": hyperintense hemorrhage, isointense necrosis, and hypointense fibrosis.

■ Additional Diagnostic Consideration

- **Desmoid tumor (aggressive fibromatosis):** This infiltrative lesion does not metastasize but may be difficult to completely resect, so recurrence is common. It is most often encountered in adolescents and young adults and may be associated with trauma or previous surgery. Usually located in muscle and adjacent fascia, it may encase nerves and vessels. MRI signal varies with cellularity, vascularity, and amount of collagen and water.

■ Diagnosis

Alveolar rhabdomyosarcoma.

✓ Pearls

- Although most pediatric soft-tissue masses are benign, risk of malignancy increases in older children and if the mass is >10 cm, deep, heterogeneous, and noncircumscribed.
- Of all soft-tissue sarcomas, synovial sarcoma most often resembles a benign lesion.
- 1/3rd of synovial sarcomas calcify, and another 1/3 show "triple signal" of hemorrhage, necrosis, and fibrosis.
- Desmoid tumor does not metastasize but is very infiltrative and hence difficult to resect.

■ Suggested Readings

Brisse HJ, Orbach D, Klijanienko J. Soft tissue tumours: imaging strategy. Pediatr Radiol. 2010; 40(6):1019–1028

McCarville MB, Spunt SL, Skapek SX, Pappo AS. Synovial sarcoma in pediatric patients. AJR Am J Roentgenol. 2002; 179(3):797–801

Roper GE, Stein-Wexler R. Soft tissue masses. In: Stein-Wexler R, Wootton-Gorges SL, Ozonoff MB, eds. Pediatric Orthopedic Imaging. Berlin Heidelberg: Springer; 2015

Case 139

Philip Granchi

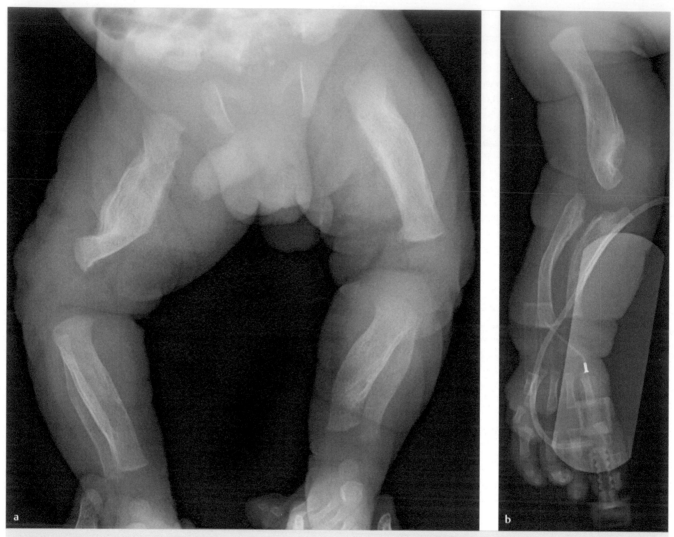

Fig. 139.1 Frontal view of both lower extremities **(a)** and frontal view of right upper extremity **(b)** show asymmetric, coarse periosteal reaction along long bones in this 4-week-old boy with irritability.

■ Clinical History

Newborn with hyperirritability (▶ Fig. 139.1).

■ Key Finding

Periosteal reaction in a newborn/infant.

■ Top 3 Differential Diagnoses

- **Physiologic periosteal reaction:** Between 1 and 6 months of age, periosteal new bone formation occurs as thin lines parallel to the cortices of long bones in about 1/3rd of all infants. Key to recognizing this process as benign is its symmetry. It commonly affects the humerus, femur, and tibia bilaterally. Follow-up films will show confluence of the periosteal reaction with the existing cortex. Physiologic periosteal bone formation will not involve the metaphyses. 1 to 6 months is the only period in which periosteal bone formation is considered physiologic.
- **Trauma:** Periosteal reaction occurs at sites of fracture from both accidental and nonaccidental trauma. In particular, nonaccidental trauma must be considered whenever periosteal reaction is identified in pediatric patients. Factors favoring a diagnosis of periosteal reaction secondary to nonaccidental trauma include multiple fractures of differing ages, as well as fractures with a high-specificity for child abuse. High-specificity fractures include posterior rib and metaphyseal corner fractures.
- **Infection:** Skeletal findings secondary to infection are diverse but a unifying element of these etiologies is the presence of lucency, either as vertical or longitudinal bands in the case of the TORCH infections, or as more poorly defined areas in osteomyelitis. The metaphyses are most commonly involved, which is a differentiating feature from normal physiologic periosteal bone formation.

■ Additional Diagnostic Considerations

- **Prostaglandin therapy:** Patients with congenital heart disease may require patency of the ductus arteriosus to provide oxygenated blood to the systemic circulation. Prostaglandin therapy is used to keep the ductus open prior to corrective surgery. Although the periosteal reaction in these patients is diffuse, the patient will have clear history of cardiac anomaly and long-term treatment (4–6 weeks) with prostaglandins.
- **Infantile cortical hyperostosis (Caffey disease):** Occurring in the first few months of life, Caffey disease presents with fever, irritability and periosteal reaction primarily involving the mandible, long bones, ribs, and scapulae. Key features that allow differentiation of Caffey disease are its coarse, irregular, and asymmetric periosteal reaction, along with the presence of soft-tissue swelling over the affected areas.

■ Diagnosis

Caffey disease.

✓ Pearls

- Physiologic periosteal reaction occurs between 1 and 6 months of age which does not involve the metaphyses.
- Trauma (accidental and nonaccidental) and infection result in localized periosteal reaction.
- Prostaglandin therapy may result in a diffuse periosteal reaction with long-term (4–6 weeks) treatment.
- Caffey disease results in a coarse, irregular, and asymmetric periosteal reaction with soft-tissue swelling.

■ Suggested Readings

Kirks D, Griscom NT. Practical pediatric imaging: diagnostic radiology of infants and children. 3rd ed. Philadelphia: Lippincott-Raven; 1998:335–336

Nistala H, Mäkitie O, Jüppner H. Caffey disease: new perspectives on old questions. Bone. 2014; 60:246–251

Swischuk LE, Ed. Imaging of the Newborn, Infant and Young Child. 5th ed. Philadelphia: Lippincott Williams and Wilkins; 2004:733

Velaphi S, Cilliers A, Beckh-Arnold E, Mokhachane M, Mphahlele R, Pettifor J. Cortical hyperostosis in an infant on prolonged prostaglandin infusion: case report and literature review. J Perinatol. 2004; 24(4):263–265

Case 140

Philip Granchi

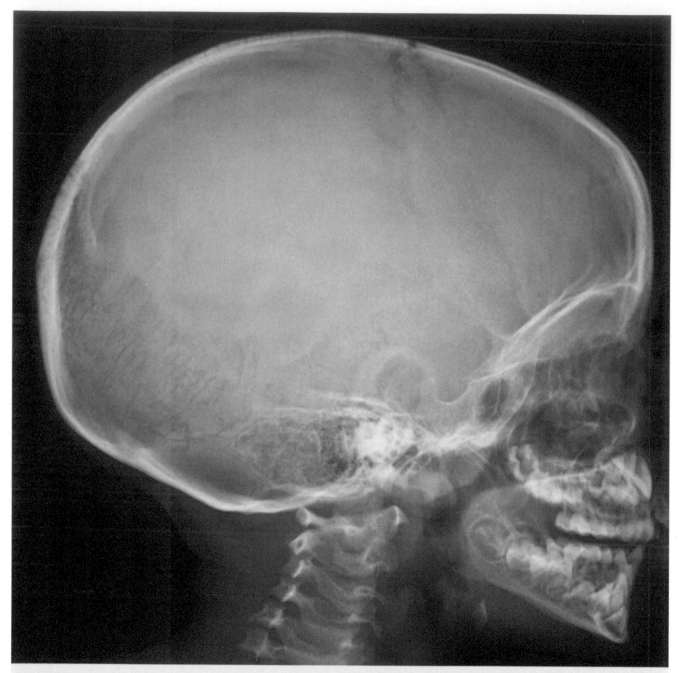

Fig. 140.1 Lateral skull radiograph reveals multiple intrasutural bones (Wormian bones) involving the squamosal and lambdoid sutures.

■ **Clinical History**

Child with facial abnormalities (▶ Fig. 140.1).

■ Key Finding

Wormian bones.

■ Top 3 Differential Diagnoses

- **Idiopathic:** Wormian bones are a descriptive designation for irregular ossicles located within the sutures of calvarium. Idiopathic Wormian bones are reported to be smaller and less numerous than those associated with an identifiable skeletal dysplasia, although no hard and fast criteria exist for this determination. Most commonly located within the lambdoid suture (50%), Wormian bones may also occur in the coronal suture (25%) and have been identified in all cranial sutures and fontanelles.
- **Osteogenesis imperfecta (OI):** Wormian bones in OI may be numerous and demonstrate a mosaic ("crazy paving")

pattern. Besides Wormian bones, other radiologic findings include osteoporosis, multiple fractures, gracile diaphysis, and scoliosis.

- **Cleidocranial dysostosis.** Cleidocranial dysostosis is a genetic disorder with abnormal membranous bone development that leads to findings of a small face, enlarged head, and hypertelorism. Wormian bones are one part of a radiographic constellation of findings that include delayed closure of sutures and fontanelles, absence or hypoplasia of the clavicles, widened symphysis pubis, and coxa vara.

■ Additional Diagnostic Considerations

- **Down syndrome:** Down syndrome (Trisomy 21) is the most common genetic cause of mental impairment in children and has been associated with an increased incidence with advanced maternal age (>35 years of age). A host of radiographic findings are associated with Down syndrome, including Wormian bones. Additional classic findings include atlantoaxial instability, 11 rib pairs, short tubular bones of the hands, flared iliac wings, hip dysplasia, and patellar dislocation.

- **Metabolic disease (hypothyroidism, rickets):** Wormian bones may be found in patients with multiple metabolic deficiencies. In rickets, Wormian bones are associated with the healing phase of the deficiency. Early findings include frayed physes and flaring (cupping) of the metaphyses. Hypothyroidism is characterized by markedly delayed skeletal maturity, "bullet" vertebrae at the thoracolumbar junction, and fragmentation of the epiphyses. Hypophosphatasia, a rare genetic defect of alkaline phosphatase, leads to rickets in the absence of dietary deficiency.

■ Diagnosis

Osteogenesis imperfecta.

✓ Pearls

- Wormian bones may be idiopathic in etiology with the lambdoid suture most commonly involved.
- Wormian bones in osteogenesis imperfecta may be numerous and demonstrate a mosaic pattern.

- Cleidocranial dysostosis presents with Wormian bones and absence or hypoplasia of the clavicles.
- Wormian bones may be found with multiple metabolic disorders.

■ Suggested Readings

Jeanty P, Silva SR, Turner C. Prenatal diagnosis of wormian bones. J Ultrasound Med. 2000; 19(12):863–869

Manaster BJ, May DA, Disler DG. Musculoskeletal imaging. The Requisites. 4th ed. Philadelphia: Mosby Elsevier; 2013

Marti B, Sirinelli D, Maurin L, Carpentier E. Wormian bones in a general paediatric population. Diagn Interv Imaging. 2013; 94(4):428–432

Paterson CR. Radiological features of the brittle bone diseases. J DiagnRadiogr Imaging. 2003; 5:39–45

Case 141

Michael A. Tall

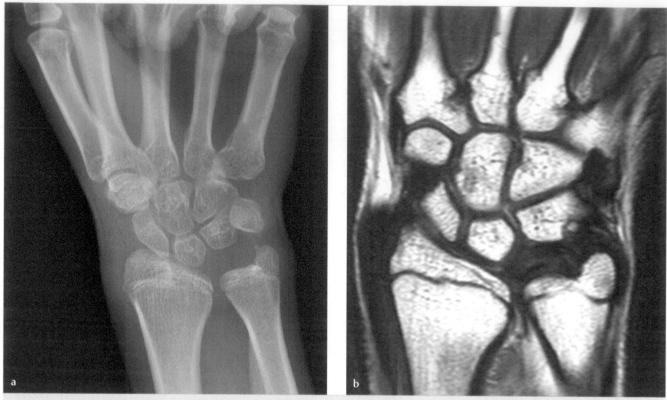

Fig. 141.1 Frontal radiograph of the wrist **(a)** and corresponding coronal proton density-weighted MRI image **(b)** demonstrate a triangular configuration of the distal radius and ulna articulation, with wedging of the proximal carpal bones between the distal radius and ulna, from Madelung deformity in this adolescent female.

■ Clinical History

A 16-year-old female with wrist pain and weakness (▶ Fig. 141.1).

■ Key Finding

Madelung deformity.

■ Top 3 Differential Diagnoses

- **Idiopathic Madelung deformity:** Idiopathic Madelung deformity often clinically manifests itself in young adulthood or adolescence and can present with visible deformity, pain, weakness, and limited range of motion. It results from premature closure of the medial volar aspect of the distal radial growth plate. Radiographic findings consist of increased inclination of the radial articular surface and volar tilt, proximal and volar migration of the lunate with triangulation of the carpus, relative ulnar lengthening and dorsal subluxation of distal ulna. The isolated form of Madelung deformity is typically bilateral, asymmetric, and more common in women.

- **Posttraumatic:** Madelung-type deformity may be secondary to trauma or infection. It can result from single or repetitive axial loading trauma, an injury frequently seen in gymnasts.
- **Skeletal dysplasias:** It is frequently associated with the Leri–Weill dyschondrosteosis, an autosomal dominant skeletal dysplasia. Patients with other osseous dysplasias, including Ollier disease, multiple epiphyseal dysplasia, and multiple hereditary exostoses may present with Madelung-type deformity. It is also seen in less than 10% of patients with Turner syndrome.

■ Diagnosis

Idiopathic Madelung deformity.

✓ Pearls

- The isolated form of Madelung deformity is typically bilateral, asymmetric, and more common in women.
- Bilateral Madelung deformities may be present in several skeletal dysplasias.

- Trauma and infection are two common causes of a unilateral Madelung deformity.

■ Suggested Readings

Ali S, Kaplan S, Kaufman T, Fenerty S, Kozin S, Zlotolow DA. Madelung deformity and Madelung-type deformities: a review of the clinical and radiological characteristics. Pediatr Radiol. 2015; 45(12):1856–1863

Peh WC. Madelung's deformity. Am J Orthop. 2001; 30(6):512

Resnick D, Kransdorf MJ. Bone and joint imaging. 3rd ed. Philadelphia, PA: Elsevier Saunders; 2005

Schmidt-Rohlfing B, Schwöbel B, Pauschert R, Niethard FU. Madelung deformity: clinical features, therapy and results. J Pediatr Orthop B. 2001; 10(4):344–348

Case 142

Eva Escobedo and Jasjeet Bindra

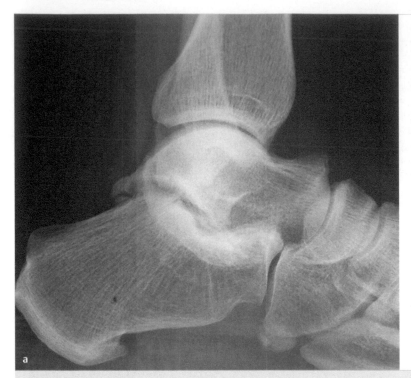
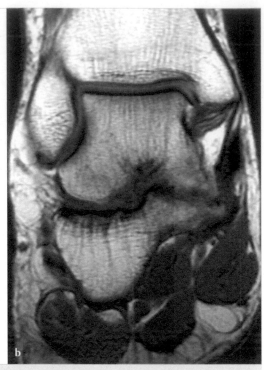

Fig. 142.1 Lateral view of the ankle **(a)** shows a curvilinear density along the inferior aspect of the subtalar joint ("continuous C" sign), an osseous projection off the dorsal aspect of the head of the talus ("talar beak"), and the middle facet of the subtalar joint is not well-visualized. T1-weighted coronal image of the ankle **(b)** shows narrowing and irregularity, with hypertrophic deformity and downward slanting of the middle subtalar joint (the "drunken waiter" sign).

■ Clinical History

A 29-year-old male with chronic foot and ankle pain
(► Fig. 142.1).

■ Key Finding

Tarsal coalition.

■ Top 3 Differential Diagnoses

- **Talocalcaneal coalition:** This is one of the most common types of tarsal coalition, which may be osseous, fibrous, or cartilaginous. The most common site of involvement is the middle subtalar joint. Radiologic signs can be direct or indirect. Direct findings demonstrate an osseous continuity between two tarsal bones in the setting of osseous coalition. Indirect signs can be subtler. In the case of nonosseous coalitions, the joint will demonstrate abnormal narrowing and irregularity, which may radiologically appear to be like osteoarthritis. The patient's age may clue in the interpreter, as most tarsal coalitions present in late childhood or early adulthood. Other signs may include a "talar beak," an osseous projection off the dorsal talar head, thought to be secondary to abnormal mechanics; the "continuous C sign" due to bony fusion or hypertrophy of the subtalar joint, and the "absent middle facet" due to narrowing or fusion of the middle subtalar joint.

Signs on MRI include the "drunken waiter sign," likened to a waiter having trouble carrying his tray, due to a dysplastic and downward medial sloping middle subtalar joint on a coronal plane.

- **Calcaneonavicular coalition:** This is as common, if not slightly more common, than talocalcaneal coalition. The majority of cases are fibrous or cartilaginous rather than osseous. Radiographic signs may include elongation of the anterior process of the calcaneus ("anteater" sign), articulation or fusion between the calcaneus and navicular, and elongation of the lateral navicular ("reverse anteater" sign). The "anteater" and "reverse anteater" signs may also be seen on MRI.
- **Talonavicular coalition:** This is the third most common type of coalition, but it is much less common than talocalcaneal or calcaneonavicular coalition.

■ Diagnosis

Talocalcaneal coalition (middle subtalar joint).

✓ Pearls

- The most common types of tarsal coalition are talocalcaneal and calcaneonavicular coalition; it is bilateral in up to half of the cases.
- Symptoms often present in the second decade, which include, pain, stiffness, decreased range of motion, flatfoot deformity, tarsal tunnel syndrome, and peroneal tendon spasm.

- Common signs noted on radiographs are the "continuous C" and "absent middle facet" with talocalcaneal coalition, the "anteater" sign with calcaneonavicular coalition, and the "talar beak" can be seen with either.
- Common signs noted on MRI include the "reverse anteater" sign in calcaneonavicular coalition, and the "drunken waiter" sign seen with talocalcaneal coalition.

■ Suggested Readings

Crim JR, Kjeldsberg KM. Radiographic diagnosis of tarsal coalition. AJR Am J Roentgenol. 2004; 182(2):323–328

Lawrence DA, Rolen MF, Haims AH, Zayour Z, Moukaddam HA. Tarsal coalitions: radiographic, CT, and MRI findings. HSS J. 2014; 10(2):153–166

Nalaboff KM, Schweitzer ME. MRI of tarsal coalition: frequency, distribution, and innovative signs. Bull NYU Hosp Jt Dis. 2008; 66(1):14–21

Case 143

Jasjeet Bindra

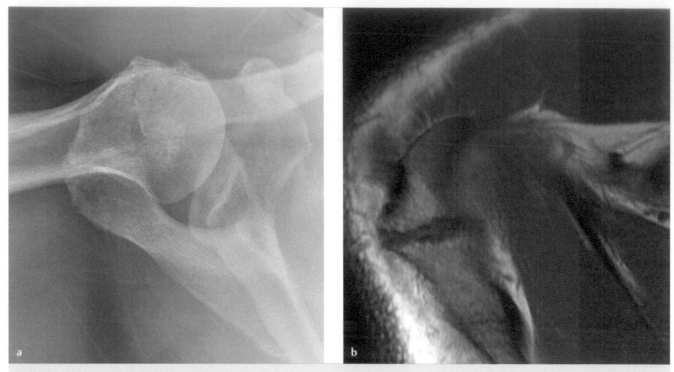

Fig. 143.1 Axillary radiograph of the shoulder **(a)** shows a triangular ossific density at the lateral aspect of acromion. Axial proton density-weighted MR image of the shoulder **(b)** demonstrates the well-corticated ossific density again.

■ Clinical History

A 56-year-old female with shoulder pain (▶ Fig. 143.1).

■ Key Finding

Well-corticated ossific density at the lateral aspect of acromion
—Roentgen classic.

■ Diagnosis

Os acromiale: Distal acromion is cartilaginous at birth. With growth, the primary ossification center or ossified plate of acromion advances anteriorly toward the acromioclavicular (AC) joint. Secondary ossification centers develop in the distal acromion by about 15 years of age and fuse by 25 years. The three potential ossification centers are called preacromion, mesoacromion and meta-acromion from anterior to posterior. An unfused secondary ossification center in people older than 25 years is termed os acromiale. It is a relatively common finding on shoulder imaging studies seen in about 5% of cases. The most common os acromiale is a relatively large, triangular mesoacromion, which has a transverse linear interface with the primary bone plate.

It is best identified on axillary shoulder radiographs and on high-axial images on MRI. Its diagnosis on coronal and sagittal images is challenging, as it bears a strong resemblance to the AC joint. Os acromiale can be symptomatic because of micromotion between the os and acromion and resultant pseudoarthrosis. It has been implicated as a risk factor for impingement syndromes. This may be due toosteophytes at the synchondrosis. Also, when the os is unstable, downward pull of deltoid on it can reduce the subacromial space and cause mass effect on the underlying rotator cuff. On MRI, edema and fluid may be seen along the synchondrosis in symptomatic cases. Most cases can be treated nonoperatively, but a variety of operative procedures have been reported in the treatment of a symptomatic osacromiale.

✓ Pearls

- The most common os acromiale is a relatively large, triangular mesoacromion.
- Axillary image on shoulder radiographs and high-axial images on MRI are the best for identifying osacromiale.
- Edema and fluid may be seen along the synchondrosis in symptomatic cases.

■ Suggested Readings

Motamedi D, Everist BM, Mahanty SR, Steinbach LS. Pitfalls in shoulder MRI: part 1–normal anatomy and anatomic variants. AJR Am J Roentgenol. 2014; 203(3): 501–507

Zember JS, Rosenberg ZS, Kwong S, Kothary SP, Bedoya MA. Normal skeletal maturation and imaging pitfalls in the pediatric shoulder. Radiographics. 2015; 35 (4):1108–1122

Case 144

Leslie E. Grissom

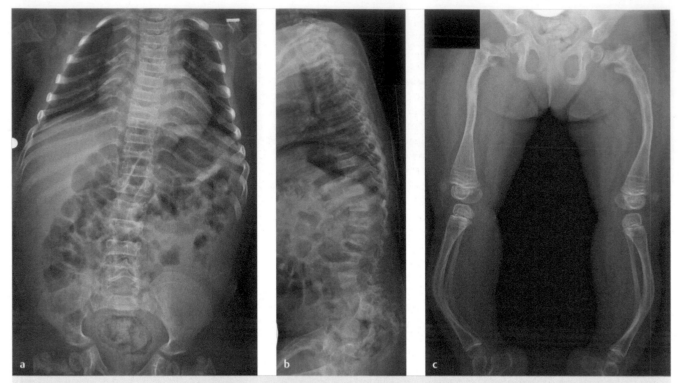

Fig. 144.1 Frontal **(a)** and lateral **(b)** views of the spine show multiple vertebral compression fractures. Lower extremities in another patient **(c)** are gracile and osteoporotic; the tibias, fibulas, and left femur are bowed, undulation and sclerosis of the right femur indicates a healed fracture, and there is bilateral coxa vara. (Images courtesy of Rebecca Stein-Wexler.)

■ Clinical History

Two patients with the same disorder (▶ Fig. 144.1).

■ Key Findings

Osteoporosis, bowing deformities, and multilevel spine fractures—Roentgen classic.

■ Diagnosis

Osteogenesis imperfecta (OI, also known as "brittle bone disease"): First described in 1788, OI is a heterogeneous group of disorders characterized by some or all of the following: osteopenia, multiple fractures, blue sclerae, hypoplastic teeth/caries, easy bruising, joint hypermobility, and premature deafness. The incidence is about 6 per 100,000 births. Various genetic defects lead to at least 16 different subtypes. Abnormal Type I collagen is seen in most of these disorders. Most cases are autosomal-dominant, but some are autosomal-recessive or result from new mutations. Types I through IV are the most common.

Patients with Type I OI, which is the most mild, may present as children or adults with fractures from insignificant trauma. Type II is lethal in the perinatal period, and these patients are frequently diagnosed in utero with multiple rib and long bone fractures, leading to severe deformities. The skull bones are very poorly ossified. Patients with Type III OI often have fractures at birth, but fractures may be delayed until the age of 2 years; they develop moderately short stature, scoliosis, and progressive deformity. Type IV is moderate in severity. Clinical features of these (and other) subtypes overlap, and therefore the disease may be described best as mild, moderate, marked and lethal.

In general, bones are osteoporotic, and trabeculae are relatively thin. Patients with the *lethal* form of OI are born with beaded ribs, crumpled, short and thick long bones, and biconcave vertebrae. Patients with *severe* OI usually have fractures at birth. Bones are gracile and somewhat short, and biconcave deformity of the vertebrae leads to severe kyphoscoliosis. Patients with *moderate* OI have moderately fragile bones, some have short stature, and ¼th have fractures at birth. Finally, those with *mild* OI have gracile bones that may be bowed; fractures are especially common in the lower extremities. Striking features of OI include excessive callus formation, popcorn calcifications about the epiphyses, large skull with frontal bossing, thin calvarium, Wormian bones, and basilar impression/invagination.

Treatment with bisphosphonates leads to thin metaphyseal bands, which resemble growth arrest lines. Intramedullary rods are commonly placed across fractures or across particularly gracile bones, and joint replacement and spine surgery may be required to preserve function.

Steroid-induced osteoporosis, idiopathic juvenile osteoporosis, metabolic bone disease, and neuromuscular disease may also lead to osteoporosis and multiple fractures, but clinical findings usually differentiate these entities from OI. Similarly, patients with dysplasias such as NF1 and camptomelic dysplasia may have bowing of the extremities, but they also have features typical of their disease. Finally, multiple fractures are seen in patients with nonaccidental trauma, but they should not have Wormian bones and, in the absence of malnutrition, bone density is normal.

✓ Pearls

- *Lethal* OI presents perinatally with beaded ribs, crumpled long bones, and biconcave vertebrae.
- Severe kyphoscoliosis develops in patients with *severe* OI, and fractures are commonly present at birth.
- Patients with *mild* OI may have gracile, bowed bones, but presentation may be delayed until childhood or early adulthood.

■ Suggested Readings

Burnei G, Vlad C, Georgescu I, Gavriliu TS, Dan D. Osteogenesis imperfecta: diagnosis and treatment. J Am Acad Orthop Surg. 2008; 16(6):356–366

Renaud A, Aucourt J, Weill J, et al. Radiographic features of osteogenesis imperfecta. Insights Imaging. 2013; 4(4):417–429

Sillence D. Osteogenesis imperfecta: an expanding panorama of variants. Clin Orthop Relat Res. 1981(159):11–25

Van Dijk FS, Pals G, Van Rijn RR, Nikkels PG, Cobben JM. Classification of osteogenesis imperfecta revisited. Eur J Med Genet. 2010; 53(1):1–5

Case 145

Rebecca Stein-Wexler

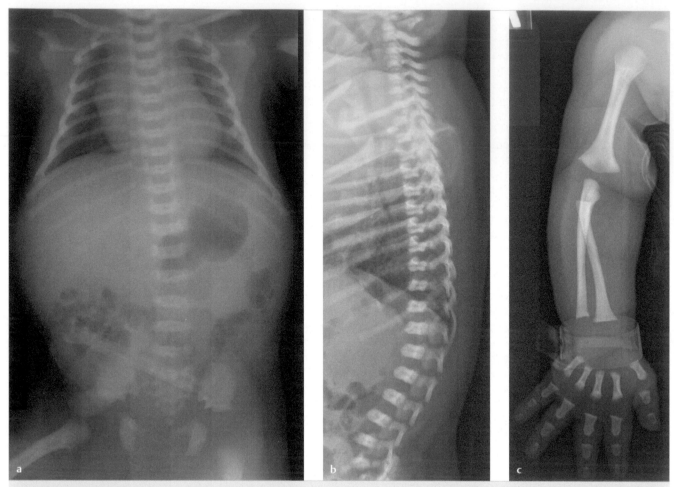

Fig. 145.1 Frontal radiograph of the chest and abdomen **(a)** shows decreased interpediculate distances at the lower lumbar spine, "tombstone" iliac bones secondary to decreased acetabular angles, and a "champagne glass" pelvic inlet. Lateral view of the spine **(b)** shows short pedicles leading to a small spinal canal. Upper extremity radiograph **(c)** shows rhizomelic (proximal) limb shortening, an unusually broad and lucent proximal humerus, and a "trident" appearance of the hand.

■ Clinical History

Infant with short stature and limb deformities (► Fig. 145.1).

■ Key Findings

Decreased lower lumbar interpediculate distances, "tombstone" iliac bones, "champagne glass" pelvic inlet, and rhizomelic limb shortening—Roentgen classic.

■ Diagnosis

Achondroplasia: The most common nonlethal skeletal dysplasia, achondroplasia, is a genetic disorder that results from autosomal-dominant inheritance or from spontaneous mutation. It is characterized by skeletal abnormalities attributable to decreased cartilage matrix production and endochondral ossification. Rhizomelic (proximal) limb shortening, metaphyseal flaring, and decreased interpediculate distance within the lower lumbar spine are typical.

Neurological problems are common. The foramen magnum and the skull base are small, which may result in brainstem compression. Restricted flow of cerebrospinal fluid (CSF) in this area sometimes causes hydrocephalus. The skull vault is large. The typical spine findings of narrow interpediculate distance and short pedicles may cause spinal cord compression. This may lead to weakness and numbness of the lower extremities.

The pelvis has a typical "tombstone" appearance due to squared iliac bones with decreased acetabular angles. The inner pelvic contour, with small sacrosciatic notches, has a "champagne glass" configuration.

The upper femurs and humeri of infants appear oval, and they are relatively lucent. Long bones are short and tubular, and the metaphyses slope more than usual. As the child matures, the tubular bones appear to become abnormally thick, although this just reflects normal width increase not lack of lengthening. Metaphyses develop irregular contour at sites of muscle insertion. Bullet-shaped phalanges of the hand taper above broad metastases. The hand has a "trident" shape.

Achondroplasia may be diagnosed by prenatal US at 25 weeks, with femur length often below the 3rd percentile, a large head, small chest, and polyhydramnios.

A less severe form of achondroplasia is termed "hypochondroplasia." In this condition, findings are mild, and sometimes limited to the spine. Patients usually present with short stature and short limbs after the age of 2 to 4 years. Vertebral abnormalities are limited to decreased lumbar interpediculate distance. Limb shortening is usually rhizomelic but may be mesomelic (middle). The skull, pelvis, and hands appear normal, unlike with achondroplasia.

It is important not to confuse achondroplasia with "pseudoachondroplasia," which is a completely unrelated syndrome that resembles multiple epiphyseal dysplasia.

✓ Pearls

- Achondroplasia shows decreased interpediculate distance, "champagne glass" pelvis, and "tombstone" iliac bones.
- The findings of hypochondroplasia are milder than with achondroplasia and may be limited to decreased lumbar interpediculate distance, although some patients have limb shortening as well.

■ Suggested Readings

Glass RB, Norton KI, Mitre SA, Kang E. Pediatric ribs; a spectrum of abnormalities. Radiographics. 2002; 22(1):87–104

Lemyre E, Azouz EM, Teebi AS, Glanc P, Chen MF. Bone dysplasia series. Achondroplasia, hypochondroplasia and thanatophoric dysplasia: review and update. Can Assoc Radiol J. 1999; 50(3):185–197

Parnell SE, Phillips GS. Neonatal skeletal dysplasias. Pediatr Radiol. 2012; 42 Suppl 1: S150–S157

Case 146

James S. Chalfant

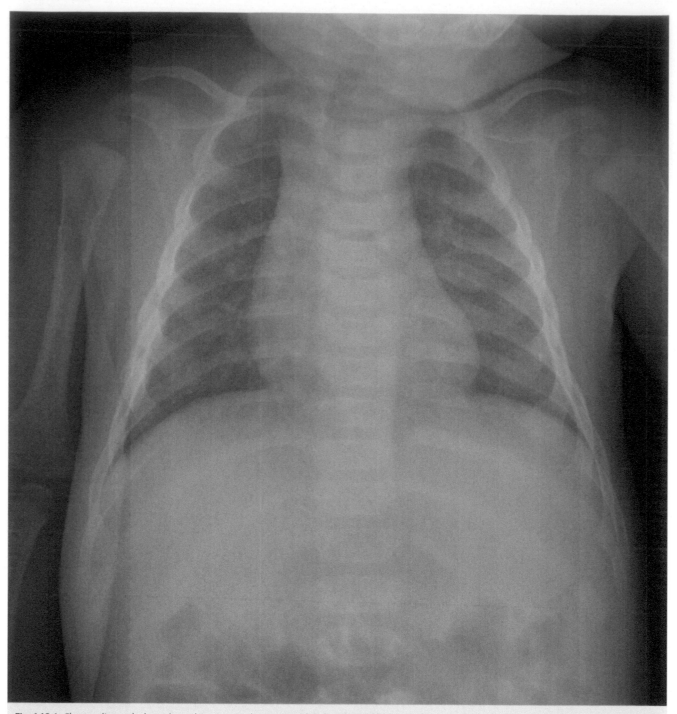

Fig. 146.1 Chest radiograph shows linear lucencies in the posterior left fourth and fifth ribs, and the posterior left sixth and seventh ribs are expanded and sclerotic. There is also expansion and sclerosis of the anterior left fifth through seventh ribs. Cloudy density surrounds the right lateral fourth through sixth ribs. The cortex of the right proximal humerus appears slightly buckled. (Image courtesy of Rebecca Stein-Wexler.)

▪ Clinical History

A 5-month-old female with cough and wheezing (▶ Fig. 146.1).

■ Key Finding

Multiple rib fractures in various stages of healing—Roentgen classic.

■ Diagnosis

Nonaccidental trauma: Fractures comprise the second most common finding in nonaccidental trauma after cutaneous injuries. While metabolic disorders, skeletal dysplasias, and birth trauma may result in fractures that mimic abuse, the presence of suspicious fractures must prompt further evaluation, at which point other etiologies may also be explored. Radiography is usually sufficient to identify osseous injuries, and multiple professional societies including the American College of Radiology have published recommended skeletal survey protocols. The value of the skeletal survey decreases with age. A more focused examination should be performed for children over 2 years of age based on clinical history, symptoms, and physical examination. A total body radiograph (babygram) is not appropriate in the evaluation of nonaccidental trauma, as it offers poor bone detail. Bone scintigraphy may augment the nonaccidental trauma workup if radiographs are negative.

For children under 3 years without significant known trauma, the positive predictive value of rib fractures for abuse is 95%. Commonly, fractures occur in the rib head or neck due to AP compression from squeezing. However, fractures due to abuse may be seen anywhere along the rib. Acute, nondisplaced fractures may be very difficult to see. Repeat imaging after 2 weeks may show sclerosis, periosteal reaction, and callus formation, and thus help identify occult fractures.

Classic metaphyseal lesions (corner and bucket handle fractures) are highly specific for abuse among children aged below 1. Transmetaphyseal disruption of trabeculi from shearing forces during shaking causes these fractures. The classically described corner and bucket handle fractures represent the same pattern of metaphyseal injury viewed in different projections. A corner fracture (triangular-shaped bone fragment) is apparent when imaged tangentially, while a bucket handle fracture (crescent-shaped bone fragment) is seen when imaged at an angle.

Long bone fractures raise concern for abuse if the patient is nonambulatory. Other fractures that are associated with abuse include scapular, spinous process, and sternal fractures. Multiple bilateral fractures, injuries incompatible with the provided history, or findings indicating delay in seeking medical attention should also raise suspicion. Fractures of different ages are worrisome, with the caveat that fracture dating may be difficult and should be done cautiously, given its role in legal proceedings. Repeat imaging may help.

Intra-abdominal injuries such as hepatic/splenic lacerations and duodenal hematomas may be seen. Nonaccidental trauma may also result in hypoxic–ischemic brain injury, along with subdural and parenchymal hemorrhage. If there is high-suspicion, cross-sectional imaging may be appropriate. While the need for cross-sectional imaging is case-based, the American College of Radiology's Appropriateness Criteria deems a noncontrast CT head as "usually appropriate" for children under 24 months with high-risk features (rib fractures, multiple fractures, facial injury, and less than 6 months), even in the absence of focal neurologic signs or symptoms.

✓ Pearls

- Rib fractures and classic metaphyseal lesions are highly specific for nonaccidental trauma.
- A complete skeletal survey is indicated for nonaccidental trauma workup in children below 2 years.
- A more focused examination can be performed for children above 2 years based on areas of suspected injury.
- Fractures in unusual locations, of different ages, or incompatibility with history should raise suspicion.

■ Suggested Readings

Kraft JK. Imaging of non-accidental injury. Orthop Trauma. 2011; 25:109–118

Offiah A, van Rijn RR, Perez-Rossello JM, Kleinman PK. Skeletal imaging of child abuse (non-accidental injury). Pediatr Radiol. 2009; 39(5):461–470

Stoodley N. Neuroimaging in non-accidental head injury: if, when, why and how. Clin Radiol. 2005; 60(1):22–30

Index

Note: Page numbers set **bold** or *italic* indicate headings or figures, respectively.

Index of Key Findings

Note: The index is ordered by case number within each part.